To my husband, Bruce, and son, Raymond,
with all my love and appreciation

KPS

To Don, David, and Ellen

DJB

Contents

Preface

Have you ever wondered how to find out about educational
programs in nursing? How to review for state board examinations? How to look up information on a clinical problem? How to write a grant proposal? How to prepare a
paper for publication? How to keep up with what is being
published in your area of expertise?

The rapid increase in materials relevant to nursing
makes a guide to finding and using them an essential item.
Overwhelmed with the bulk of materials that are available
when we enter a library, many of us fail to utilize the existing resources to full advantage.

Our goal is to familiarize users with both the basic
and specialized tools in libraries as well as their usefulness
to the nursing profession. Whether one has access to a
large medical or university library or to a small public
library, many of the materials discussed here will be available. While we realize that library orientations and tours
are essential for first-time users, this guide is designed to
provide the information needed when time has passed since
one's last major use of a library, if a new area is being ex-
plored, or to help one employ the librarian's services more
effectively.

This book is for all persons involved in nursing: students, practitioners, teachers, researchers, and administrators. Librarians will also find it indispensable in assist-
ing them to serve the needs of this segment of their user
population. Not to be overlooked is the utility of this

resource to other health-related disciplines such as allied health personnel and medical social workers. Teachers of courses in nursing research will find this book particularly useful as a text since students are often unfamiliar with the library resources they will need. It is also appropriate as a text and reference in formal and informal library orientation courses for nursing students and personnel. Nurses involved in inservice education in a variety of health care agencies can use the text to select materials as well as to assist their consumers to find appropriate resources.

The authors are a nursing faculty member with extensive experience in nursing—practice, teaching, and research—and a librarian with experience in a separate school of nursing library and several health sciences libraries.

Section I opens with a brief chapter which discusses some general reference sources and moves on to annotated listings of books in various areas of nursing as well as listings of pertinent periodicals. Section II provides an introduction to the library as well as miscellaneous library information on computerized literature searches and other selected topics.

The Guide to Library Resources for Nursing is the result of experience with and comments from people like you, and we hope this book will be a guide to help you find the information which you will need throughout your career. We also hope that it will make your next library visit a little more fun and a lot more profitable.

Acknowledgments

We would like to acknowledge the help and cooperation we received from the library staffs at the Medical University of South Carolina Library in Charleston, S.C. and from the Duke University Medical Center Library and the Duke University School of Nursing in Durham, N.C. In addition, without the encouragement and support of our families, this book would not be a reality.

Thank you one and all.

Introduction

Because of the large volume of new literature that is con-
tinually being published in nursing, it is impossible to compile an exhaustive bibliography of all the up-to-date, pertinent materials now available to the nurse or the student of
nursing. It has been our aim, rather, to locate book and
journal resources in most of the areas of nursing and to put
under one cover a resource that would be useful to nurses,
nursing students, administrators, librarians, and other
health professionals interested in the subject of nursing.
We realize that there are many useful resources which we
may not have included in this compilation, and we hope that
users of this book will inform us of omissions so that we
can include them in future editions of this work.

Several guidelines were followed in the presentation
of the sources listed in the following pages. We list these
guidelines below with the hope that they will facilitate the
use of this volume.

1. In general, books have been listed alphabetically by
   author. In some cases, it was appropriate to list
   items under title, when the author was not clearly
   identifiable, or when there were too many major
   authors to list practicably.
2. We have tried to note authors of special chapters when
   this was highlighted on the title page of the book.
3. Special attention has been paid to the inclusion of

bibliographies, indexes, appendixes, glossaries, and the like.

4.   In very few cases have we included materials specifically for practical or associate degree nurses since we believe that most of the material included would also be useful to this category of nurse.

5.   In general, we have not included British texts since in most areas there are comparable American texts. One notable area of exception was midwifery.

6.   Series have been noted when we could locate a notation of this on the book.

7.   Only selected publications of the National League for Nursing, the American Nurses' Association, and the U.S. government and its agencies have been included in this compilation, since a bibliography of the works of these agencies would fill a book in itself.

8.   Regrettably, a standardized subject vocabulary could not be used in entering the materials in this compilation, because of the specialized nature of the different chapters. However, the indexes have been prepared with the recognition that readers will look for sources in a variety of ways.

9.   The number of books entered under a particular heading in this resource was governed by what was available as well as by what we judged to be the prominence of the subject in the literature.

10.   In many cases, we have capitalized words or phrases which denote the actual chapter, unit, or section headings in a book or we have quoted from the preface of materials. Our aim has been to give a meaningful annotation that would allow the user of this book to determine as closely as possible the areas covered by a specific resource. In most cases, we were careful not to make value judgments since the usefulness of a particular resource depends largely on why it is being sought.

11.   The city of publication is that actually given in the book itself. Thus, there is some variation among books from the same publisher, particularly when the publisher has moved or comprises publishing divisions located in different cities.

12.   A maximum of three authors has been listed per book.
        In the case of four or more authors, this has been in-
        dicated by "et al."

13.   In some cases, we have had to note the existence of
        a subsequent edition of a book when we were unable to
        locate a copy for the purpose of a current annotation.

14.   Books located or published after the original compila-
        tion are included in a supplement at the back of this
        volume (pp. 491-509) and are listed alphabetically by
        author under the appropriate chapter headings. These
        items, unfortunately, could not be listed in the author,
        title, and subject indexes.

Guide to Library Resources
for Nursing

I

ANNOTATED LISTINGS

1
General Reference Sources

The reference collection in a library contains useful materials designed to be consulted briefly rather than read from cover to cover. A library's reference collection is traditionally contained in a separate place from the rest of the collection, may have its own designation, often has a separate card catalog listing the materials in the collection, and cannot be taken out of the library.

This chapter lists the types of materials in the reference collection: gazetteers, atlases, dictionaries, encyclopedias, etc., for both non-medical and medical categories. On the whole, we have included sources which are difficult to fit into the other chapters because of their all-encompassing nature.

ATLASES AND GAZETTEERS

An atlas is a compilation of maps of various regions of a given geographic area, for example, the United States or the world. Atlases usually contain some factual explanation, but are primarily composed of maps or charts. Gazetteers, on the other hand, are alphabetical listings of places giving geographical information on such places, including location and the like.

1.1   Columbia-Lippincott Gazetteer of the World (With 1961
       Supplement). Edited by Leon E. Seltzer, et al. New York:
       Columbia University Press, 1962.
              Cities, states, countries, regions and the like are
              listed in alphabetical order. Includes pronunciation,
              and brief information (e.g., population, history,
              battles, etc.) concerning each location. Comprehen-
              sive.

1.2   National Geographic Atlas of the World, 4th ed. Edited by
       Melville B. Grosvenor, et al. Washington, D.C.: National
       Geographic Society, 1975.
              Maps of geographic regions with many essays preced-
              ing them. Has sections on oceans, volcanoes, earth-
              quakes, etc. Well indexed.

1.3   Webster's New Geographical Dictionary, rev. ed. Spring-
       field, Mass.: Merriam Co., 1977.
              Contains 47,999 entries and 2,167 maps. For cities,
              states, dependencies, etc., arranged alphabetically.
              Includes information on pronunciation, location, size,
              etc. Not quite as comprehensive as the Columbia-
              Lippincott Gazetteer.

BIBLIOGRAPHIES

Bibliographies are listings of materials such as books,
articles, audiovisuals, and pamphlets, usually on specific
topics. Bibliographies give you the information you need to
retrieve the items listed, i.e., author, title, place of publication, publisher, date, etc. Annotated bibliographies give
a brief summary of the content of a particular item and as
such may give you evaluative information on the items listed.

Non-Medical

1.4   Books in Print, 1979-80. 4 vols. New York: R.R. Bowker
       Co., 1979.
              Published annually, this is an alphabetic listing of

books available primarily from U.S. publishers. Two
volumes list the books by author and two list the books
by title. Each book listed gives author, title, publisher, date of publication, edition, series, standard book
number, price if available, etc. At the end of the
second volume of the title listing there is an alphabetical list of publishers with their addresses and telephone numbers. This is an excellent resource for or-
dering a specific title.

1.5   Cumulative Book Index, World List of Books in the English
Language. New York: H.W. Wilson Co., 1898 to date.
Published monthly (except August) and cumulated yearly. More comprehensive than Books in Print since it
lists books in the English language, not just books published in the United States. Gives author-title-subject
listing in a single alphabet. Also includes "Directory
of Publishers and Distributors" at end of each volume
or issue.

1.6   Subject Guide to Books in Print, 1979-80. 2 vols. New
York: R.R. Bowker Co., 1979.
Gives a detailed breakdown of the titles listed in
Books in Print by subject.

1.7   Ulrich's International Periodicals Directory, A Classified
Guide to Current Periodicals, Foreign and Domestic 1979-80,
18th ed. New York: R.R. Bowker Co., 1979.
Published every two years. Lists current periodicals
which come out more than once a year and are published at regular intervals. Arranged by subject, the
information given includes title of journal, publisher,
subscription price, year first published, frequency,
editor, address, and other miscellaneous facts. Includes index by periodical titles.

Medical and Nursing

1.8   Catalog of the Sophia F. Palmer Memorial Library. 2 vols.
Compiled by Sophia F. Palmer Library, American Journal
of Nursing. Boston: G. K. Hall, 1973.

A listing of the materials owned by this major nursing library. Authors, titles, and subjects are arranged as in a dictionary. Very useful but limited for current information because of its 1973 publication date.

1.9   Medical Books and Serials in Print 1979; An Index to Literature in the Health Sciences. New York: R.R. Bowker Co., 1979.

Lists books and serials in the medical fields, including nursing, dentistry, psychology, psychiatry, medicine, etc. Begins with a preface and an introduction on how to use the volume, then lists books by subject and author in two separate sections and serials by subject and title in two separate sections. For the most part, contains information on materials which are published by the standard trade publishers. Includes price, address of publishers in a separate section, and bibliographic information.

1.10 U.S. National Library of Medicine. Current Catalog. Bethesda, Md., 1966 to date.

Published quarterly, cumulated annually. A listing by "main entry" and subject of materials received by the National Library of Medicine in Bethesda. Useful in locating what has been published on a given subject.

1.11 U.S. National Library of Medicine. List of Journals Indexed in Index Medicus. Bethesda, Md., 1980.

Annually published both separately and as a part of Part   of the January Index Medicus, the major medical index. Lists journals alphabetically by title, title abbreviation, and subject. Gives only the journal title and its abbreviation, yet is useful in locating names of periodicals on particular subjects. Lists "Special List Nursing" journals as well (journals indexed in the International Nursing Index primarily).

1.12 U.S. National Library of Medicine. Medical Subject Headings, 1980. U.S. Department of Health, Education, and Welfare, Public Health Service, National Institutes of Health, National Library of Medicine, 1980.

Comes out annually as part of the January Index
Medicus. Contains alphabetical and categorized lists
of approved subject headings used in the Index Medicus.

BIOGRAPHICAL DICTIONARIES, INDEXES

A biographical dictionary gives information on a specific
group of persons, usually including their birth dates and
death dates (if applicable), degrees, general information,
and the like. A biographical index tells where information
on a specific person is located; it does not contain the information itself.

Non-Medical

1.13 Biography Index, A Cumulative Index to Biographical
      Material in Books and Magazines. New York: Wilson,
      1947 to date.
            Quarterly with annual cumulations. Indexes biographi-
            cal information which appears in books, magazines,
            etc. A good source for current biographical informa-
            tion.

1.14 Current Biography. New York: Wilson, 1940 to date.
            Published monthly (except August) and cumulated year-
            ly. Includes one- to two-page biographies on well-
            known persons or persons in the news. Often includes
            a picture and sources of other information on the
            person.

1.15 Webster's Biographical Dictionary, rev. ed. Springfield,
      Mass.: Merriam, 1976.
            A good one-volume source of information on persons
            who are no longer living. Gives name, pronunciation,
            birth and death dates, occupation, and brief biographi-
            cal information.

1.16 Who's Who: An Annual Biographical Dictionary. London:
      Black; New York: St. Martin's Press; 1849 to date.

Published annually. Lists prominent people from all over the world, but emphasis is given to the British.

1.17   Who's Who in America, 1978-79, 40th ed. 2 vols. Chicago: Marquis Who's Who, 1978.
Published since 1898, now published every two years. Includes persons notable in government, business, education, religion, athletics, art, music, and science. For each entry, gives full name, current position, date of birth, education, marital status, children, activities (career and civic), publications, and home and/or office addresses. This is supplemented by the Who's Who in the various regions, such as Who's Who in the East, Who's Who in the Midwest, etc.

1.18   World Who's Who in Science, A Biographical Dictionary of Notable Scientists from Antiquity to the Present. Edited by Allen G. Debus. Chicago: Marquis Who's Who, 1968.
"A component volume of the Marquis Biographical Library." Lists some 30,000 outstanding scientists (living and dead) all over the world. Gives place and date of birth, family, education, experience, publications, date of death (if applicable), current address, etc.

Nursing

1.19   International Directory of Nurses with Doctoral Degrees. New York: American Nurses' Foundation, 1973.
The only substantial source for biographical information about nurses with their doctorates. Gives educational background, subject area, title of dissertation. Has also been published and updated in Nursing Outlook.

Medical

1.20   American Medical Directory, 27th ed. 4 vols. Chicago: American Medical Association, 1979.

Began publication in 1907; now published irregularly. Volume I is an alphabetical listing of physicians with their geographic locations noted. Volumes II-IV arrange physicians by states, giving their address, type of practice, medical school, Board certification, etc.

1.21 American Men and Women of Science, 14th ed. 8 vols. (including index volume). Edited by The Jaques Cattell Press. New York: R.R. Bowker Co., 1979.

To date, this edition includes physical and biological sciences only. Publication of social and behavioral sciences section is pending. Gives biographical data on some 130,500 notable men and women in the physical and biological sciences. In alphabetical order by name, with discipline and geographic index volume.

1.22 Directory of Medical Specialists, 1979-80, 19th ed. 3 vols. Chicago: Marquis Who's Who, 1979.

First published in 1940. Lists physicians with American Specialty Boards' certification. Arranged alphabetically by specialty board, then by state and city. For each physician, gives birth date, educational and work background, etc. Indexed by the name of the physician. Contains information on the specialty boards as well. Not as comprehensive as the American Medical Directory since not all doctors choose to be board certified.

DICTIONARIES

A dictionary is an alphabetical listing of words, including their definition and usually giving their syllabification, pronunciation, and often their derivation.

Non-Medical

1.23 Acronyms, Initialisms, and Abbreviations Dictionary: A Guide to Alphabetic Designations, Contractions, Acronyms,

Initialisms, Abbreviations, and Similar Condensed Appella-
tions, 6th ed. 3 vols. Edited by Ellen T. Crowley, et al.
Detroit: Gale Research Company, 1978.
> Lists well over 100,000 abbreviations, acronyms and
> the like, dealing not only with medical topics, but also
> education, media, etc. Includes some foreign entries.

1.24 The American Heritage Dictionary of the English Language.
Edited by William Morris. New York: American Heritage,
1973.
> A moderately long dictionary with many black and white
> sketches. Gives standard dictionary information on
> words (syllabification, pronunciation, etc.).

1.25 The New Cassell's French Dictionary: French-English,
English-French. Completely revised by Denis Girard, et al.
New York: Funk and Wagnalls, 1977.
> Cassell's dictionaries also cover Dutch, German,
> Italian, Latin, Spanish, and other languages. The first
> section is an alphabetical listing of French words with
> the English translation and the second section is a list-
> ing of English words with the French translation.
> Covers the entire language, not just medical or tech-
> nical terms. There are many similar dictionaries and
> this is intended only to give you an example of this
> type of reference tool.

1.26 Roget's Thesaurus of English Words and Phrases, new ed.,
completely rev. and modernized. Edited by Robert A.
Dutch. New York: St. Martin's Press, 1965.
> First published in 1852. Contains a listing of syno-
> nyms for the words included. An indispensable tool,
> particularly for writing.

1.27 Van Nostrand's Scientific Encyclopedia, 5th ed.
Edited by Douglas M. Considine. New York: C. Van
Nostrand Reinhold Co., 1976.
> A comprehensive volume which has short definitions
> and discussions of topics in all areas of the sciences.

1.28 Webster's Third New International Dictionary of the English
      Language, Unabridged. Edited by Philip B. Gove, et al.
      Springfield, Mass.: G. & C. Merriam Co., 1976.
          The archetypical dictionary. Contains some 450,000
          entries. Includes many illustrations, tables, color
          plates.

Medical and Nursing

1.29 Abbreviations and Acronyms in Medicine and Nursing.
      Edited by Solomon Garb, Eleanor Krakauer, and Carson
      Justice. New York: Springer Publishing Co., 1976.
          A list of abbreviations in medicine and nursing. In-
          cludes the Greek alphabet and some symbols with their
          meanings.

1.30 Abbreviations in Medicine, 4th ed. Edited by Edwin B.
      Steen. London: Ballière Tindall, 1978.
          Includes all sorts of abbreviations relevant to medi-
          cine. Has symbols and abbreviations of principal
          medical journals as well.

1.31 Dorland's Illustrated Medical Dictionary, 25th ed. Phila-
      delphia: Saunders, 1974.
          With Stedman's (1.34), among the major medical dic-
          tionaries. Inclusive and excellent definitions.

1.32 Elsevier's Medical Dictionary in Five Languages: English/
      American, French, Italian, Spanish and German, 2d rev. ed.
      Amsterdam: Elsevier, 1975.
          Lists the English word and its counterparts in the
          other five languages in tabular form. Gives strictly
          one-word translations. Includes an index for each
          language.

1.33 Encyclopedia and Dictionary of Medicine, Nursing, and
      Allied Health, 2d ed. Edited by Benjamin F. Miller and
      Claire Brackman Keane. Philadelphia: Saunders, 1978.

Written by a physician and a nurse, this is an excellent
resource for nurses and other health professionals.
Definitions include pronunciations and often are more
extensive than in a traditional dictionary, hence the
use of the word "encyclopedia." Sometimes includes
patient care category under definitions. Appendixes
cover weights for boys/girls, men/women; patient education materials information; conversion information.

1.34 Stedman's Medical Dictionary: A Vocabulary of Medicine
and Its Allied Sciences, with Pronunciations and Derivatives,
23d ed. Baltimore: Williams & Wilkins, 1976.
See Dorland's (1.31).

1.35 Taber's Cyclopedic Medical Dictionary, 13th ed. Edited by
Clayton L. Thomas. Philadelphia: Davis, 1977.
A good, large-sized pocket dictionary. Definitions
are briefer than Stedman's (1.34) or Dorland's (1.31).

DIRECTORIES

Directories list information, principally about organizations,
giving background, purpose, etc.

General

1.36 Encyclopedia of Associations, 14th ed. 3 vols. Edited by
Margaret Fisk, et al. Detroit: Gale Research Company,
1980.
Arranged by broad subject categories initially. This
source lists primarily U.S. organizations and international organizations of interest to Americans. Includes
indexes by the name of the organization, geographic
regions, and executives. Periodically updated with
loose-leaf publications. For the organizations listed
gives address, phone number, founding date, chief
official, number of members, description of publications, convention/annual meeting information, etc.

Useful for many things, particularly names and addresses of organizations for patients or information concerning publications or meetings of a specific association.

1.37 The World of Learning, 1979-80, 30th ed. 2 vols. London: Europa Publications, 1979.

For international associations, gives information on goals, budget, persons responsible, publications, etc. For the countries of the world (arranged in alphabetical order), gives population, educational institutions, libraries, museums, etc. Includes address, persons in charge, publications. Has an index to the institutions. Information for this is gathered from mailings to the various institutions covered.

Medical and Nursing

1.38 American Hospital Association. Guide to the Health Care Field. Chicago: American Hospital Association, 1979.

Index and index to advertisers.

Published annually. Four main sections include: information on U.S. health care institutions (hospitals in the United States, those outside the United States with U.S. association, U.S. government hospitals, long-term care facilities which are accredited); members of the American Hospital Association (officers, various categories of members); health organizations, (international, national, and regional) agencies, and educational programs in health; and a buyer's guide arranged by subject with manufacturers' names, addresses, and telephone numbers. The hospital section gives the address of each hospital, telephone number, administrator, accreditation, types of facilities, control of the facility (government, private, etc.), number of beds, expense figures, number of personnel, and the like.

1.39 Health Organizations of the United States, Canada, and Internationally: A Directory of Voluntary Associations, Professional Societies, and Other Groups Concerned with Health
and Related Fields, 4th ed. Edited by Paul Wasserman and
Jane K. Bossart. Ann Arbor: Edwards Brothers for
Anthony T. Kruzas Associates, 1977.
> Brief descriptions of unofficial and non-government
> associations, societies, and the like in health and re-
> lated fields. Covers the United States and Canada as
> well as international organizations. Data were com-
> piled from questionnaires and are arranged by name
> of organization as well as by subject field.

ENCYCLOPEDIAS

Encyclopedias give background information on a wide variety
of topics. They contain much valuable information though
the extent to which they can explore a subject is limited by
space. Encyclopedias usually contain references for further
research and are often excellent resources to begin study of
a topic.

1.40 The Encyclopedia Americana, International edition. 30 vols.
New York: Americana Corp., 1979.
> With The Encyclopaedia Britannica, one of the major
> encyclopedias.

1.41 The New Columbia Encyclopedia, 4th ed. Edited by William
H. Harris and Judith S. Levey. New York: Columbia University Press, 1975.
> A short-entry encyclopedia with information on a wide
> variety of subjects. Entries are arranged alphabeti-
> cally. Includes cross references, maps, diagrams,
> and bibliographies.

1.42 The New Encyclopaedia Britannica, 15th ed. 30 vols.
[Propaedia, 1 vol.; Micropaedia, 10 vols.; Macropaedia,
19 vols.] Chicago: Encyclopaedia Britannica, 1979.

Format changed with this edition. Propaedia presents an outline of knowledge in one volume; Micropaedia, "ready reference and index," goes into more detail; and Macropaedia, "knowledge in depth," gives even more information.

HANDBOOKS

Handbooks are small books which usually deal with a topic in brief fashion.

1.43 Familiar Quotations: A Collection of Passages, Phrases and Proverbs Traced to Their Sources in Ancient and Modern Literature, 14th ed., rev. and enl. Compiled by John Bartlett. Edited by Emily Morrison Beck. Boston: Little, Brown, 1968.
    A listing of authors and their quotations in chronological order. Has indexes by author and subject.

1.44 Harbrace College Handbook, 8th ed. By John C. Hodges and Mary E. Whitten. New York: Harcourt Brace Jovanovich, 1977.
    A basic book of grammatical rules and styles for use in writing.

INDEXES AND ABSTRACTS

Indexes are by far the single most important item in any reference collection. Indexes do not provide information in themselves; they simply indicate where information can be located. The card catalog is the index to the books in a particular library. It tells you if the library has a particular book or a particular item on a specific subject, and where it can be found. Books usually have indexes which tell whether a specific concept or word is mentioned in them. Indexes are usually arranged in alphabetical order by subject and cover a specific period of time. Probably most indexes with which one is familiar are those for journals or periodicals, which list articles in specific journals on specific topics. However, many indexes deal not only with journals, but also with books, audiovisuals, newspapers, short stories, essays, etc. Needless to say, indexes allow you to find certain sorts of information much more quickly than you could by looking through individual magazines.

Abstracts (or abstracting services) perform the same function as indexes except they contain a summary of the item they are indexing and as such give information which may help you decide if you need to consult that item. Because it usually takes longer to prepare abstracts than to prepare indexes, abstracts may not be as current as indexes.

General

1.45 New York Times Index. Microfilming Corporation of America, 1620 Hawkins Avenue, P.O. Box 10, Sanford, N.C. 27330. Twice monthly. 1913 to date.

1.46 *Readers' Guide to Periodical Literature. H.W. Wilson Co., 950 University Avenue, Bronx, N.Y. 10452. Twice monthly September to June, monthly July and August; annual cumulations. 1900 to date.

Nursing

1.47 *Cumulative Index to Nursing and Allied Health Literature. Glendale Adventist Medical Center Publications Service, Box 871, Glendale, Calif. 91209. Every 2 months with yearly cumulation. 1961 to date. (Former title: Cumulative Index to Nursing Literature.)

1.48 *Hospital Literature Index. American Hospital Association, 840 N. Lake Shore Drive, Chicago, Ill. 60611. Monthly with annual and 5-year cumulations. 1945 to date.

---

*See Chapter 16 for detailed explanation of these indexes.

1.49   *International Nursing Index. American Journal of Nursing Co., 10 Columbus Circle, New York, N.Y. 10019. (For the American Nurses' Association and the National League for Nursing) Quarterly; annual cumulations. 1966 to date.

Medical

1.50   *Abridged Index Medicus. National Library of Medicine, 8600 Rockville Pike, Bethesda, Md. 20209. Monthly with an annual cumulation. 1970 to date.[†]

1.51   *Index Medicus. National Library of Medicine, 8600 Rockville Pike, Bethesda, Md. 20209. Monthly with an annual cumulation. 1960 to date.[†]

YEARBOOKS

Yearbooks are defined as books which "give the year in review," i.e., tell what has occurred in a given year.

1.52   The World Almanac and Book of Facts, 1980. New York: Newspaper Enterprise Association, 1979.
        Comes out every November. One of the single most important available sources of factual information. Has an index in the front of the volume.

CONCLUSION

We have listed items and categories of items in this chapter as a starting point for study. There are, of course, other categories of materials in reference collections, for example, pamphlets or "vertical files" containing information with a brief time span of usefulness. Also, other librarians or libraries may group items differently from the manner in which we have grouped them above.

---

*See Chapter 16 for detailed explanation of these indexes.
[†]Order from Superintendent of Documents, Washington, D.C. 20402.

2
Fundamentals of Nursing

In this chapter, we have grouped general books on the fundamentals of nursing care in the first section; then books dealing with the nursing process in particular: patient education, physical assessment, infection control, and the problem-oriented system. A listing of relevant periodicals is included at the end of the chapter.

FOUNDATIONS OF NURSING CARE

2.1   Brill, Esther Levine; Kilts, Dawn F.   Foundations for Nursing.   New York: Appleton-Century-Crofts, 1980.
>   848 pp.   Cloth.   Index.   Reading lists.
>   Comprehensive textbook emphasizing both theory and skills.   Strong in the areas of physical assessment. Unique in its inclusion of change theory and change skills.   Uses a health maintenance approach, organized around human needs.   Strong growth and development charts throughout.   Teacher's manual available. Case studies and clinical examples included in text.

2.2   Brunner, Lillian Sholtis; Suddarth, Doris Smith; et al.   The Lippincott Manual of Nursing Practice, 2d ed.   Philadelphia: Lippincott, 1978.
>   1868 pp.   Cloth.   Index.   Bibliographies.

An extensive reference work which covers the major
concepts of clinical nursing practice in succinct, outline form with illustrations where appropriate. Divided into three parts: Medical-Surgical Nursing,
Maternity Nursing, and Pediatric Nursing.

2.3   Byrne, Marjorie L.; Thompson, Lida F.   Key Concepts for
the Study and Practice of Nursing, 2d ed.   St. Louis:
Mosby, 1978.
   150 pp.   Paper.   Index.   References.   Additional readings.   Glossary.
   The authors provide a perspective and framework for
   understanding those faced with the threat of illness,
   that is, a way to organize concepts and theories from
   the natural and behavioral sciences into a framework
   for nursing practice.   Their assumptions and beliefs
   about human beings, health, and the recipients of
   health care are made clear in the introduction.   Concepts included are: basic human needs, patterns of
   behavior and levels of instability, and assessment of
   variables likely to influence the nurse-patient interaction, levels of wellness, stress, prediction of consequences, position and role, and the nurse-client
   relationship.

2.4   Campbell, Claire.   Nursing Diagnosis and Intervention in
Nursing Practice.   New York: Wiley, 1978.
   1928 pp.   Cloth.   Nursing diagnoses alphabetical index,
   nursing diagnoses subject index, nursing interventions
   alphabetical index, nursing interventions subject index.   References.
   "This book is devoted to the nursing process and emphasizes the development and identification of nursing
   diagnoses and interventions." (p. v.) Stresses nursing, rather than medical, problems.   Part One goes
   into theory and Parts Two and Three deal with specific
   nursing diagnoses and interventions.   "The book is
   intended to be a quick, practical source from which
   patient care plans can be made and is applicable to
   the Problem-Oriented Record System." (p. v.) An
   extensive textbook for reference.

2.5   Coffey, Lou. Modules for Independent-Individual Learning
in Nursing. Philadelphia: Davis, 1975.
>389 pp. Paper. References. Additional readings.
>An outgrowth of collaboration between teachers and
>students in the United States and Canada, this book is
>designed to be a less traditional means of learning, to
>help the student become a "self-directed learner."
>The three parts present first, a guide to development
>and implementation of an independent-individualized
>learning approach; second, actual modules on nursing
>activities (e.g., bedmaking, nurse-patient relations,
>asepsis, etc.); and third, other materials which may
>be needed (e.g., audiovisual resources). Modules
>contain the following elements: guiding principles,
>general and specific objectives, vocabulary, sugges-
>tions for learning activities and experiences, and
>readings.

2.6   Dison, Norma. Clinical Nursing Techniques, 4th ed.
St. Louis: Mosby, 1979.
>491 pp. Paper. Index. Selected references.
>Glossary.
>Using text and illustrations, explains selected tech-
>niques viewed as basic to nursing practice. Included
>are personal hygiene, infection control, safety, ad-
>ministration of drugs, irrigations, and others.

2.7   DuGas, Beverly W. Introduction to Patient Care: A Comprehensive Approach to Nursing. 3d ed. Philadelphia:
Saunders, 1977.
>686 pp., Cloth. Index. Suggested readings.
>Glossary.
>Provides an introduction to the practice of nursing as
>part of the total health care system. Introduces the
>basic skills in using the nursing process. Units cover:
>The Role of the Nurse in Health Care; The Nursing
>Process; Helping People Meet Basic Health Needs;
>Common Health Problems in Practice. Includes stu-
>dent objectives, guides to the assessment of patient
>status, evaluating the effectiveness of nursing action,

vocabulary, and study situations for most chapters.
Appendixes include listings of prefixes, suffixes.

2.8   Gooding, Marion Brown. Techniques for Utilizing Nursing
Principles. St. Louis: Mosby, 1972.
    163 pp. Paper. Index.
    Emphasizes the principles behind nursing care func-
    tions, using examples throughout. Chapters include:
    Why Teach Nursing Principles?; A Philosophy of Nurs-
    ing; Relationship of Nursing to Other Theory; The
    Process of Identifying Nursing Principles; Techniques
    for Coring Nursing Content; Lecture and Laboratory
    Applications. Aimed at the nurse educator. Appendix
    includes samples for teacher planning (nursing care
    plan, teaching plan, etc.).

2.9   Henderson, Virginia; Nite, Gladys. Principles and Practice
of Nursing, 6th ed. New York: Macmillan, 1978.
    2119 pp. Cloth. Index. References. Additional
    readings.
    For students in their first nursing course as well as
    later ones. Looks at the place of nursing in the health
    field; the role of the nurse in meeting patients' health
    needs; fundamentals of nursing, therapeutic measures,
    procedures, and techniques; and common problems in
    nursing. Includes comprehensive information on pri-
    mary care, health as well as illness, and the family
    and community. Well documented; seventeen contrib-
    utors add depth from their clinical expertise.

2.10   King, Eunice M.; Wieck, Lynn; Dyer, Marilyn. Illustrated
Manual of Nursing Techniques. Philadelphia: Lippincott,
1977.
    432 pp. Cloth. Index. Bibliography.
    A basic book concerning nursing care given by all
    levels of nurses. Presents factual material in two
    major units: Techniques Related to General Nursing
    and Techniques Related to Obstetrical and Newborn
    Nursing. Each technique presented includes: defini-
    tion, terminology, rationale for nursing action,

nursing objectives, equipment, and nursing intervention (including therapeutic, communicative, teaching, and evaluative aspects). Examples of techniques covered are bathing, catheterization, restraints, breast care, weighing of the newborn, etc.

2.11 Kozier, Barbara; Erb, Glenora Lea. Fundamentals of Nursing: Concepts and Procedures. Menlo Park, Ca.: Addison-Wesley, 1979.
        980 pp. Cloth. Index. Suggested readings. References. Glossary.
        A comprehensive fundamentals of nursing text. Seven units cover: Nursing and Health Needs; Integrating Concepts; Integrating Skills; Therapeutic Communication; Physiologic Needs, Psychosocial Needs; Special Nursing Measures. Each chapter includes an outline, objectives at the beginning, a summary, and potential activities. Appendixes include abbreviations, prefixes and suffixes, etc.

2.12 Lewis, LuVerne Wolff. Fundamental Skills in Patient Care. Philadelphia: Lippincott, 1976.
        495 pp. Paper. Index. References. Glossaries.
        "The purpose of this book is to present basic nursing skills which every nurse needs to know, regardless of the type of educational program in which she is enrolled—practical, associate degree, or baccalaureate." (p. v.) Each chapter includes an outline, and a listing of behavioral objectives. Includes extensive illustrative material and charts. Second edition due 1980.

2.13 Little, Dolores E.; Carnevali, Doris L. Nursing Care Planning, 2d ed. Philadelphia: Lippincott, 1976.
        325 pp. Paper. Index. References.
        Instead of merely discussing "the techniques of writing care plans," the second edition examines "how one must think in order to begin to write or report on plans of care." (pp. vii-viii.) Chapters discuss nursing care, the nursing care plan, nursing assessment,

nursing diagnosis, nursing prescription, evaluation of
nursing care, etc. This change in the focus of the text
was dictated by the new identity of the nursing profession as more than a "physician extender service."
(p. vii.)

2.14 Marram, Gwen; Barrett, Margaret W.; Bevis, Em O.
Primary Nursing: A Model for Individualized Care, 2d ed.
St. Louis: Mosby, 1979.
216 pp. Paper. Index. References.
Discusses ways of organizing work to deliver individualized nursing care. For nursing students, educators,
and nurses in practice, this book focuses on primary
nursing and related research. Primary nursing is
proposed as a way to deliver high quality care in a
humanistic, holistic manner. Major sections are:
Evolution of Nursing Care Modalities, Nature and
Scope of Primary Nursing, and Evaluating the Effects
of Primary Nursing.

2.15 Massachusetts General Hospital, Department of Nursing.
Manual of Nursing Procedures. Boston: Little, Brown,
1975.
389 pp. Paper (spiral bound). Index.
A reference book for nursing procedures, including
procedures carried out at the Massachusetts General
Hospital. Includes General Procedures; Fundamental
Nursing; Diagnostic Tests and Procedures; Care of
Patients Receiving Radioactive Materials; Isolation
Techniques; General Therapeutic Measures; General
Preoperative and Postoperative Care; "Line" Ther-
apy—IV, CVP, Hyperalimentation, and Arterial Lines;
Cardiac Nursing Care, Including Cardiopulmonary
Resuscitation; Respiratory Nursing Care; Urological/
Renal Nursing Care; Ostomy Nursing Care; Neurologi-
cal Nursing Care; Orthopedic Nursing Care; Eye, Ear,
and Nose Nursing Care; Burn Nursing Care; and Psychiatric Nursing Care. An abbreviations list is at the
back of the book. Lists equipment, procedure, and
points of emphasis for each procedure.

2.16 Mitchell, Pamela Holsclaw. Concepts Basic to Nursing,
      2d ed. New York: McGraw-Hill, 1977.
            575 pp. Cloth. Name and subject indexes. Refer-
            ences.
            Provides an in-depth discussion for beginning students
            on the role of nursing in health care and the process of
            diagnosis and decision-making in patient care as well
            as providing content for specific areas (e.g., environ-
            ment, nutrition, behavior, temperature, sleep, etc.).
            Each chapter opens with a "Data to be Assessed"
            section.

2.17 Murray, Malinda. Fundamentals of Nursing. Englewood
      Cliffs: Prentice-Hall, 1976.
            530 pp. Cloth. Index. Selected bibliographies.
            Glossary.
            For beginning nursing students in any program, bac-
            calaureate, associate, or diploma. Designed to de-
            velop basic abilities (interpersonal, intellectual, and
            psychomotor) necessary for good nursing care. In
            seven parts, deals with: nursing and the nurse; the
            nursing process; psychosocial concerns and commu-
            nication in nursing; the health care environment;
            assessment of human needs in the health care system;
            nursing intervention in certain situations (e.g., pain,
            rehabilitation); and finally, the future in nursing.
            Includes marginal notes and study questions after each
            chapter. Second edition due 1980.

2.18 Murray, Ruth Beckmann; Zentner, Judith Proctor; et al.
      Nursing Concepts for Health Promotion, 2d ed. Englewood
      Cliffs: Prentice-Hall, 1979.
            525 pp. Cloth. Index. References.
            Looks at materials needed for an integrated approach
            to nursing in any setting. The book examines the
            factors affecting a person as a member of a pluralis-
            tic society as well as considerations related to health
            promotion. The goal of the authors is to give nurses
            and nursing students the broad conceptual base needed
            to promote comprehensive health. Chapters in Unit I

look at health and illness, health care delivery, communication, and other topics. Unit II includes cultural
and environmental influences and the family unit.

2.19 Orem, Dorothea E. Nursing: Concepts of Practice. New
York: McGraw-Hill, 1971.
>237 pp. Cloth. Index. Bibliographies.
"Designed to aid nursing students and nurses . . . by
providing general guides for use in understanding the
relationship between health states and health care
problems of patients and nursing action." (p. vii)
Deals with Nursing and Society; Dimensions of Nursing;
Nursing and Health Care; Variations in Nursing Situations; The Process of Nursing the Individual Patient;
Nursing and the Law. Designed to provide a base;
students should go to items referenced for further
reading.

2.20 Paterson, Josephine G.; Zderad, Loretta T. Humanistic
Nursing. New York: Wiley, 1976.
>141 pp. Cloth. Index. Bibliography.
A philosophy-of-nursing book that deals with humanistic nursing in general and then specific applications of
the theory, including case situations. By the authors'
definition, "[humanistic nursing] . . . focuses on the
meaning and means of nursing's particular mode of
interhuman caring." (p. x)

2.21 Riley, Mary Ann K. Case Studies in Nursing Fundamentals.
New York: Macmillan, 1979.
>302 pp. Paper. Bibliographies.
A workbook for the nursing student that contains simulated case studies. Chapters cover the nursing process, nurse-patient relationships, safety, stress,
nutrition, pain, wound care, patient education, etc.
Prior to going through the workbook on a given topic,
students are to read designated chapters in recommended texts. Each chapter in this workbook contains
objectives, situations (except for the beginning exercises), study exercises, or other type of exercise.

The author advocates problem analysis via the SOAP method (Subjective, Objective, Assessment, and Plan).

2.22 Rines, Alice R.; Montag, Mildred. Nursing Concepts and Nursing Care. New York: Wiley, 1976.
    431 pp. Cloth. Index. Bibliographies.
    Designed "to give the beginning student of nursing a good grasp of nursing fundamentals." (p. v) Nine parts contain chapters on the following: Social Influence, The Nursing Process, Human Needs, Cultural Beliefs, Behavior Patterns, Wellness, Protection, Oxygenation, and Body Defenses.

2.23 Roy, Callista. Introduction to Nursing: An Adaptation Model. Englewood Cliffs: Prentice-Hall, 1976.
    402 pp. Cloth. Index. References. Glossaries.
    This book poses the Roy Adaptation Model as a means to develop a conceptual framework of nursing knowledge. Original papers by varied authors focus on Introduction to the Roy nursing model; basic physiologic and psychological needs, including self concept; role function; interdependence; and minority cultures. Appendixes include assessment and nursing interventions based on the Roy Adaptation Model. Most chapters include summaries.

2.24 Saxton, Dolores F.; Hyland, Patricia A. Planning and Implementing Nursing Intervention: Stress and Adaptation Applied to Patient Care, 2d ed. St. Louis: Mosby, 1979.
    195 pp. Paper. Index. Bibliography. Glossary.
    This text is designed to help the nursing student plan and implement interventions based on an understanding and recognition of a person's varying adaptations to stress. The two parts give, first, a theoretical base for interventions, and, second, applications based on specific patient care problem situations (e.g., regulatory, emotional, elimination, fluid and electrolyte, etc.).

2.25 Sorensen, Karen Creason; Luckmann, Joan. Basic Nursing:
A Psychophysiologic Approach. Philadelphia: Saunders,
1979.
>1311 pp. Cloth. Index. Bibliographies.
>A comprehensive fundamental nursing textbook de-
signed to be used separately or together with Medical-
Surgical Nursing: A Psychophysiologic Approach
(3.10). Units cover Unifying Concepts Basic to
Nursing Practice; Basic Concepts of Stress,
Homeostasis, Health and Illness; Understanding the
Existence of the Ill; Establishing Medical and Nursing
Diagnosis; Planning and Providing Care; Introduction
to Legal Concepts; Application of Biomechanics to
Nursing; Providing Food and Fluids; Basic Clinical
Considerations; Advanced Clinical Considerations;
Caring for Persons with Special Needs, etc. Includes
highlighted information in italics and enclosed in
boxes, along with an overview and a study guide (with
objectives) for most chapters. The appendix includes
normal value tables.

2.26 Sutterley, Doris Cook; Donnelly, Gloria Ferraro. Perspectives in Human Development: Nursing Throughout the Life
Cycle. Philadelphia: Lippincott, 1973.
>331 pp. Cloth. Index. References.
Bibliographies.
>One of the first books which was "designed to intro-
duce the student to a more unified approach to the
study of man." (p. ix)   Chapters discuss nursing in
today's health care environment, systems theory,
growth, communication, sexuality, and the like. In
an attempt to look at human beings holistically, the
authors have used an integrated approach viewing the
person as a "psychophysical" entity.

2.27 University of Kansas Medical Center, Department of Nursing Education, Kansas City, Kansas. Case Studies of
Nursing Intervention. New York: McGraw-Hill, 1974.
>245 pp. Paper. Selected readings.

These case studies were developed for a clinical
course at the University of Kansas, Department of
Nursing Education. The cases include all age groups
and many common patient care problems, e.g., child
abuse, cystic fibrosis, toxemia, abortion, alcoholism,
burns, mastectomy, depression, myocardial infarct,
cataracts, etc. Each case includes background information, patient history, nurses' and/or doctors'
orders, notes or actions, study guide questions.

2.28 Watson, Jean. Nursing, the Philosophy and Science of Car-
      ing. Boston: Little, Brown, 1979.
          321 pp. Cloth. Index. References.
          Discusses the caring relationship in nursing in order
          to promote better communication between nurse and
          client and, therefore, provide better nursing care.
          Chapters are organized around three parts: Nursing
          as the Science of Caring; Assistance with the Gratifi-
          cation of Human Needs; and Application of the Carative
          Factors to Situations that Affect Health-Illness. Each
          chapter includes a summary.

2.29 White, Dorothy T.; Rubino, Edith; DeLorey, Philip E.
      Fundamentals: The Foundation of Nursing. Englewood
      Cliffs: Prentice-Hall, 1972.
          281 pp. Cloth. Index. Bibliographies.
          Glossary.
          The aim of this book is "to bring alive a multifaceted
          concept of nursing for the novice." (p. xix) The book
          has an open, readable, non-textbook approach to
          nursing and contains many humorous and informative
          drawings. Chapters discuss people, the nurse-patient
          relationship, the nurse's role in patient care, the
          hospital environment, and specific nursing tasks,
          e.g., aseptic procedures, administering medications,
          etc. The discussion on tasks describes the nursing
          actions and the reasons for those actions, as well as
          listing the equipment needed, when applicable. In-
          cludes an alphabetical list of suffixes and tables and
          charts.

2.30 Wolff, LuVerne; Weitzel, Marlene H.; Fuerst, Elinor V.
Fundamentals of Nursing: The Humanities and the Sciences
in Nursing, 6th ed. Philadelphia: Lippincott, 1979.
>512 pp. Cloth. References.
>Glossaries.
>Presents concepts basic to nursing practice, including
>units on Nursing and the Consumer of Health Services,
>The Methodology of Nursing, Environmental Consider-
>ations in the Practice of Nursing, and Technical Skills
>In and Underlying the Principles of the Practice of
>Nursing. Primarily for the nursing student. Each
>chapter includes behavioral objectives and questions
>for further work by the student.

2.31 Wood, Lucile A.; Rambo, Beverly J., eds. Nursing Skills
for Allied Health Services, rev. ed. Philadelphia:
Saunders, 1977.
>752 pp. Paper. Index.
>Contains 37 instructional units on nursing procedures,
>e.g., handwashing, positioning, baths, vital signs,
>charting, preoperative and postoperative care, re-
>straints, spiritual care, cardiopulmonary resuscita-
>tion, etc. Each unit consists of objectives, vocabu-
>lary, information, and a post-test with answers. The
>information presented is basic and brief and is de-
>signed for all levels of nursing personnel, from nurs-
>ing assistants to RN's.

THE NURSING PROCESS

2.32 Burgess, Ann Wolbert. Nursing: Levels of Health Intervention. Englewood Cliffs: Prentice-Hall, 1978.
>809 pp. Cloth. Index. Bibliography. Glossary.
>A basic text for nursing students in their first profes-
>sional nursing course. Five parts address the basis
>for nursing practice, a system model for nursing,
>the nursing process, nursing intervention at different
>levels, and procedures for nurses.

2.33 Documenting Patient Care Responsibly. [Nursing '78 Skill-
      book Series.] Horsham, Pa.: Intermed Communications,
      1978.
             191 pp. Cloth. Index. Bibliography.
             Shows the interrelationship between charting and the
             nursing process in a readable, practical form. Di-
             vided into five basic parts: How to Make the Most of
             the Nursing Process; How to Collect and Document
             Data; How to Identify Your Patient's Problems and
             Plan His Care; How to Record Your Patient's Prog-
             ress; and How to Evaluate Your Care and Protect
             Yourself Legally. Chapters within each section in-
             clude reminders at the end of each chapter. Each
             section ends with a skillcheck, in the form of several
             multiple choice questions applying concepts learned in
             the earlier chapters. Answers are included at end of
             the book. Appendixes include examples of a nursing
             data base (assessment), a patient care plan, 50 com-
             monly confused abbreviations, and a brief guide to
             assessment.

2.34 Eckelberry, Grace K. Administration of Comprehensive
      Nursing Care: The Nature of Professional Practice. New
      York: Appleton-Century-Crofts, 1971.
             175 pp. Paper. Index. References.
             Three parts discuss the Nature of Comprehension:
             How It Is Changed; The Nursing Process; Providing
             for Nursing Care. Includes a brief summary for each
             chapter. The book gives a framework for evaluating
             nursing processes with examples of actual nursing
             care situations.

2.35 Johnson, Mae M.; Davis, Mary Lou C. Problem Solving in
      Nursing Practice, 2d ed. [Foundations of Nursing Series]
      Dubuque: Brown, 1975.
             142 pp. Paper. Index. Bibliographies.
             A presentation of problem solving as it fits in with the
             entire nursing care plan. Chapters deal with problem
             solving in general, discovering the problem, assess-

ment, statement of the problem, and solution of the problem. The appendix includes a brief discussion of terminology in nursing, guides to assessment of patient needs, nursing admission interview guide, and an example of problem solving in a specific nursing care situation.

2.36 La Monica, Elaine Lynne. The Nursing Process, A Humanistic Approach. Menlo Park, Ca.: Addison-Wesley, 1979.
527 pp. Paper. Index. References.
Through the use of the humanistic nursing process, this book helps the nurse (student or otherwise) take the behavior learned in the theory behind the nursing process and apply it. Five parts are included: Methods of the Nursing Process; Skills and Competencies; Quality Systems in Nursing Practice; Theory and Strategies for Facilitating Practice in the Clinical Environment; and Nursing: A Helping Profession. Each section includes information and papers, some reprinted from other sources, as well as humanistic exercises. The appendix includes abbreviations.

2.37 Lewis, Lucile. Planning Patient Care, 2d ed. [Foundations of Nursing Series] Dubuque: Brown, 1976.
209 pp. Paper. Index. Bibliographies.
A concise, handy little book organized around the nursing process (including assessment, intervention, evaluation, especially). Stress is on the theory behind nursing practice, but also includes practical descriptions of items such as a nursing history, a nursing care plan, nursing orders, etc.

2.38 Marriner, Ann. The Nursing Process, A Scientific Approach to Nursing Care, 2d ed. St. Louis: Mosby, 1979.
276 pp. Paper. Index. Suggested readings.
"This book presents a compilation of various theoretical concepts concerning the four phases of the [nursing] process: assessment, planning, implementation,

and evaluation." (p. v) Each chapter includes pertinent selected readings reprinted from other sources.

2.39   Mayers, Marlene Glover. A Systematic Approach to the
Nursing Care Plan, 2d ed. New York: Appleton-Century-
Crofts, 1978.
    341 pp. Paper. Index. References.
    Presents a method of patient care planning related to
a systematic problem-solving approach. After discussing current care planning, chapters address problem solving in the nursing process, including stating
the problem, the expected outcome, the nursing action,
and the response of the patient. Next, the book addresses the use of this approach in all types of settings, e.g., hospitals, the community, nursing education. Also includes material on the data base and
quality assurance.

2.40   Yura, Helen; Walsh, Mary B. The Nursing Process:
Assessing, Planning, Implementing, Evaluating, 3d ed.
New York: Appleton-Century-Crofts, 1978.
    266 pp. Paper. Index. Bibliography.
References.
    The third edition addresses the nursing process'
historical development, theories and the nursing
process, the components of the process, situations in
which the nursing process is applied, and future directions for the process. Appendixes include the
American Nurses' Association Code for Nurses, and
the Guide for Nursing Observations Using the Four
Senses.

2.41   Yura, Helen; Walsh, Mary B.; eds. Human Needs and the
Nursing Process. New York: Appleton-Century-Crofts,
1978.
    330 pp. Paper. Index. References.
    "The purpose of this text is to present human needs as
the territory for the utilization of the nursing process." (p. xi) Needs addressed include nutrition,
territoriality, air, love, tenderness, activity, sleep.

Each need is developed using the nursing process
(assessing, planning, implementing, evaluating) on
two levels, wellness and illness. Chapters are by
different experts in the field of nursing.

PATIENT EDUCATION

2.42 Narrow, Barbara W. Patient Teaching in Nursing Practice:
A Patient and Family-Centered Approach. New York:
Wiley, 1979.
> 219 pp. Paper. Index. Annotated bibliography.
> A text for undergraduate nursing students as they
> learn to incorporate patient teaching into the nursing
> process. Divided into two parts: I. Concepts Basic
> to Teaching and Learning, and II. The Teaching-
> Learning Process. Provides a conceptual framework
> and a practical guide for patient teaching.

2.43 Redman, Barbara Klug. The Process of Patient Teaching
in Nursing, 3d ed. St. Louis: Mosby, 1976.
> 272 pp. Paper. Index. References.
> Chapters cover teaching in nursing, the teaching/
> learning process, readiness for learning, behavioral
> objectives, learning theory, teaching theory, printed
> and nonprinted tools in teaching, planning and carry-
> ing out teaching, evaluation of teaching in health, and
> developing and carrying out patient education. Most
> chapters include a summary and study questions. The
> approach is practical as well as theoretical. The
> appendix includes sample answers to study questions,
> case studies, and questions on patient teaching.

2.44 Zander, Karen S.; Bower, Kathleen A.; Foster, Susan D.;
et al.; eds. Practical Manual for Patient-Teaching. St.
Louis: Mosby, 1978.
> 394 pp. Paper. Bibliographies.
> Contains actual protocols developed by nurses at the
> Tufts-New England Medical Center Hospital for use in
> teaching patients in different areas. The protocols

were developed to help provide documentation of patient education activities in a non-cumbersome fashion. After a general chapter on patient teaching, the book goes on to include teaching plans and guidelines for disorders of interrelated systems: the cardiovascular system, the endocrine system, the gastrointestinal system, the genitourinary system, the musculoskeletal system, the neurological system, and the respiratory system.

PHYSICAL ASSESSMENT

2.45 Assessing Vital Functions Accurately [Nursing '79 Skillbook Series] Horsham, Pa.: Intermed Communications, 1978.
136 pp. Cloth. Index.
An excellent discussion of physical assessment that includes both "how to" material and theory. Could serve as a baseline for information; its purpose is to increase the nurse's clinical judgment. Moves from the basics to assessing the various functions: respiratory, cardiac, cranial, etc. Includes skillchecks and answers in addition to charts, diagrams, vocabulary, color photos of skin conditions, and other materials. Useful as a review book as well.

2.46 Bates, Barbara. A Guide to Physical Examination, 2d ed. Philadelphia: Lippincott, 1979.
440 pp. Cloth. Index. Bibliographies.
This is an extensively illustrated text for beginning students and practitioners. For each region or system of the body, it gives the anatomy and physiology, techniques of examination, and tables of related abnormalities. Includes a special chapter on the pediatric exam by Robert A. Hoekelman, M.D. Also available from the publisher are twelve sound motion pictures which reflect the textual content.

2.47 Brown, Marie Scott; Hudak, Carolyn M.; Brenneman, Janice; et al. Student Manual of Physical Examination. Philadelphia: Lippincott, 1977.

251 pp. Paper. References.
Designed for nurse practitioner students for use in a
core course of physical assessment of the adult, the
pregnant woman, and the child. Basic knowledge, inspection, palpation, percussion, and auscultation are
included under each specific part of the examination.
Student objectives, learning activities, and review
questions facilitate learning. Includes illustrations
and answers to questions.

2.48 DeGowin, Elmer L.; DeGowin, Richard L. Bedside Diagnostic Examination, 3d ed. New York: Macmillan, 1976.
952 pp. Cloth. Index. Procedures in examination
index. References.
A compact reference book that deals with the physical
examination, examination of the skin, the thorax and
cardiovascular system, the neurologic exam, etc.
Includes a chapter on diagnosis in specific diseases.

2.49 Hobson, Lawrence B. Examination of the Patient: A Text
for Nursing and Allied Health Personnel. New York:
McGraw-Hill, 1975.
456 pp. Cloth. Index.
Designed for non-medical students to introduce them
to skills needed in examining patients. Divided into
three parts: I. Basic Examination of Patients (medical
history, the physical exam); II. Advanced Examination
of Patients (builds on part one and explains some more
complicated procedures, e.g., the use of the ophthal-
moscope); and III. Basis for Findings in Health and
Disease (anatomical, functional, and pathological).
Includes exercises throughout for the student.

2.50 Judge, Richard D.; Zuidema, George D., eds. Methods of
Clinical Examination: A Physiologic Approach, 3d ed.
Boston: Little, Brown, 1974.
439 pp. Cloth. Index. References.
Glossaries.
A succinct, clear text on the physical examination in-
tended primarily for the medical student. After an

introduction and a chapter on the problem-oriented
system, chapters proceed to examination of the skin,
eyes, respiratory system, breasts, etc. Includes
chapters on The Acutely Injured Patient and the Pediatric Examination. The appendix includes examples
from the problem-oriented system.

2.51 Malasanos, Lois; Barkauskas, Violet; Moss, Muriel; et al.
      Health Assessment. St. Louis: Mosby, 1977.
          526 pp. Cloth. Index. Bibliographies.
          Glossary.
          Written for beginning practitioners as they learn to
          assess the health status of the client through taking a
          health history and performing a physical examination.
          An appropriate text for a course that includes structured practice with preceptors, especially those preparing for roles in primary care or health maintenance. The focus is on health, the normal state.
          Selected problems are used to demonstrate deviations,
          early detection, prevention of more serious problems,
          and disability. A very useful book with good charts,
          clear diagrams and illustrations, and helpful hints to
          organize data.

2.52 Prior, John A.; Silberstein, Jack S.; et al. Physical Diagnosis: The History and Examination of the Patient, 5th ed.
      St. Louis: Mosby, 1977.
          504 pp. Cloth. Index. Bibliography.
          Besides chapters on diagnosis and taking medical histories, the book has sections on physical diagnosis in
          each of the body systems (eyes, cardiovascular, etc.),
          pediatric examination, and a brief chapter on reassuring the patient.

2.53 Sana, Josephine M.; Judge, Richard D., eds. Physical
      Appraisal Methods in Nursing Practice. Boston: Little,
      Brown, 1975.
          402 pp. Paper. Index. References. Suggested
          readings. Glossaries.

Designed to help the nurse whose expanding role makes it important that she have experience and knowledge in this area. The authors are a nurse and a physician. Three sections discuss trends in physical appraisal (problem-oriented documentation, use of computers, etc.); appraisal of adults (appearance, vision, hearing, reproductive and other systems, etc.); and, finally, appraisal of various age groups (newborn, elderly, etc.).

2.54 Sauvé, Mary J.; Pecherer, Angela. Concepts and Skills in Physical Assessment. Philadelphia: Saunders, 1977.
     424 pp. Paper. Bibliography.
     A self-instructional book that may be used with a variety of physical assessment texts and audiovisual materials. Contains guidelines and objectives, learning activities. Pre- and post-tests are included with each unit. Performance guides are printed on heavy paper in the appendix and can be removed for use in the clinical area. A clinical practicum with validation by a preceptor is important to successful use of this text. Answers to test questions are included.

2.55 Sherman, Jacques L., Jr.; Fields, Sylvia Kleiman. Guide to Patient Evaluation: History Taking, Physical Examination, and the Problem-Oriented Method, 3d ed. Garden City: Medical Examination, 1978.
     360 pp. Paper (spiral bound). Index. References.
     This book describes a sound basic examination. The focus is on principles and techniques. Other texts must be consulted for details of anatomy, physiology, psychology, and pathophysiology. Includes assessment of the newborn through the elderly. Designed for the non-medical student learner of physical assessment. Meant to be used with a classroom instructor and a clinical preceptor.

INFECTION CONTROL

2.56 American Hospital Association. Infection Control in the
      Hospital, 4th ed. Chicago: American Hospital Association,
      1979.
         242 pp. Paper. Index. Bibliographies. Glossary.
         This manual gives "an account of practical manage-
         ment of infection problems within hospital units and
         . . . [presents] essential features as succinctly and
         explicitly as possible." (p. xi) Chapters cover
         introduction to infection; occurrence of infec-
         tions; reporting regarding infections; responsibilities
         concerning infection within hospital departments; con-
         trol of infection; procedures and areas causing infec-
         tion; and the like. Includes sample reports, floor
         plans, etc. Appendixes include guidelines for specific
         procedures relating to infection.

2.57 Benenson, Abram S., ed. Control of Communicable Dis-
      eases in Man, 12th ed. Washington: American Public
      Health Association, 1975.
         413 pp. Paper. Index.
         Presents essential facts needed by public health work-
         ers to control communicable diseases. Provides a
         central source of information to be used as a refer-
         ence or supplemental text. Gives recognition and
         treatment data.

2.58 Bennett, John V.; Brachman, Philip S., eds. Hospital In-
      fections. Boston: Little, Brown, 1979.
         542 pp. Cloth. Index. References.
         Edited by two physician/epidemiologists with the
         Center for Disease Control in Atlanta who have in-
         cluded original papers by physicians, epidemiologists,
         and nurses. "The book not only provides useful in-
         formation for controlling and preventing hospital in-
         fections but also comprehensively discusses each

problem and its solution, incorporating epidemiologic,
clinical, and laboratory aspects of nosocomial infections, with emphasis on the former." (pp. xv-xvi)
Part I gives basic information about hospital infections (epidemiology, hospital personnel and infection
control, investigation of infections, areas of particular concern regarding infection, e.g., the intensive
care unit, the pharmacy, the operating room, etc.,
isolation, legal considerations and the like). Papers
in part II discuss infections relating to various organ
systems and procedures.

2.59 Burke, John F.; Hildick-Smith, Gavin Y., eds. The
Infection-Prone Hospital Patient. Boston: Little, Brown,
1978.
> 252 pp. Cloth. Index. References.
> Contains papers presented at a symposium that fo-
> cused on the altered resistance of patients to infection.
> The nature of the host defense mechanisms as well as
> the problems in specific conditions are included. Of
> special interest are leukemia, protein-calorie malnu-
> trition, immunosuppression, and trauma.

2.60 Dubay, Elaine C.; Grubb, Reba Douglass. Infection: Prevention and Control, 2d ed. St. Louis: Mosby, 1978.
> 179 pp. Paper. Index. Resources (readings and
> audiovisual educational materials). Glossary.
> Addresses the problem of infection in the health care
> environment. Chapters discuss microorganisms and
> infection; infection control structure and organization
> (committees, persons responsible for it, etc.); poli-
> cies and procedures for prevention and control of
> infection; education (for infection control); the isola-
> tion patient; legal aspects of hospital-associated in-
> fections, etc. Written in a semi-outline format for
> ease of reference, clarity.

2.61 Kolff, Cornelis A.; and Sanchez, Ramon C. Handbook for
Infectious Disease Management. Menlo Park, Ca.:
Addison-Wesley, 1979.

280 pp. Paper. Index. References.
Written for health professionals in a primary care
setting, this book contains an approach and a set of
guidelines with the critical information needed to
diagnose, treat, and contain an infectious disease.
Discusses disease entities, antimicrobial agents,
laboratory techniques, and infectious disease control
measures.

THE PROBLEM-ORIENTED SYSTEM

2.62 Berni, Rosemarian; Readey, Helen. Problem-Oriented
Medical Record Implementation, Allied Health Peer Review,
2d ed. St. Louis: Mosby, 1978.
   186 pp. Paper. Index. References.
   Because competent health care documentation is necessary, the authors have developed guidelines for the use
   of the problem-oriented medical record by allied
   health professionals. Includes examples of implementation by many disciplines and in many health care
   settings. Major sections deal with system description,
   implementation, evaluation, modification, and com-
   puterization. A syllabus containing an implementation
   model is included. The appendix contains examples of
   flowsheets, order sheets, progress notes, and summary sheets.

2.63 Hurst, J. Willis; Walker, H. Kenneth, eds. The Problem-
Oriented System. [Medcom Medical Update Series] New
York: Medcom Press, 1972.
   287 pp. Paper. References.
   A collection of original papers by different authors
   giving the background of the problem-oriented record,
   practical considerations of the problem-oriented record, education and the problem-oriented system,
   nursing and the problem-oriented system, ambulatory
   care and the problem-oriented system, the system in
   other applications (e.g., private practice, continuing
   education), computers and the system, and finally, a
   look toward the future. The editors stress the use of

the system as a tool to assess what is being done and
not as something that will solve all problems by itself.

2.64 Larkin, Patricia; Backer, Barbara. Problem-Oriented
Nursing Assessment. New York: McGraw-Hill, 1977.
   190 pp. Paper. Bibliography.
   An introduction to the nursing process and health status assessment for use as a supplement to classes and
   other texts. Looks at "problem solving, process recordings, and the problem-oriented health records."
   (p. vii) Includes assessment guides for areas such as
   Mobility/Rest/Comfort and Nutrition/Elimination.
   Assessment practice sheets are included in appropriate chapters.

2.65 Vaughan-Wrobel, Beth C.; Henderson, Betty. The Problem-
Oriented System in Nursing, A Workbook. St. Louis:
Mosby, 1976.
   152 pp. Paper. Bibliography.
   This workbook is designed to aid practicing nurses and
   nurse/educators devise a system of health care management. Divided into three units: Applying the
   Problem-Oriented System (the system explained and
   its use in nursing and in nursing documentation); Implementing the Problem-Oriented Record (includes
   exercises in using the problem-oriented system); and
   Evaluating the Problem-Oriented Record (answers
   given to the exercises in Unit Two). Punched for in-
   sertion into a notebook; perforated pages for tearing
   out for grading.

2.66 Walker, H. Kenneth; Hurst, J. Willis; Woody, Mary F.,
eds. Applying the Problem-Oriented System. [Medcom
Medical Update Series] New York: Medcom Press, 1973.
   472 pp. Paper. References.
   This book evolved from two conferences in Atlanta on
   the problem-oriented system and is designed for anyone involved in health care delivery. Emphasis is on
   how to apply the problem-oriented system in many
   different settings, so the book is organized by the

location of care rather than by who is giving the care.
There are ten parts: Introduction; Problem-Oriented
Practice in Vermont; Problem-Oriented Practice in
Hampden Highlands, Maine; Community Health Care
Delivery: People and Techniques; A Review; Quality
Control in Health Care Delivery; Education; Hospital
and Specialty Practice; Pathology; Psychiatry and
Psychosocial Aspects. Two of the editors are physi-
cians and the other a master's-prepared RN.

2.67 Woolley, F. Ross; Warnick, Myrna W.; Kane, Robert L.;
et al. Problem-Oriented Nursing. New York: Springer
Publishing, 1974.
  167 pp. Cloth. References.
  A background text on the problem-oriented record.
  Encompasses an explanation of the system, auditing
  the system, using the system, etc. Has a review sec-
  tion, a look at the future, and appendixes, including
  Joint Commission on the Accreditation of Hospitals'
  Medical Records Standards and Data Base for the
  Problem-Oriented Record.

PERIODICALS

2.68 American Journal of Nursing. American Journal of Nursing
Co., 10 Columbus Circle, New York, N.Y. 10019. (For
the American Nurses' Association). Monthly. 1900 to date.

2.69 Canadian Nurse. Canadian Nurses' Association, 50 The
Driveway, Ottawa K2P 1E2, Ontario, Canada. Monthly.
1905 to date.

2.70 Nursing . . . [current year]. Intermed Communications,
Inc., 132 Welsh Road, Marion, Ohio 43302. Monthly.
1971 to date.

2.71 Nursing Clinics of North America. W. B. Saunders Co.,
Washington Square, Philadelphia, Pa. 19105.
Quarterly. 1966 to date.

2.72 Nursing Forum. Nursing Publications, Inc., Box 218,
      Hillsdale, N.J. 07642. Quarterly. 1961 to date.

2.73 Nursing Times. Macmillan Journals, Ltd., 4 Little Essex
      Street, London WC2R 3LF, England. Weekly. 1905 to date.

2.74 R.N., National Magazine for Nurses. Medical Economics
      Co., 680 Kinderkamack Rd. , Oradell, N.J. 07649.
      Monthly. 1937 to date.

3

Medical-Surgical Nursing

One of the basic divisions of nursing practice, medical-
surgical nursing, contains such a broad spectrum of components that two chapters are devoted to it. Chapter Three
includes general, broad-based texts. Chapter Four includes
those books which focus on specialty areas.

The chapter begins with general texts for nursing,
medicine, and surgery and continues with books related to
chronic illness, emergency care, pain, and rehabilitation and
physical disability. Finally, periodicals are listed at the
end of the chapter.

GENERAL

Nursing

3.1　Barber, Janet Miller; Stokes, Lillian Gatlin; Billings,
　　　Diane McGovern. Adult and Child Care, A Client Approach
　　　to Nursing, 2d ed. St. Louis: Mosby, 1977.
　　　　　　1036 pp. Cloth. Index. Bibliography.
　　　　　　"This text is an integrated approach to nursing care of
　　　　　adults and children and is organized in accordance with
　　　　　basic human needs." (p. ix) Seven units deal with:
　　　　　The Nursing Client and the Family—Growth and Devel-
　　　　　opmental Considerations; Life Crises—The Nurse in
　　　　　the Helping Relationship; Safety and Security; Activity
　　　　　and Rest; Sexual Role Satisfaction; Nutrition and

Elimination; The Need for Oxygen. Suggested readings follow each unit. Appendixes deal with appraisal
of health hazards, infectious diseases, etc. Uses the
word <u>client</u> as opposed to <u>patient</u>.

3.2   Beland, Irene L.; Passos, Joyce Y. Clinical Nursing, Patho-
.physiological and Psychosocial Approaches, 3d ed. New
York: Macmillan, 1975.
1120 pp. Cloth. Index. References.
For nursing students in medical-surgical nursing.
This text uses an "integrated comprehensive problem-
oriented approach" that is most compatible with many
of the integrated nursing curricula in effect today.
The first chapters look at nursing and patient needs
broadly—health-illness spectrum, control of infections, and defenses against and responses to injury,
among other things. Other chapters cover nursing
problems such as problems with nutrition and dis-
turbance in fluid and electrolyte balance, rather than
specific diseases.

3.3   Beyers, Marjorie; Dudas, Susan. The Clinical Practice of
Medical-Surgical Nursing. Boston: Little, Brown, 1977.
1234 pp. Cloth. Index. References. Bibliographies.
A comprehensive medical-surgical nursing text. The
first section deals with health and disease states and
fluid and electrolyte balance. The second section goes
into nursing care and assessment of patients with specific medical-surgical disorders; e.g., eye dysfunction, gastrointestinal system dysfunction, and so forth.
Key terminology is written throughout the text in bold
print and the bibliographies at the end of each chapter
are extensive.

3.4   Clark, Carolyn C. Nursing Concepts and Processes.
Albany: Delmar, 1977.
547 pp. Paper. Index. Suggested Readings. Glossary.
Part of a series for nursing students in two-year nursing programs. Integrates medical-surgical and
psychiatric-mental health concepts while developing

the themes of the health-illness continuum and developmental stages. Contains student objectives, summaries, activities and discussion topics, and review
questions.

3.5   Corbett, Nancy H.; Beveridge, Phyllis. Clinical Simulations
in Nursing Practice. Philadelphia: Saunders, 1980.
332 pp. Paper. References.
A programmed text of simulations of clinical nursing
situations that provides the opportunity to practice
making nursing decisions and evaluating them. Six
situations include: patients with a symptom (indiges-
tion), disease (diabetes, liver disease), and facing
specific situations (terminal illness, first hospitalization, and surgery). The simulation data are followed
by chart material and discussion.

3.6   Johnston, Dorothy F.; Hood, Gail H. Total Patient Care:
Foundations and Practice, 4th ed. St. Louis: Mosby, 1976.
617 pp. Cloth. Index. References. Glossary.
A text written for students in a course in medical-
surgical nursing or in a one-year nursing program.
Each chapter contains a summary outline, review
questions, and annotated films. Includes chapters on
traditional medical-surgical nursing topics such as
nursing the geriatric patient, preoperative and postoperative care, rehabilitation in nursing, nursing the
patient with diseases and disorders of the cardiovascular system and others.

3.7   Jones, Dorothy A.; Dunbar, Claire F.; Jirovec, Mary M.
Medical-Surgical Nursing: A Conceptual Approach. New
York: McGraw-Hill, 1978.
1418 pp. Cloth. Index. Bibliographies.
A medical-surgical text that considers nursing prac-
tice with adults in both acute and non-acute settings.
The authors use the conceptual framework, human-
environment interaction, as the organizing framework.
Stresses nursing assessment throughout. Covers four
levels of nursing intervention: first, identification and

prevention of problems; second, care of community-
based persons; third, acute care of hospitalized patients; fourth, rehabilitation in hospital and community. Discusses disruptions of health in terms of
major biophysical concepts: cellular growth prolifera-
tion, inflammation and immunity, fluid and electrolyte
dynamics, metabolism, oxygenation, and perception
and coordination. Discussions include psychosocial
and cultural aspects as well as current research.

3.8   Keane, Claire B. Essentials of Medical-Surgical Nursing,
rev. ed. Philadelphia: Saunders, 1979.
721 pp. Cloth. Index. References.
A text for students new to nursing. The author has
taught in diploma and practical nursing programs.
Major sections open with a perspective on nursing,
effects of disease-producing factors, the internal
environment, and medical-surgical problems.

3.9   Kintzel, Kay C., ed. Advanced Concepts in Clinical Nursing,
2d ed. Philadelphia: Lippincott, 1977.
784 pp. Cloth. Index. References. Bibliography.
A supplementary text for undergraduate and graduate
nursing students and nurses in practice. Focuses on
physiological and psychosocial processes in health and
disease. The many contributors provide the strength
and breadth. Includes an assortment of topics and approaches, some general, e.g., the nursing process,
providing for health maintenance, assessment of physical health, health in varying ages; some specialized,
e.g., intensive care nursing; some focused on body
systems, e.g., kidney, heart, central nervous system.

3.10 Luckmann, Joan; Sorensen, Karen Creason. Medical-
Surgical Nursing; A Psychophysiologic Approach, 2d ed.
Philadelphia: Saunders, 1980.
2276 pp. Cloth. Index. References.
A basic medical/surgical nursing text which is divided
into three sections. Section 1 covers unifying, basic
concepts in nursing practice such as adaptation, health,

and disease. Section 2 covers psychosocial factors
and physical assessment. Section 3 deals with nursing
of patients with specific medical/surgical problems,
e.g., surgery, neoplastic disorders, pain, kidney and
urinary tract dysfunction, integumentary system problems, eye, ear, and nose disturbances, and the like.
Chapters focus on nursing care, often including questions, points to remember, highlighted sections,
charts, tables, and illustrations.

3.11 Phipps, Wilma J.; Long, Barbara C.; Woods, Nancy Fugate.
Medical-Surgical Nursing: Concepts and Clinical Practice.
St. Louis: Mosby, 1979.
1634 pp. Cloth. Index. References. Selected
readings.
Presents information relevant to the practice of
medical-surgical nursing for nursing students and
nurses in practice. Part 1. Perspectives for Nursing
Practice looks at sociocultural and environmental aspects and concepts and processes widely used in nursing today. Part 2. Stress and Adaptation includes relevant concepts. Part 3. Clinical Management of Persons
with Medical-Surgical Problems includes common problems with a systems approach to assessment and management. The last section comprises two-thirds of the
book and looks at the failure of integrative mechanisms;
problems of sensorimotor systems, gas transport,
elimination, nutrition, sexuality and reproduction, impaired protective mechanisms; and critical care nursing.

3.12 Putt, Arlene M. General Systems Theory Applied to Nursing.
Boston: Little, Brown, 1978.
195 pp. Cloth. Index. Bibliography. Glossary.
For the nurse educator or practitioner as well as nursing students. Presents the application of general systems theory to nursing, specifically to areas of
medical-surgical nursing. Topics include theory structure and development, living systems, assessment of
social systems, and nursing care plans using general
systems concepts.

3.13 Scherer, Jeanne C. Introductory Medical-Surgical Nursing,
2d ed. Philadelphia: Lippincott, 1977.
690 pp. Cloth. Index. References. Glossary.
For students in their first medical-surgical course.
The focus is on clinical practice using pathophysio-
logical and psychosocial concepts to teach the nursing
management of patients with medical-surgical problems. Stresses pharmacology and nutrition where
appropriate. Includes chapter objectives and lab
values in the appendix. The first edition, entitled
Nursing of Adults, was authored by D. W. Smith and
C. P. Germain.

3.14 Watson, Jeannette E. Medical-Surgical Nursing and Related
Physiology, 2d ed. Philadelphia: Saunders, 1979.
1043 pp. Cloth. Index. References.
A text for students and graduates of nursing programs
that provides basic information for patient care. Includes brief reviews relevant to pathophysiology when
appropriate. Provides chapters on general topics such
as rehabilitation, infection, and cancer in addition to
those focused on major body systems. Contains many
charts, tables, and illustrations.

Medicine

3.15 Beeson, Paul B.; McDermott, Walsh; Wyngaarden, James B.;
eds. Textbook of Medicine, 15th ed. 2 vols. Philadelphia:
Saunders, 1979.
2357 pp. Cloth. Index. References.
A medical text that is a classic resource for management and treatment of disorders of body systems.
Also discusses genetic principles, environmental factors in disease, and normal laboratory values and
their clinical importance. Formerly authored by
Russell L. Cecil and Robert F. Loeb.

3.16 Lambert, Edward C. Modern Medical Mistakes. Blooming-
ton: Indiana University Press, 1978.
190 pp. Cloth. References.

Major errors in twentieth-century medical treatment
and how they were detected are the topics of this small
book written for the physician and layman alike. Discusses methods to evaluate modes of therapy. The
errors selected for inclusion here are classified as
errors of concept, laboratory mistakes and accidents,
side effects of drugs, overdose, and possible errors—
not proven. The last section, lessons, discusses the
manner in which therapies are accepted or discarded.
Some of the errors examined are x-ray of infant's
thymus, gluing of fractures, freezing of stomachs,
coated KCl tablets, hexachlorophene, synthetic hor-
mones, thalidomide, oxygen excess in premature infants. Scientific studies before release and careful
monitoring are suggested.

3.17 The Merck Manual of Diagnosis and Therapy, 13th ed.
Rahway: Merck Sharp & Dohme Research Laboratories, 1977.
    2165 pp. Cloth. Index.
    "One of the world's most widely used medical text-
    books." (p. v) Chapters are grouped by type of
    disorder (e.g., Infectious and Parasitic Diseases,
    Hematologic Disorders, Pulmonary Disorders,
    Dental and Oral Disorders). Within each chapter, dis-
    orders are listed with etiology, signs and symptoms,
    variations and complications, prognosis, treatment,
    and the like. Includes chapters on pharmacology and
    poisoning as well as a ready reference section. Suc-
    cinct and compact.

3.18 Thorn, George W.; Adams, Raymond D.; Braunwald, Eugene;
et al.; eds. Harrison's Principles of Internal Medicine, 8th
ed. 2 vols. New York: McGraw-Hill, 1977.
    2088 pp. Cloth. Index. Bibliography.
    An excellent medical reference. Organized as follows:
    the physician and the patient; manifestations and ap-
    proach to disease; biological considerations; nutritional,
    hormonal, and metabolic considerations; chemical and
    physical agents; biologic agents; and diseases of organ
    systems. Earlier editions by T. R. Harrison. Ninth
    edition due 1980.

Surgery

3.19 Bunker, John P.; Barnes, Benjamin A.; Mosteller,
      Frederick, eds. Costs, Risks, and Benefits of Surgery.
      New York: Oxford University Press, 1977.
          401 pp. Cloth. Index. References.
          This book looks at surgical therapy, its discreteness,
          accomplishments, and costs. Makes an attempt to do
          a cost-benefit analysis and to measure the "quality of
          life." Examines the moral and economic implications
          of modern surgery.

3.20 Rhodes, Marie J.; Gruendemann, Barbara J.; Ballinger,
      Walter F. Alexander's Care of the Patient in Surgery, 6th
      ed. St. Louis: Mosby, 1978.
          886 pp. Cloth. Index. References.
          A well-illustrated, basic reference for nursing care of
          persons undergoing operative procedures. Opens with
          a discussion of basic concepts, administrative con-
          cerns, physical layout and environmental concerns,
          asepsis, positioning, and instruments. Most of the
          book is concerned with specific types of surgery in-
          cluding anatomy and physiology and nursing considera-
          tions. A recent revision of a standard text. Formerly
          authored by Edythe L. Alexander.

3.21 Sabiston, David C., Jr., ed. Davis-Christopher Textbook
      of Surgery: The Biological Basis of Modern Surgical Prac-
      tice, 11th ed. Philadelphia: Saunders, 1977.
          2465 pp. Cloth. Index. References. Annotated
          bibliographies.
          A definitive text and reference for medical students,
          residents, practicing surgeons, and teachers of sur-
          gery. The focus is on the "biological basis of modern
          surgical practice." Contributors are well-known
          authorities. General topics such as shock, fluid and
          electrolyte management, and preoperative preparation
          are followed by trauma, surgical complications, and
          surgery of specific body parts.

3.22 Sabiston, David C., Jr.; Spencer, Frank C., eds. Gibbon's
Surgery of the Chest, 3d ed. Philadelphia: Saunders, 1976.
1592 pp. Cloth. Index. References.
A classic in the field of cardiovascular and thoracic
surgery. Discusses a wide variety of procedures and
practices.

Surgical Nursing

3.23 Atkinson, Lucy Jo; Kohn, Mary Louise. Berry & Kohn's
Introduction to Operating Room Technique, 5th ed. New
York: McGraw-Hill, 1978.
558 pp. Paper. Index. Bibliographies.
For all learners of operating room techniques. The
focus is on total patient care and the contributions of
each member of the health team in the operating room
setting. The first part of the book looks at the setting,
the team, the patient, asepsis and all the related activities, and anesthesia. General surgical methods
and then surgical specialties complete the book. Surgical complications and legal aspects are included.

3.24 Brooks, Shirley M. Fundamentals of Operating Room
Nursing, 2d ed. St. Louis: Mosby, 1979.
198 pp. Paper. Index. References.
Gives a basic introduction to operating room nursing,
including photographs. Five units cover: Terminology; Preoperative Preparation; Intraoperative Care;
Immediate Postoperative Care; and Accepted Techniques. Unit 5 (Accepted Techniques) is a "photo quiz"
for review of material presented earlier. Each chapter includes objectives.

3.25 Brooks, Shirley M. Instrumentation for the Operating Room:
A Photographic Manual. St. Louis: Mosby, 1978.
413 pp. Paper. References.
Commonly used surgical and diagnostic instruments
are pictured both individually and in complete setups
for various procedures. A useful reference for nurse
or technician.

3.26 Crooks, Lois C., ed. Operating Room Techniques for the
      Surgical Team. Boston: Little, Brown, 1979.
            459 pp. Cloth. Index. Suggested readings. Glossary.
            A text for nurses, nursing and medical students, and
            surgical residents that includes theory and principles,
            and techniques relevant to the operating room. Chap-
            ters on aseptic techniques, sterilization, and anes-
            thesia are followed by chapters which discuss surgery
            of major body areas. Does not cover orthopedic,
            urologic, or neurosurgical procedures. Illustrated.

3.27 Desharnais, Anna. Review of Surgical Nursing. New York:
      McGraw-Hill, 1979.
            228 pp. Paper. Bibliography.
            Has some 600 multiple-choice questions with answers,
            reasons, and pertinent references for each question.
            Comprised of 14 units, each with cognitive behavioral
            objectives. Units cover   stress, general care of the
            surgical patient, the burn patient, care of patients with
            dysfunctions (e.g., reproductive, cerebral, motor,
            endocrine, respiratory, urinary, etc.).

3.28 Gruendemann, Barbara J.; Casterton, Shirley B.; Hesterly,
      Sandra C.; et al. The Surgical Patient: Behavioral Con-
      cepts for the Operating Room Nurse, 2d ed. St. Louis:
      Mosby, 1977.
            190 pp. Paper. Index. Bibliography.
            Incorporates the Association of Operating Room Nurses'
            Standards of Nursing Practice: Operating Room and
            gives ideas for implementing the nursing process in
            the surgical setting. It includes behavioral concepts,
            not just technical procedures. Written for both the
            practicing nurse and the nursing student.

CHRONIC ILLNESS

3.29 Brown, Marie S. Distortions in Body Image in Illness and
      Disease. New York: Wiley, 1977.
            116 pp. Paper. References.
            Discusses the nursing process in relation to distor-

tions and changes in body image. Problems that cause
major alterations in body image are integrated with
the situations of persons of varying ages, e.g., the
school age child and burns; the adult with a myocardial
infarction, cancer, or personality distortion. A Wiley
nursing concept module for self-instruction.

3.30 Cohen, Stuart J., ed. New Directions in Patient Compliance.
      Lexington, Mass.: Heath, 1978.
          167 pp. Cloth. Index. References.
          This book includes a series of papers from a confer-
          ence that focused on a major concern of persons asso-
          ciated with chronic illness: patient noncompliance with
          regimens prescribed for them. Becker discusses the
          health belief model; Hackett summarizes compliance
          research; Dunbar focuses on assessment of compliance;
          Barofsky and others look at the patient's quality of life;
          R. Caplan discusses factors in adherence; and other
          chapters discuss problems related to research in com-
          pliance.

3.31 Moos, Rudolf H., ed. Coping with Physical Illness. New
      York: Plenum, 1977.
          440 pp. Cloth. Subject and author indexes. References.
          Focuses on the personal crisis of illness, how people
          cope with serious physical illness or injury. Contains
          a conceptual model of the process of coping, basic
          adaptive tasks, and types of coping skills. Material is
          relevant for schools of nursing, medicine, and public
          health. Major segments deal with specific kinds of ill-
          ness, response to treatment, death and fear of dying.
          Of special interest are the sections on unusual hospital
          environments, dialysis, transplantation, and stresses
          on the staff.

3.32 Strauss, Anselm L. Chronic Illness and the Quality of Life.
      St. Louis: Mosby, 1975.
          160 pp. Paper. Index. Bibliography.
          Written for health professionals who work with the
          chronically ill. Three major sections cover major
          complications and problems of living with a chronic

illness, studies of chronic conditions with their specific implications, and the health care system and chronic illness.

EMERGENCY CARE

3.33 American College of Surgeons. Early Care of the Injured Patient, 2d ed. Philadelphia: Saunders, 1976.
        443 pp. Cloth. Index. References.
        Discusses current concepts in the care of the injured patient from primary assessment to legal aspects and disaster planning. Includes material on CPR, shock, head injuries, traumatic amputations, etc. Good use of charts, illustrations, lists.

3.34 Barry, Jeanie, ed. Emergency Nursing. New York: McGraw-Hill, 1978.
        491 pp. Cloth. References. Bibliography.
        Written for an emergency medical services (EMS) program, the book has a clear, helpful format, is well illustrated, and builds on basic nursing preparation. Part 1. The Biologic Bases of Emergency Nursing discusses major body systems and physiologic processes. Part 2. The Psychosocial Bases of Nursing discusses communication, stress, anxiety, death, and dying. Part 3. Pathophysiology: Theory and Emergency Treatment includes emergency assessment, legal aspects, and specific emergencies.

3.35 Cosgriff, James H., Jr. An Atlas of Diagnostic and Therapeutic Procedures for Emergency Personnel. Philadelphia: Lippincott, 1978.
        315 pp. Cloth. Index. Bibliography.
        Includes 70 procedures commonly used for the acutely ill or injured patient. Examines the use, equipment, involved anatomy, and step-by-step techniques for each procedure. Includes airway management, arteriograms, venous cutdown, central venous catheterization, nasogastric-intestinal tubes, nerve blocks, thoracentesis, emergency maternity care, and others. Well illustrated.

3.36 Cosgriff, James H., Jr.; Anderson, Diann Laden. The
      Practice of Emergency Nursing. Philadelphia: Lippincott,
      1975.
           488 pp. Cloth. Index. Bibliography.
           An introduction to emergency room nursing practice,
           its roles and functions. Includes legal aspects; assess-
           ment; priorities; specific situations; death, shock,
           wounds and bites, drug reactions, selected body sys-
           tem problems; and emergency care of the child. Or-
           ganized to include observations, identification, clinical
           signs and symptoms, life threatening situations, life
           support measures for the critically ill, injured patient.
           Includes appendixes.

3.37 Emergency Department Nurses' Association. Emergency
      Department Nurses' Association Continuing Education Cur-
      riculum. East Lansing: EDNA, 1975.
           179 pp. Paper.
           Developed by EDNA, this collection of modules has a
           set of objectives, content delineation, a suggested
           teaching/learning experience, methods of evaluation,
           and possible resource materials for problems dealing
           with clinical assessment and priority setting, psycho-
           logical intervention, fluid and electrolyte/IV therapy,
           shock, legal considerations, clinical modules, multiple
           trauma patient, management, and other situations.

3.38 Lanros, Nedell E. Assessment and Intervention in Emer-
      gency Nursing. Bowie, Md.: Brady, 1978.
           486 pp. Cloth. Index. Bibliography.
           A manual for the preparation and continuing education
           of those nurses who specialize in emergency nursing.
           Three sections look at Assessment and Triage, Emer-
           gency Intervention and Care, and Management Areas.
           Each section begins with key concepts and ends with a
           review. The physical assessment by systems is very
           helpful. The emergencies included range from shock
           to airway problems to burns and fractures. Pediatric
           problems are also addressed. Legal problems and
           disaster plans are discussed in the last section.

3.39 Oaks, Wilbur W.; Bharadevaja, Krishan; Hertz, Lee, eds.
Emergency Care. New York: Grune & Stratton, 1979.
    243 pp. Cloth. Index. Bibliography.
    Problems and emergencies of the practicing physician
are discussed in this report of a symposium which
focused on emergency room care. Included are surgical, medical, pediatric, obstetric-gynecologic, and
given to emergency room organization and legal aspects.

3.40 Stephenson, Hugh E., Jr., ed. Immediate Care of the
Acutely Ill and Injured, 2d ed. St. Louis: Mosby, 1978.
    346 pp. Paper. Index. Bibliography. Suggested
readings.

    Written for medical students, this book has been found
useful by nurses and those in emergency medical training programs. It covers what to do during the first
few minutes of medical emergencies. Major divisions
are: Diagnostic Challenges, Pathophysiology of
Trauma, Reaching the Victim, Cardiopulmonary
Emergencies, Emergencies Involving Environmental
Excess, Pharmacologic Excess, Physical Trauma,
Special Considerations (pediatric, obstetric-gynecologic, etc.), Psychiatric Emergencies, Prevention,
and Medicolegal Considerations. Each chapter has
questions for the reader.

3.41 Warner, Carmen G., ed. Emergency Care, 2d ed. St.
Louis: Mosby, 1978.
    537 pp. Cloth. Index. Bibliography.
    A comprehensive text for the diverse kinds of person-
nel involved in emergency care, both pre-hospital and
in-hospital. Topics include emergency medical system, legal aspects, emergency nursing, triage, shock,
endocrine emergencies, poisons, life support in an
emergency department, child abuse, and others.

PAIN

3.42 Fagerhaugh, Shizuko Y.; Strauss, Anselm. Politics of Pain
Management: Staff-Patient Interaction. Menlo Park, Calif.:
Addison-Wesley, 1977.
> 323 pp. Paper. Index. References.
> Concepts and theories are presented as case studies
> and histories for those health professionals and fami-
> lies who work with patients in pain. Three themes are
> presented: Organizational settings affect behavior;
> Political processes influence pain management; Acute
> care model is inadequate for chronic pain. Based on
> the report of extensive field studies, this book goes
> beyond the traditional approaches to pain management.

3.43 Jacox, Ada K., ed. Pain: A Source Book for Nurses and
Other Health Professionals. Boston: Little, Brown, 1977.
> 535 pp. Cloth. Index. Bibliography.
> Contributors from a variety of scientific and profes-
> sional disciplines present a "comprehensive overview
> of the many dimensions of pain." (p. xiii) A useful
> book for those in the health professions interested in
> learning about clinical pain.

3.44 LeRoy, Pierre L., et al., eds. Current Concepts in the
Management of Chronic Pain. New York: Stratton Inter-
continental, 1977.
> 192 pp. Cloth. Index. References. Glossary.
> Provides up-to-date knowledge and recent advances in
> the evaluation and management of chronic pain syn-
> drome that is not relieved by conventional methods.
> Discusses theories of pain, the treatment of chronic
> pain, and intractable pain states. Includes a directory
> of pain centers. Proceedings of Postdoctoral Pro
> Dolore Pain Symposium, University of Delaware, 1976.

3.45 McCaffery, Margo. Nursing Management of the Patient with
Pain, 2d ed. Philadelphia: Lippincott, 1979.

338 pp. Paper. Index. References. Bibliography.
Written by a nurse, this book provides the nursing
practitioner and student with a reasonable approach to
caring for patients with pain. Chapters cover pain
from the nursing standpoint, nursing assessment of
pain behaviors, nursing diagnosis of patients in pain,
nursing intervention with the pained patient, pain-
relief measures, and the aftermath of pain. Appendixes include assessment tools and addresses for books
and audiovisuals, clinics, equipment, and so on.

REHABILITATION AND PHYSICAL DISABILITY

3.46 Albrecht, Gary L. , ed. The Sociology of Physical Disability and Rehabilitation. [Contemporary Community Health
Series.] Pittsburgh: University of Pittsburgh Press, 1976.
303 pp. Cloth. Index. Bibliography.
A collection of essays that review much of what is
known about physical disability and its social, psychological, economic, and political aspects.

3.47 Boroch, Rose M. Elements of Rehabilitation in Nursing:
An Introduction. St. Louis: Mosby, 1976.
316 pp. Paper. Index. References.
Care within both in-patient and ambulatory care set-
tings, focusing on returning people to their highest
level of function, is the subject of this text. Presents
the principles of rehabilitation in four parts: Part I:
Concepts in Rehabilitation, Part II: Physical and
Psychosocial Functions, Part III: Nursing Process,
Part IV: Patterns of Care.

3.48 Christopherson, Victor A.; Coulter, Pearl Parvin; Wolanin,
Mary Opal, eds. Rehabilitation Nursing; Perspectives and
Applications. New York: McGraw-Hill, 1974.
586 pp. Paper. References.
A collection of papers, primarily reprinted from other
sources, dealing with rehabilitation. Five parts include psychological and cultural considerations; the

nurse's role in teaching and in prevention of disability;
rehabilitation nursing in situations that are not life-
threatening (arthritis, amputation, pain, etc.); rehabilitation nursing in situations that are life-threatening (cardiovascular problems, malignancy, geriatrics,
etc.); and, finally, the nurse's rehabilitative role with
alcoholics and drug abusers.

3.49 Goldenson, Robert M.; Dunham, Jerome R.; Dunham,
Charlis S., eds. Disability and Rehabilitation Handbook.
New York: McGraw-Hill, 1978.
846 pp. Cloth. Index. Selected references.
Discusses the rehabilitative process and gives detailed
information on particular disabilities. The broad
range of disabilities included makes it a comprehensive resource. Describes the contributions of various
professions involved in providing rehabilitative services. Part 1—Foundations of Rehabilitation, Part 2—
Disabling Disorders, Part 3—Cases, Facilities, and
Professions, Part 4—Data Bank. Examples of disabilities discussed are alcoholism, cancer, mental
illness, ostomies, stroke, and venereal disease. Part
4 lists voluntary organizations, federal organizations,
periodicals, directories, and other sources of information.

3.50 Marinelli, Robert P.; Dell Orto, Arthur E., eds. The
Psychological and Social Impact of Physical Disability. New
York: Springer Publishing, 1977.
414 pp. Cloth. Index. Bibliography.
Written by rehabilitation counselors, the book dis-
cusses Perspectives on Disability; Disability: The
Child and the Family; Personal Impact of Disability;
Interpersonal Impact of Disability; Attitudes Toward
Disabled Persons; Sexuality and Disability; The Rights,
Contributions, and Problems of Disabled Consumers;
and Helping Persons with Disabilities. The appendixes
contain lists of books, journals, and organizations related to the disabled. A structured group experience
in rehabilitation is also included.

3.51 Meislin, Jack. Rehabilitation Medicine and Psychiatry.
      Springfield, Ill.: Thomas, 1976.
>   526 pp. Cloth. Subject and author indexes.
>   Bibliography.
>   A comprehensive text with contributions by 28 special-
>   ists in mental health and rehabilitation. Rehabilitation
>   in mental health is part of the plan of treatment. Ef-
>   forts are made to maximize the patient's capacity for
>   social adjustment and productive living in society.
>   Major topics include rehabilitation of the mentally ill,
>   research in this area, mental retardation, alcoholism,
>   community programs, and the psychosocial aspects of
>   rehabilitation of the physically disabled.

3.52 Roessler, Richard; Bolton, Brian. Psychosocial Adjustment
      to Disability. Baltimore: University Park Press, 1978.
>   184 pp. Paper. Author and subject indexes.
>   References.
>   This report of empirical research and training pack-
>   age development on the psychosocial adjustment strate-
>   gies in rehabilitation focuses on effects of disablement
>   on personality, process of adjustment to disability,
>   and techniques and strategies for enhancing psycho-
>   social adjustment to disability. Disablement may be
>   physical, psychological, intellectual, or social. The
>   training packages discussed are Personal Achievement
>   Skills, Physical Fitness Training, and Behavioral
>   Analysis Training. The book has a practical orienta-
>   tion and contains reviews and summaries of relevant
>   research.

3.53 Shestack, Robert. Handbook of Physical Therapy, 3d ed.
      New York: Springer Publishing, 1977.
>   216 pp. Paper. Index. Bibliography.
>   A concise reference to the " most common indications
>   for physical therapy and modalities in current use. "
>   (p. v). For the professional and paraprofessional health
>   worker in the general hospital. The book opens with gen-
>   eral considerations. Discussion of the modalities of
>   therapy is followed by the conditions frequently treated.
>   Includes a special section on geriatric patients.

3.54 Sine, Robert D.; Liss, Shelley E.; Roush, Robert E.; et al.,
eds. Basic Rehabilitation Techniques: A Self-Instructional
Guide. Germantown, Md.: Aspen Systems Corp., 1977.
  228 pp. Paper. Index. Bibliography.
  Written primarily for nurses, this book is helpful for
  any health professional who works with disabled clients.
  Each chapter has objectives and a post-test. Skillful
  use of illustrations enhances the usefulness of the text.
  Topics include, among others, common disability syndromes, psychosocial aspects of rehabilitation, identification and management of bowel and bladder problems,
  and pressure sores.

3.55 Stryker, Ruth P. Rehabilitative Aspects of Acute and
Chronic Nursing Care, 2d ed. Philadelphia: Saunders, 1977.
  272 pp. Cloth. Index. Bibliography.
  Basic rehabilitation concepts that are necessary in all
  nursing settings are made applicable to adults and elderly people with neuromuscular-skeletal disorders.
  After an overview of basic concepts, the author discusses the psychological reactions to physical disability, essential nursing skills, and plans for return to
  the community.

PERIODICALS

Nursing

3.56 ANA Clinical Sessions. American Nurses Association, 2420
Pershing Rd., Kansas City, Mo. 64108. Biannually.
(Alternates with ANA Clinical conferences) 1966 to date.

3.57 AORN Journal. Association of Operating Room Nurses, Inc.,
10170 East Mississippi Avenue, Denver, Colo. 80231.
Monthly. 1963 to date.

3.58 ARN Journal; Official Journal of the Association of Rehabilitation Nurses. ARN, 1701 Lake Ave., Glenview,
Ill. 60025. Bimonthly. 1975 to date.

3.59 Current Concepts in Clinical Nursing. C.V. Mosby Co.,
      11830 Westline Industrial Drive, St. Louis, Mo. 63141.
      Biannually. 1967 to date.

3.60 JEN; Journal of Emergency Nursing. Emergency Depart-
      ment Nurses Association, Box 1566, 3900 Capital City
      Boulevard, Lansing, Mich. 48906. Bimonthly.
      1975 to date.

3.61 Topics in Clinical Nursing. Aspen Systems Corporation,
      20010 Century Boulevard, Germantown, Md. 20767. Quar-
      terly. 1979 to date.

Medical

3.62 American Journal of Physical Medicine. Williams & Wilkins
      Co., 428 E. Preston Street, Baltimore, Md. 21202. Every
      two months. 1921 to date.

3.63 Journal of the American Medical Association. American
      Medical Association, 535 N. Dearborn Street, Chicago, Ill.
      60610. Weekly. 1848 to date.

3.64 New England Journal of Medicine. Massachusetts Medical
      Society, 10 Shattuck Street, Boston, Mass. 02115. Weekly.
      1812 to date.

4
Medical-Surgical Nursing Specialties

As nursing has developed, many areas of specialization have arisen to parallel the medical specialties. In addition, in recent years specialties like oncology and critical care have evolved that cut across the boundaries of the traditional specialties.

This chapter is subdivided into nursing areas of both kinds. Major headings are: cancer; cardiovascular; critical care; dermatologic; endocrine; eye, ear, nose, and throat; gastrointestinal; neurologic; orthopedic; renal; respiratory; and urologic nursing.

CANCER (ONCOLOGIC) NURSING

4.1 Aker, Saundra; Tilmont, Gail; Harrison, Vangee. A Guide to Good Nutrition during and after Chemotherapy and Radiation. Seattle: Medical Oncology Unit, 1976.

117 pp. Paper.
A guide to help clients eat the right foods in the right amounts. Addresses major problems of weight loss, nausea, vomiting, sore mouth, constipation, adequate nourishment. Includes recipes that use commercial high-calorie products.

4.2 Baldonado, Ardelina A.; Stahl, Dulcelina A. Cancer Nursing: A Holistic Multidisciplinary Approach. [Nursing Outline Series.] Garden City: Medical Examination, 1978.

287 pp. Paper (spiral bound). Index. Bibliography.
A concise yet comprehensive review of current concepts for students, nurses, and other health care professionals. Uses an outline format with references,
review questions, and reading for each chapter. Considers pathology, management, diagnostic tests,
treatment, and related nursing care.

4.3   Bouchard, Rosemary; Owens, Norma F. Nursing Care of
the Cancer Patient, 3d ed. St. Louis: Mosby, 1976.
313 pp. Paper. Index. Bibliography. Glossary.
Discusses aspects of prevention, detection, diagnosis,
therapy, rehabilitation, and terminal care of oncologic
patients. Includes general approaches to care and
specific nursing needs. For nursing students and
graduates, whatever the setting for their practice.

4.4   Burkhalter, Pamela K; Donley, Diana L.; eds. Dynamics of
Oncology Nursing. New York: McGraw-Hill, 1978.
490 pp. Cloth. Index. References. Bibliography.
Five parts cover   The Nature of Cancer, the Role of
the Nurse in Cancer Management, Psychosocial Implications of Oncological Nursing, Unique Roles in Oncological Nursing, and Educational Aspects of Oncological Nursing.

4.5   Cassileth, Barrie R., ed. The Cancer Patient; Social and
Medical Aspects of Care. Philadelphia: Lea & Febiger,
1979.
332 pp. Paper. Index. References.
Contributions from clinical oncology, psychiatry,
epidemiology, ethics, rehabilitation, nutrition, pas-
toral counseling, social work, and nursing are included in this book that focuses on cancer and the care
of the cancer patient. Major sections are   Social and
Cultural Dimensions; Management Issues; and the
Human Dimension: Patients, Families, Staff, and
Students.

4.6   Dodd, Marylin J. Oncology Nursing, Case Studies. Garden
       City: Medical Examination Co., 1978.
             248 pp. Paper (spiral bound). Index.
             References.
             Includes 54 case studies with questions (multiple-
             choice, fill-in-the-blank, essay) and appropriate
             answers after each case study. Written by a nurse
             primarily for nursing students and practitioners, and
             the like.

4.7   Donovan, Marilee I.; Pierce, Sandra G. Cancer Care Nurs-
       ing. New York: Appleton-Century-Crofts, 1976.
             272 pp. Paper. Index. References.
             One goal of this monograph is to promote a more posi-
             tive attitude among nurses who work with oncology
             patients and their families. Includes approaches to
             managing general categories of problems that occur in
             these patients. Addresses the areas of dying, pain,
             infection, nutrition, elimination, and identity and body
             image.

4.8   Downie, Patricia A. Cancer Rehabilitation: An Introduction
       for Physiotherapists and the Allied Health Professions.
       London: Faber and Faber, 1978.
             205 pp. Cloth. Index. Bibliography. Glossary.
             Written for the physiotherapist, this book includes an
             overview of diagnosis and therapy as well as of the
             role of the physical therapist in chemotherapy and
             radiotherapy. Provides information on patients with
             specific disorders. Stresses the psychological im-
             pact of cancer and the importance of nutrition in re-
             habilitation. Lists the addresses of useful cancer
             organizations in Canada and the United States.

4.9   Leahy, Irene M.; St. Germain, Jean M.; Varricchio,
       Claudette G. The Nurse and Radiotherapy: A Manual for
       Daily Care. St. Louis: Mosby, 1979.
             171 pp. Paper. Index. References. Glossary.
             Focuses on the uses of radiation therapy, radiation
             protection, and the associated nursing implications.

Explores the fundamentals of radiation therapy as a base for nursing care for patients receiving external and internal sources of radiation.

4.10 Pitot, Henry C. Fundamentals of Oncology. New York: Marcel Dekker, 1978.

192 pp. Paper. Index. References.
A text for a first course in oncology. Focuses on the basic concepts of the science of this disease, including terminology, etiology, pathogenesis, biochemical aspects, and immunobiology, all as related to cancer.

4.11 Weisman, Avery D. Coping with Cancer. New York: McGraw-Hill, 1979.

138 pp. Paper. Index. Bibliography.
By the author of On Dying and Denying. This book examines the nature of coping as observed in cancer patients, including the intrapersonal and interpersonal aspects, and introduces the concept of psychosocial staging. The book is based on substantial psychosocial research and clinical studies.

4.12 Whelan, Elizabeth M. Preventing Cancer. New York: Norton, 1977.

285 pp. Cloth. Index. References.
The author considers what is known about the causes of cancer and concentrates on primary prevention. Discusses those high risk factors that are more within the control of an individual than others. Includes types of evidence and how scientists have reached their conclusions about cancer causation. A readable text for layman and professional.

4.13 White, Linda N.; Patterson, Judy E.; Cornelius, Janet L.; et al. Cancer Screening and Detection Manual for Nurses. New York: McGraw-Hill, 1979.

163 pp. Paper. Index. References. Glossary.
Presents the specific knowledge, skills, and techniques needed for cancer screening and detection. After a discussion of the general medical history,

introduces guidelines for screening individuals for
cancer in specific areas, including skin, head and
neck, abdomen, lung, breast, genitourinary system,
female genital tract, and rectum.

4.14   Wollard, Joy J., ed. Nutritional Management of the Cancer
Patient. New York: Raven Press, 1979.
   204 pp. Cloth. Index. References.
   Written for all the professionals involved in the care
   of cancer patients. Examines "the metabolic stress
   of cancer . . . interactions between food and drugs
   received by the cancer patient . . . significant aspects
   of nutritional care" throughout therapy (p. v). Discusses general principles and then covers specific
   problem areas (patient with colostomy, leukemia, the
   pediatric patient, etc.). Reports a symposium sponsored by the University of Texas System Cancer Center, M. D. Anderson Hospital and Tumor Institute.

CARDIOVASCULAR NURSING

4.15   Andreoli, Kathleen G.; Fowkes, Virginia Hunn; Zipes,
Douglas P.; et al. Comprehensive Cardiac Care: A Text for
Nurses, Physicians, and Other Health Practitioners, 4th ed.
St. Louis: Mosby, 1979.
   398 pp. Paper. Index. References.
   A basic text for health professionals involved in caring
   for cardiac patients. Chapters discuss   Anatomy and
   Physiology of the Heart; Coronary Artery Disease;
   Assessment of Patients with Coronary Artery Disease;
   Introduction to Electrocardiography; Arrhythmias;
   Artificial Cardiac Pacemakers; and Care of the Car-
   diac Patient. Includes appendixes on cardiovascular
   drugs, chest pain.

4.16   Chow, Rita K. Cardiosurgical Nursing Care: Understand-
ings, Concepts, and Principles for Practice. New York:
Springer Publishing Co., 1976.
   386 pp. Cloth. Index. Bibliography.
   This report on the nursing care of cardiovascular sur-

gical patients provides a review for the nurse experienced in this area and serves as a text for nursing students. Uses a systems approach to explore eight important patient care problems in detail: blood imbalances; hematologic disorders; water, electrolyte, acid-base balance alterations; circulatory failure; respiratory insufficiency or failure; renal insufficiency or failure; pain; and cerebral damage. Theoretical guides outline basic knowledge of physiology, specific knowledge of pathophysiologic considerations, manifestations, and nursing assessment and intervention.

4.17 Conover, Mary H. Cardiac Arrhythmias: Exercises in Pattern Interpretation, 2d ed. St. Louis: Mosby, 1978.
267 pp. Paper. Index. References.
Provides practical experience for those persons learning to identify arrhythmias. The author advocates step-by-step deductive reasoning. Each example is followed by a careful analysis. Includes suggestions for additional reading.

4.18 Cromwell, Rue L.; Butterfield, Earl C.; Brayfield, Frances M.; et al. Acute Myocardial Infarction: Reaction and Recovery. St. Louis: Mosby, 1977.
224 pp. Cloth. Index. References.
The book reports a major study of stress, personality, and nursing care factors involved in recovery from acute myocardial infarction. It is written for nurses, physicians, research scientists, psychologists, other health professionals, and the educated layman. Discusses the psychological understanding and treatment of the coronary patient and prevention of coronaries.

4.19 Croog, Sydney H.; Levine, Sol. The Heart Patient Recovers: Social and Psychological Factors. [Health Services Series.] New York: Human Sciences Press, 1977.
432 pp. Cloth. Subject and author indexes. Bibliography.
A long-term report on social and psychological aspects of heart attacks for patients, physicians, health planners, and nurses.

4.20 Donoso, Ephraim; Lipski, Janet, eds. Acute Myocardial
      Infarction. [Current Cardiovascular Topics, IV.] New
      York: Stratton Intercontinental, 1978.
           248 pp. Cloth. Index. References.
           Written for the continuing education of the general
           physician as well as the cardiovascular specialist.
           Focuses on evolving concepts and principles and the
           associated practical details.

4.21 Dubin, Dale. Rapid Interpretation of EKG's: A Programmed
      Course, 3d ed. Tampa, Fla.: Cover Publishing, 1974.
           295 pp. Paper. Index.
           A programmed course which covers the interpretation
           of the electrocardiogram using Dr. Dubin's rapid,
           systematic method. Designed to be followed in logical
           sequence, this text consists of illustrations and brief-
           ly stated factual information. Sentences below the fac-
           tual information contain blanks to be filled in, with
           answers provided. Sections progress from the basic
           principles to heart rate, rhythm, hypertrophy, etc.
           Includes reference sheets for a small notebook and a
           section of EKG tracings. Editions are available in
           French, Spanish, Japanese, Serbo-Croatian, German,
           Portuguese, and Persian.

4.22 Finlayson, Angela; McEwen, James. Coronary Heart
      Disease and Patterns of Living. New York: Prodist, 1977.
           222 pp. Cloth. Index. References.
           Explores important aspects of living after a myocar-
           dial infarction and makes suggestions for research
           and intervention studies. For students and workers
           in the health professions and social services.

4.23 Fletcher, Gerald F.; Cantwell, John D. Exercise and Coro-
      nary Heart Disease; Role in Prevention, Diagnosis, and
      Treatment, 2d ed. Springfield, Ill.: Thomas, 1979.
           340 pp. Cloth. Subject and author indexes.
           References.

Discusses the place of exercise in the prevention, diagnosis, treatment, and rehabilitation of coronary artery disease patients. The text is written for those in primary care practice.

4.24 Garcia, Rebecca M. Rehabilitation after Myocardial Infarction. [Continuing Education in Cardiovascular Nursing, Series 1: Myocardial Infarction, Unit 2.] New York: Appleton-Century-Crofts, 1979.
    83 pp. Paper. References. Bibliography.
    The book opens with the ANA's Standards for Cardiovascular Nursing Practice. Topics covered are rehabilitation, enhancing learning, plans for learning, physical reconditioning. Each unit has objectives, study guide, text, references, and a self-examination. A post-test concludes the book. Appendixes include classification, heart disease, lesson plans, and materials for patients. ing program, and materials for patients.

4.25 Gentry, W. Doyle; Williams, Redford B., Jr., eds. Psychological Aspects of Myocardial Infarction and Coronary Care, 2d ed. St. Louis: Mosby, 1979.
    162 pp. Paper. Index. References.
    Looks at the psychological involvement in both the etiology of and the adaptation to myocardial infarction. For nurse specialists, physicians, psychiatrists, and psychologists. The contributors are representatives from these fields. The major sections are Etiology, Acute Care, Rehabilitation, and Intervention. References to basic research studies as well as the inclusion of clinical material add depth to the book. Of special interest are chapters on critical life events and coronary disease, psychological aftermaths, vocational rehabilitation, and sexual counseling.

4.26 Glass, David C. Behavior Patterns, Stress, and Coronary Disease. Hillsdale: Lawrence Erlbaum Associates, 1977.
    217 pp. Cloth. Index. References.
    Presents experimental findings that reflect the interplay of uncontrolled stress and the coronary prone Type A behavior pattern.

4.27 Holland, Jeanne M. Cardiovascular Nursing: Prevention,
Intervention, and Rehabilitation. Boston: Little, Brown,
1977.
    233 pp. Paper. Index. References.
    Written for the nurse returning to practice or moving
    to the special area of cardiovascular nursing. In-
    cludes selected aspects of physiology and pathophysiol-
    ogy. Emphasizes prevention, patient education, and
    rehabilitation. Contains a patient teaching guide.

4.28 Meltzer, Lawrence E.; Pinneo, Rose; Kitchell, J. Roderick.
Intensive Coronary Care: A Manual for Nurses, 3d ed.
Bowie, Md.: The Charles Press, 1977.
    280 pp. Cloth. Index. Bibliography.
    A standard text for coronary care nursing, presented
    with simplicity, clarity, scope, and depth. Includes
    pathophysiology, pharmacology, hemodynamic moni-
    toring, and management of acute myocardial infarction.
    Much of the book is in outline format and is well illus-
    trated.

4.29 Pinneo, Rose. Congestive Heart Failure. [Continuing Education in Cardiovascular Nursing, Series I: Myocardial Infarction, Unit 1.] New York: Appleton-Century-Crofts,
1978.
    70 pp. Paper. Bibliography.
    A teaching-learning module on congestive heart failure
    with objectives, study guides, bibliographies, and self-
    examinations. Topics include: pathology and etiology,
    compensatory mechanisms, clinical assessment, and
    management of patients. The book ends with a post-
    test (answers included).

4.30 Sweetwood, Hannelore M. The Patient in the Coronary Care
Unit. New York: Springer Publishing, 1976.
    465 pp. Cloth. Index. References.
    Written for nurses in community hospitals with coro-
    nary care units where frequently no physician is in
    attendance. Includes discussions of selected heart

diseases, anatomy and physiology of the heart, arrhythmias, monitoring, cardiac arrest, prevention of psychological problems, and others.

4.31   Wenger, Nanette K.; Hellerstein, Herman K.   Rehabilitation of the Coronary Patient.   New York: Wiley, 1978.
323 pp.   Cloth.   Index.   References.   Glossary.
An accepted part of medical practice, rehabilitation includes physical activity, functional evaluation, prescriptive training, patient and family education, and psychosocial and vocational counseling.   This book focuses on physiologic, medical, and social problems associated with myocardial infarction and a realistic approach to patients after myocardial infarction.   Written for the primary care physician and other members of the health team.

CRITICAL CARE NURSING

4.32   Abels, Linda F.   Mosby's Manual of Critical Care.   St. Louis: Mosby, 1979.
430 pp.   Paper.   Index.   Bibliography.
This text is "a basic technical reference for those individuals providing care for the critically ill patient." (p. vii)   Includes theories and procedures used in all kinds of critical care settings.   Major segments are: Physical Assessment of the Critically Ill Patient, Life Maintenance, Infection Control, Critical Care and Other Health Delivery Systems, and Disaster Planning in Critical Care.   A series of appendixes provides useful summaries of drugs.   Illustrations and marginal headings increase the book's usefulness as a reference.

4.33   Adler, Diane C.; Shoemaker, Norma J., eds.   AACN [American Association of Critical Care Nurses] Organization and Management of Critical Care Facilities.   St. Louis: Mosby, 1979.
214 pp.   Cloth.   Index.   References.   Bibliography.
The development, organization, and management of a critical care facility is discussed in the context of the

essential interdisciplinary team approach to the care
of patients in such units. Sections include Formation
Stages, Designing and Equipping the Facility, Policies
and Procedures, Development of Nursing Personnel,
and Considerations for Patient Care.

4.34 Burrell, Zeb L., Jr.; Burrell, Lenette Owens. Critical
Care, 3d ed. St. Louis: Mosby, 1977.
>427 pp. Cloth. Index. Bibliography.
>A presentation of essential information needed by prac-
>titioners who care for critically ill persons. Basic
>principles and concepts are combined and simplified in
>order to explain the rationale of treatment. Organized
>by major body systems. The book also has a chapter
>on equipment and drugs. First and second editions
>entitled Intensive Nursing Care.

4.35 Hazzard, Mary E. Critical Care Nursing. [Nursing Outline
Series.] Garden City: Medical Examination, 1978.
>202 pp. Paper (spiral). Index. Bibliography.
>For study or review of critical care nursing. In out-
>line format with review questions and suggested read-
>ings. Uses a general systems approach. Three parts
>contain 1) philosophy of care and basic concepts, 2) con-
>ditions common to a number of critical care situations,
>and 3) common problems (medical-surgical, psychiat-
>ric, maternity and infant). The third section, which
>comprises more than half the book, includes brief re-
>views of anatomy, physiology, assessment, and inter-
>vention.

4.36 Holloway, Nancy M. Nursing the Critically Ill Adult. Menlo
Park, Calif.: Addison-Wesley, 1979.
>598 pp. Cloth. Index. References.
>For nursing students and graduates who are interested
>in critical care nursing. The book builds on the basics
>of nursing and includes cardiac assessment, arrhyth-
>mias, and failure; shock; fluid and electrolyte and acid
>base imbalances; renal problems; thermal problems;
>respiratory problems; nutrition; communication; and
>activity needs.

4.37 Hudak, Carolyn M.; Lohr, Thelma "Skip"; Gallo, Barbara M.
      Critical Care Nursing, 2d ed. Philadelphia: Lippincott,
      1977.
          562 pp. Cloth. Index. References.
          The aim is to assist the "critical care nurse practi-
          tioner to acquire the knowledge base necessary to
          carry out the responsible role of patient guardian and
          advocate." (p. viii) Unit I: New Horizons in Critical
          Care Nursing; Unit II: Holistic Approach to Critical
          Care Nursing; Unit III: Core Body Systems; Unit IV:
          Specific Crisis Situations; and Unit V: Professional
          Practice in the Critical Care Unit. Continues the
          holistic approach of the first edition and the emphasis
          on the interrelatedness of body systems.

4.38 Waisbren, Burton A. Critical Care Manual: A Systems
      Approach Method, 2d ed. Flushing, N.Y.: Medical Exam-
      ination, 1977.
          256 pp. Cloth. Drug index. Bibliography.
          A guide for paramedical personnel in administering
          medications upon receipt of critical lab values. In-
          cludes flowsheets. Has helpful summaries of particu-
          lar drug problems, i.e., interactions, toxicities.

4.39 Wilmore, Douglas W. The Metabolic Management of the
      Critically Ill. New York: Plenum, 1977.
          262 pp. Cloth. Index. References.
          A handbook for physicians who care for the critically
          ill that has an organized approach to the metabolic sup-
          port plan through the use of a metabolic and nutritional
          worksheet. Copies of these materials are in the appen-
          dix and a copy of the support plan is in a pocket on the
          back cover. Focuses on five major areas: Energy
          and Energy Balance; Control of Body Temperature;
          Relationships with Metabolic Control; Hormonal Con-
          trol of Body Fluids; Alterations in Intermediary
          Metabolism; and Feeding the Patient.

HYPERTENSION

4.40 Kaplan, Norman M. Clinical Hypertension, 2d ed.
Baltimore: Williams & Wilkins, 1978.
> 405 pp. Cloth. Index. References.
> A book (for medical practitioners, students, and
> house officers) that focuses on a practical, rational
> approach to the management of the hypertensive patient.

4.41 Margie, Joyce D.; Hunt, James C. Living With High Blood
Pressure: The Hypertension Diet Cookbook. Bloomfield,
N.J.: HLS Press, 1978.
> 309 pp. Cloth. Index.
> Modification of diet is one part of an effective blood
> pressure control program and this very well done cook-
> book is designed to assist the patient and his family
> make the necessary modifications. Part 1 explains
> what high blood pressure is and discusses the plan for
> the diet needed. Part 2 includes the recipes. Part 3
> has eight appendixes that list nutritive values of food
> and how to plan meals, calculate nutritive values,
> modify sodium intake, eat away from home, and find
> sources for special dietary foods.

4.42 U.S. National Institutes of Health. Guidelines for Educating
Nurses in High Blood Pressure Control. DHEW Publication
No. (NIH) 77-1241. Washington: Government Printing Of-
fice, 1977.
> 24 pp. Paper. Bibliography.
> Written by the Task Force on the Role of Nursing in
> High Blood Pressure Control, National High Blood
> Pressure Education Program, National Heart, Lung
> and Blood Institute. Contains guidelines for basic,
> graduate, and continuing education and in-service edu-
> cation to pretest performance and cognitive skills, to
> select content and teaching methods, and to evaluate
> outcomes.

DERMATOLOGIC NURSING

4.43   Huckbody, Eileen. Nursing Procedures for Skin Diseases.
Edinburgh: Churchill Livingstone, 1977.
>135 pp. Paper. Index.
>Includes a series of short chapters on selected skin
>conditions and, more importantly, on procedures that
>may need to be modified or are particular to the patient
>with the skin condition. The former range from admis-
>sion to vaginal exams and the latter from a biopsy of
>the skin to treatment of warts and molluscum con-
>tagiosum. Has some illustrations.

4.44   Jacoby, Florence G. Nursing Care of the Patient with Burns,
2d ed. St. Louis: Mosby, 1976.
>185 pp. Paper. Index. References.
>Written by a burn nurse clinician, this book presents
>fundamental knowledge of pathologic, physiologic, and
>psychologic changes that occur in patients with burns.
>A useful outline summary of burn therapy is located in
>an appendix.

ENDOCRINE NURSING

General

4.45   Bacchus, Habeeb. Metabolic and Endocrine Emergencies:
Recognition and Management, 2d ed. Baltimore: University
Park Press, 1977.
>233 pp. Paper. Index. References.
>Designed for the clinician who faces such emergencies
>and is concerned with rapid recognition and manage-
>ment. Includes discussions of clinical information,
>mechanisms of the disorders, and rationale for the
>emergency regimen. Also discusses clinical manifes-
>tations, clinical laboratory confirmation, recognition,
>therapy, causes, and treatment. After a general ap-
>proach, the remaining chapters focus on specific
>problems.

4.46 Hershman, Jerome M. Endocrine Pathophysiology: A
Patient-Oriented Approach. Philadelphia: Lea & Febiger,
1977.
358 pp. Paper. Index. Bibliography.
Written for medical students, this monograph has a
limited review of basic endocrinology in each chapter.
Included are testing of function, signs and symptoms,
principles of therapy, and relevant clinical pharmacology. Provides patient presentations and questions in
each chapter. Useful for other learners who wish a
succinct review of current concepts in clinical endocrinology.

4.47 Krueger, Judith A.; Ray, Janis C. Endocrine Problems in
Nursing: A Physiologic Approach. St. Louis: Mosby, 1976.
165 pp. Paper. Index. Bibliography.
Discusses each gland, anatomy and physiology, associated diseases, assessment of function, and treatment. Presents nursing care in tables in each chapter. Well illustrated with photographs, charts,
drawings.

4.48 Watts, Nelson B.; Keffer, Joseph H. Practical Endocrine
Diagnosis, 2d ed. Philadelphia: Lea & Febiger, 1978.
123 pp. Paper. Index. Bibliography.
A manual to assist in the diagnosis of endocrine problems with an emphasis on hormone measurement.
Limited discussion of nonhormonal aspects of the disease. Tabbed dividers list summary points for major
endocrine glands.

Diabetes Mellitus

4.49 Blevins, Dorothy R. The Diabetic and Nursing Care. New
York: McGraw-Hill, 1979.
366 pp. Cloth. Index. References.
A text on the care of persons with diabetes for nursing
students and practitioners. The first part of the book
looks broadly at cultural, psychosocial dimensions of

the nursing care and response of the diabetic patient
to chronic illness. Specific nursing care requirements
for diabetics of various ages and with various problems (hospitalization, pregnancy) are considered in the
latter part of the book. The emphasis on teaching is
clear.

4.50 Bonar, Jeanne R. Diabetes: A Clinical Guide. Flushing,
N.Y.: Medical Examination, 1977.
> 354 pp. Paper (spiral bound). Index. Bibliography.
> A medical text that presents facts in a controversial
> area. The focus is on physician self-education,
> patient education, and the responsibility of both the
> physician and the patient.

4.51 Guthrie, Diane W.; Guthrie, Richard A., eds. Nursing Management of Diabetes Mellitus. St. Louis: Mosby, 1977.
> 283 pp. Paper. Index. References. Glossary.
> Current information and resources for health profes-
> sional students and practitioners. Includes definition,
> management, acute and chronic care, special prob-
> lems, and education and research. Appendixes contain
> a suggested course outline, organizations and other
> sources for information and services, and a revised
> exchange list.

4.52 Krail, Leo P., ed. Joslin Diabetes Manual, 11th ed.
Philadelphia: Lea & Febiger, 1978.
> 324 pp. Paper. Index. Bibliography.
> Update of a classic on diabetes for the physician and
> the patient. Diabetes is defined, treatment is de-
> scribed, and living with it is discussed. Material in
> the appendixes includes useful addresses and sugges-
> tions for diet and medication. Twelfth edition due 1980.

4.53 Managing Diabetics Properly. [Nursing '77 Skillbooks.]
Horsham, Pa.: Intermed Communications, 1977.
> 233 pp. Cloth. Index.
> This book includes basic knowledge needed to care for
> patients with diabetes; discusses their major problems;

and considers the effect of diabetes as an additional
problem to other major medical illnesses. Content
is followed by skillchecks.

EYE, EAR, NOSE AND THROAT NURSING

4.54 Adams, George L.; Boies, Lawrence R.; Paparella,
Michael M. Boies's Fundamentals of Otolaryngology: A
Textbook of Ear, Nose, and Throat Diseases, 5th ed.
Philadelphia: Saunders, 1978.
>764 pp. Cloth. Index. References.
>A text for the health professional on head and neck
>diseases. Has been a standard text for medical stu-
>dents for years. Part 1: History and Examination;
>Part 2: The Ear; Part 3: The Nose and Paranasal
>Sinuses; Part 4: The Oral Cavity and Pharynx; Part 5:
>The Larynx; Part 6: Related Head and Neck Topics.

4.55 Goodhill, Victor. Ear: Diseases, Deafness, and Dizziness.
Hagerstown: Harper & Row, 1979.
>781 pp. Cloth. Index. References. Suggested readings.
>The author and 14 contributors discuss the ear from
>the basic anatomy and physiology and examination tech-
>niques to the disorders of the internal and external ear.
>Of special interest are the chapters on hearing losses
>(child and adult) and education of the deaf. The book
>is written for the clinical otologist and for the physi-
>cian who must deal with ear problems. Includes a
>glossary of abbreviations.

4.56 Saunders, William H.; Havener, William H.; Keith, Carol
F.; et al. Nursing Care in Eye, Ear, Nose, and Throat
Disorders, 4th ed. St. Louis: Mosby, 1979.
>520 pp. Cloth. Index. References. Glossary.
>A well known text for the student and practitioner of
>nursing that focuses on pathophysiology, significant
>signs and symptoms, treatments, and prevention of
>eye, ear, nose, and throat problems. Well illustrated.

GASTROINTESTINAL NURSING

4.57 Berk, J. Edward, ed. Developments in Digestive Diseases:
Clinical Relevance. Philadelphia: Lea & Febiger, 1977.
194 pp. Cloth. References.
First of a series of volumes that review newer
developments in gastroenterology. The focus is on
the relevance for clinical practice. Topics in this
volume include endoscopy, duodenal ulcer management, hepatitis viruses, and others.

4.58 Given, Barbara A.; Simmons, Sandra J. Gastroenterology
in Clinical Nursing, 3d ed. St. Louis: Mosby, 1979.
378 pp. Paper. Index. References.
Written for practitioners and students to provide a
base for nursing care of patients with the more common gastrointestinal disorders. After a discussion of
general aspects of care, chapters focus on preoperative
and postoperative care, and disorders related to components of the gastrointestinal tract.

4.59 Gribble, Helen E. Gastroenterological Nursing. Baltimore:
Williams & Wilkins, 1977.
309 pp. Paper. Index.
For the senior nursing student or the new graduate,
this book discusses common disorders of the gastrointestinal tract. Problems are developmental, trau-
matic, infective, inflammatory, and neoplastic. Diagnostic tests and medical and surgical treatment are
also included. Discusses specific nursing care in
each section.

4.60 May, Harriett J. Enterostomal Therapy. New York: Raven
Press, 1977.
274 pp. Paper. Index. Bibliography. Further readings. Glossary.
This text builds on the basic education of a nurse to
develop competencies needed in enterostomal therapy.
Focuses on the physical and emotional needs of the
patients. Specific topics include: ostomy functions,
teaching, principles of ostomy appliances, and diet.

4.61 Vukovich, Virginia C.; Grubb, Reba D. Care of the Ostomy
Patient, 2d ed. St. Louis: Mosby, 1977.
150 pp. Paper. Index. Suggested references.
Glossary.
Written for hospital personnel, students, and others
interested in improving service to ostomy patients.
Detailed explanations and instructions make this useful
as a text or reference. Pragmatic, procedural material is combined with conceptual material. Includes
sources for educational materials.

NEUROLOGIC NURSING

4.62 Baer, William P. The Aphasic Patient: A Program for
Auditory Comprehension and Language Training. Clinician's
edition. Springfield, Ill.: Thomas, 1976.
135 pp. Cloth.
A practical, useful program to assist language-
impaired patients to improve their understanding of
spoken language. Provides vocabulary and activity
sequence pages that help the patient learn to understand and signal that he does so before he is expected
to make verbal responses. A patient's edition is also
available.

4.63 Conway, Barbara L. Carini and Owens' Neurological and
Neurosurgical Nursing, 7th ed. St. Louis: Mosby, 1978.
640 pp. Cloth. Index. Bibliography. Glossary.
Long a standard text, this edition is updated with increased depth in anatomy and physiology, pathophysiology, and patient assessment. Its holistic approach includes a chapter on sexuality. The goal is optimal
care with a focus on rehabilitation. The fifth and sixth
editions were authored by Esta Carini and Guy Owens.

4.64 Davis, Joan E.; Mason, Celestine B. Neurologic Critical
Care. New York: Van Nostrand Reinhold, 1979.
291 pp. Cloth. Index. Bibliography.
Written for nurses involved in the critical care setting.

Topics included are: anatomy and physiology, assessment, diagnosis, trauma, injury, tumors, infection,
and vascular problems. The last section has case
situations for test and review.

4.65 Hoppenfeld, Stanley. Orthopaedic Neurology: A Diagnostic
Guide to Neurologic Levels. Philadelphia: Lippincott, 1977.
131 pp. Cloth. Index. Bibliography.
Excellent illustrations add to the clarity of this text
which focuses on crucial concepts of examination and
diagnosis of problems of the spinal cord and nerve
roots. The neurological levels and their significance
are made clear.

4.66 Howe, James R. Patient Care in Neurosurgery. Boston:
Little, Brown, 1977.
228 pp. Paper (spiral bound). Index. Bibliography.
Although this monograph is directed primarily to house
officers assigned to neurosurgery, practicing neuro-
surgeons, clinical nursing specialists, and medical
students may also find it helpful. It focuses on the
"practical description of considerations specific to the
care of the neurosurgical patient." (p. vii) The high-
lights of patient care include both pre- and postoperative care. Not for the beginning student.

4.67 Plum, Fred; Posner, Jerome B., eds. The Diagnosis of
Stupor and Coma, 2d ed. Philadelphia: Davis, 1972.
286 pp. Cloth. Index. Bibliography.
A monograph on the diagnostic problems associated
with stupor and coma. Includes pathology, physiology,
signs and symptoms, specific lesions, metabolic and
psychogenic problems, and brain death.

4.68 Roaf, Robert; Hodkinson, Leonard J. The Paralyzed Patient.
Oxford: Blackwell, 1977.
293 pp. Paper. Index. Bibliography. Glossary.
Considers the interdisciplinary approach to the care of
the paralyzed patient. Diagrams and illustrations are
helpful.

4.69 Swift, Nancy; Mabel, Robert M. Manual of Neurological
       Nursing. Boston: Little, Brown, 1978.
              201 pp. Paper. Index. References.
              A brief, up-to-date guide to neurologic nursing for
              nursing students and graduates. Includes chapters on
              observation, general problems, diagnostic studies,
              and specific neurologic disorders. The final chapter
              looks at neuropsychology and rehabilitation.

4.70 Wilson, Susan F. Neuronursing. New York: Springer
       Publishing, 1979.
              272 pp. Cloth. Index. Bibliography.
              A text on neurological and neurosurgical nursing care
              for students and nurses in practice. The book looks
              first at anatomy and physiology and assessment related
              to the nervous system. The next chapters look at nurs-
              ing care of the unconscious patient, and the patient who
              has increased intracranial pressure, seizures, or
              aphasia. Diagnostic tests and then specific diseases
              are considered in the last half of the book. Stresses
              nursing care and its rationale.

ORTHOPEDIC NURSING

4.71 Aston, J. N. A Short Textbook of Orthopaedics and Trauma-
       tology, 2d ed. Revised by Sean Hughes. Philadelphia:
       Lippincott, 1976.
              302 pp. Paper. Index.
              A text written for medical students in a concise, up-
              to-date, and authoritative manner. It focuses on the
              locomotor system, one subject to injuries. The first
              section discusses trauma to each body part and the
              second section focuses on orthopedic problems. Illus-
              trations and chapter summaries are helpful.

4.72 Brunner, Nancy A. Orthopedic Nursing; A Programmed
       Approach, 3d ed. St. Louis: Mosby, 1979.
              263 pp. Paper. References.
              Using a nursing process approach, this programmed
              text is for nursing students who are learning to care

for the patient with a fracture or one who is undergoing
orthopedic surgery. Major parts are Introduction to
Orthopedic Nursing; Treatment of Orthopedic Conditions; Principles of Nursing Care of the Surgical Orthopedic Patient; and Principles of Nursing Care of the
Nonsurgical Orthopedic Patient. Has useful illustrations.

4.73 Donahoo, Clara A.; Dimon, Joseph H., III. Orthopedic
Nursing. Boston: Little, Brown, 1977.
        256 pp. Cloth. Index.
        A supplemental text that presents material pertinent to
        the daily practice of orthopedic nursing. The intended
        audience is the orthopedic nurse practitioner but stu-
        dents and graduates will find it useful. Discusses the
        most common clinical problems but purposefully omits
        the psychosocial aspects of orthopedic nursing. Major
        headings are 1) nursing assessment, 2) trauma,
        3) common disease processes and conditions, and 4)
        plans for nursing care. Contains helpful illustrations:
        X-rays, photographs of injuries, congenital conditions,
        disease conditions, orthopedic equipment, casting tech-
        niques, and crutch walking diagrams.

4.74 Farrell, Jane. Illustrated Guide to Orthopedic Nursing.
Philadelphia: Lippincott, 1977.
        242 pp. Paper. Index. Bibliography.
        The author sees the orthopedic nurse as having a
        unique responsibility in the rehabilitation team's ef-
        forts. Emphasizes the inclusion of the patient and
        family in plans and interventions. The focus is on the
        adult orthopedic patient in the hospital setting. In-
        cludes factors that influence adjustment, behavior,
        and recovery as well as practical suggestions for re-
        turn to the home.

4.75 Larson, Carroll B.; Gould, Marjorie. Orthopedic Nursing,
9th ed. St. Louis: Mosby, 1978.
        496 pp. Cloth. Index. Bibliography.
        Updates a classic in this field. It continues to empha-

size the fundamentals of care and adds to the nurse's
ability in the assessment, planning, implementation,
and evaluation of holistic nursing care. Opening chapters discuss general considerations and subsequent
chapters focus on nursing patients with musculoskeletal problems, orthopedic surgery, and rehabilitative
needs.

4.76 Lewis, Royce C., Jr. Handbook of Traction, Casting, and
Splinting Techniques. Philadelphia: Lippincott, 1977.
129 pp. Cloth. Index.
This handbook includes principles, indications, and
methods for traction, casting, and splinting. Useful
illustrations, diagrams, and photographs.

4.77 Rowe, Joyce W.; Dyer, Lois, eds. Care of the Orthopaedic
Patient. Oxford: Blackwell, 1977.
421 pp. Cloth. Index. References.
A comprehensive text that is patient rather than
condition-centered. For nurses studying orthopedic
nursing and other members of the orthopedic team.
It includes chapters on diagnosis, hospital care, traction, casting, orthotics, the paralyzed patient, children in hospitals, physiotherapy, occupational therapy,
and frequently used medicines. Many good illustrations.

RENAL NURSING

4.78 Anderton, J. L.; Parsons, F. M.; Jones, D. E., eds.
Living With Renal Failure. Baltimore: University Park
Press, 1978.
281 pp. Cloth. Index. References.
Report of an interdisciplinary symposium held in Scot-
land in 1977 that looked at many of the problems related
to the treatment of chronic renal failure by dialysis and
transplantation. Considered are the selection of patients, economics and limited care, selected clinical
problems, psychological and personal aspects, and
practical management.

4.79 Brundage, Dorothy J. Nursing Management of Renal Prob-
     lems, 2d ed. St. Louis: Mosby, 1980.
          232 pp. Paper. Index. References.
          Discusses conservation of renal function. Normal
          function is considered first, followed by material on
          the prevention, detection, and management of renal
          disease. Nutritional aspects and acute renal failure
          close the first section. The second section focuses on
          the restoration of renal function. The treatment modal-
          ities, dialysis and transplantation, are discussed in de-
          tail. The approach used is more conceptual and theo-
          retical than procedural and provides a base for nurs-
          ing interventions.

4.80 Cameron, J. Stewart; Russell, Alison M. E.; Sale,
     Diana N. T. Nephrology for Nurses: A Modern Approach
     to the Kidney, 2d ed. [Modern Nursing Series.] Flushing,
     N.Y.: Medical Examination, 1976.
          330 pp. Paper (spiral bound). Index. Bibliography.
          Glossary.
          A concise text covering the kidneys and various diseases
          of the kidneys (uremia, nephritis, renal failure, etc.).

4.81 Coe, Fredric L. Nephrolithiasis: Pathogenesis and Treat-
     ment. Chicago: Year Book, 1978.
          235 pp. Cloth. Index. References.
          Written for physicians, this book discusses the main
          factors related to stone formation, and the diagnosis
          and treatment of the condition.

4.82 Coggins, Cecil H.; Cummings, Nancy B., eds. Prevention
     of Kidney and Urinary Tract Diseases. DHEW Publication
     no. (NIH) 78-855. [Fogarty International Center Series on
     Preventive Medicine, vol. 5.] Bethesda, Md.: National In-
     stitutes of Health, 1978.
          297 pp. Cloth. Index. References.
          Focuses on current knowledge of and efforts toward
          prevention of kidney and urinary tract diseases. Em-
          phasis is on the few renal diseases that may be pre-
          vented, and on areas that should be studied. The

diseases selected affect large numbers of patients and
may be prevented by newer approaches to research. One
chapter summarizes findings and recommendations.

4.83 Hekelman, Francine P.; Ostendarp, Carol A. Nephrology
Nursing: Perspectives of Care. New York: McGraw-Hill,
1979.
   326 pp. Cloth. Index. References.
   A text for those planning to specialize in the care of
   patients with renal problems. Includes anatomy and
   physiology, diagnostic tests, disease conditions, medical management, and suggestions for teaching patients
   and staff. Looks at dialysis and transplantation and
   closes with standards of care. Each chapter has suggestions for "active learning."

4.84 Kagan, Lynn W. Renal Disease; A Manual of Patient Care.
New York: McGraw-Hill, 1979.
   288 pp. Cloth. Index. References.
   For students: nursing, physician's associates, and dialysis technicians. Section 1: The Normal Kidney looks
   at anatomy, physiology, and diagnostic assessment.
   Section 2: Renal Failure discusses acute and chronic
   failure and its causes. Section 3: Intervention Modalities deals with conservative management, dialysis,
   and transplantation. Materials in the appendixes include physiologic values, drug dosage in renal disease,
   and general references. Each chapter has review
   questions and there is a series of case studies for a
   final self-assessment.

4.85 Massry, Shaul G.; Sellers, Alvin L., eds. Clinical Aspects
of Uremia and Dialysis. Springfield, Ill.: Thomas, 1976.
   746 pp. Cloth. Subject and author indexes.
   Bibliography.
   Presents detailed coverage of selected aspects of
   uremia and dialysis for students, clinicians, and in-
   vestigators. Contributors are well known in nephrology. Major topics include: pathogenesis, diagnosis,
   clinical features, treatment, dialysis: patients and
   technical aspects.

4.86 Sachs, Bonnie L. Renal Transplantation: A Nursing Perspective. Flushing, N.Y.: Medical Examination, 1977.
     189 pp. Paper (spiral bound). Index. References.
Provides basic information for nurses, written by a
clinical nurse specialist in the area of renal transplantation. Includes historical, ethical, and rehabilitative aspects as well as pre- and postoperative care.
One section presents multidisciplinary views and another presents the words of patients.

4.87 Uldall, Robert. Renal Nursing, 2d ed. Oxford: Blackwell,
1977.
     271 pp. Paper. Index.
Written by a physician for nurses who look after patients with renal disease. Chapters cover the following topics: physiology, tests, kidney diseases, renal
failure, peritoneal dialysis, hemodialysis, poisoning,
and renal transplantation.

RESPIRATORY NURSING

4.88 Cherniack, Reuben M. Pulmonary Function Testing. Philadelphia: Saunders, 1977.
     291 pp. Paper. Index. Bibliography.
Pulmonary function testing is an important part of
clinical assessment of respiratory problems. Written
for both allied health professionals and physicians,
this book includes both simple and complex measures.
Covers the background information needed to understand normal and disturbed pulmonary function. Each
chapter has self-assessment questions and several
have case examples.

4.89 Egan, Donald F. Fundamentals of Respiratory Therapy,
3d ed. St. Louis: Mosby, 1977.
     551 pp. Cloth. Index. References.
A text for the respiratory therapy student, therapist,
and technician, but also useful to nurses, house staff,
pulmonary fellows, and other physicians. Chapters

discuss the following topics: gases, ventilation, blood gases and acid-base balance, gas therapy, chronic care and rehabilitation of respiratory failure, and others.

4.90 Sweetwood, Hannelore M. Nursing in the Intensive Respiratory Care Unit, 2d ed. New York: Springer Publishing, 1979.
> 486 pp. Cloth. Index. Bibliography.
> Written for the beginning practitioner, this book emphasizes physiology and basic principles of care. Major sections are: basic science, patient assessment, treatment modalities, and patient care. The basic science section looks at anatomy and physiology of the respiratory system, blood gases, acid-base and fluid and electrolyte balance. The modalities of treatment include drugs, O_2, ventilators. Nursing care focuses on the major respiratory problems. Makes good use of charts, illustrations, and outlines.

4.91 Wade, Jacqueline F. Respiratory Nursing Care: Physiology and Technique, 2d ed. St. Louis: Mosby, 1977.
> 231 pp. Paper. Index. Bibliography.
> For professional practitioners with a broad need for knowledge of respiratory care, especially in nursing specialty areas. The second edition increases the emphasis on respiratory physiology and its application in bedside monitoring, physical assessment of the chest, and interpreting chest X-ray films. Chapter topics include laboratory findings, respiratory diseases, therapy, and intensive care.

UROLOGIC NURSING

4.92 Harrison, J. Hartwell; Gittes, Ruben F.; Perlmutter, Alan D.; et al.; eds. Campbell's Urology, 4th ed. Philadelphia: Saunders, 1978-79.
> 3 vols.   Cloth. Index. References.
> Includes physiology, pathophysiology, diagnosis, treatment of problems of the urinary tract. A classic medical text. Previous editions edited by M. F. Campbell.

4.93   Winter, Chester C.; Morel, Alice. Nursing Care of Patients
with Urologic Diseases, 4th ed. St. Louis: Mosby, 1977.
    366 pp. Paper. Index. Bibliography.
    For nurses in urologic units. Discusses urologic anat-
omy, physiology, examination equipment (with pictures),
ostomy care and appliances, renal disorders, the
adrenals. Includes a chapter on patient's age and influencing factors. Each chapter includes a brief outline at the beginning and review questions at the end.

PERIODICALS

4.94   AANA Journal. American Association of Nurse Anesthetists,
Suite 929, 111 E. Wacker Drive, Chicago, Ill. 60601.
Bimonthly. 1933 to date.

4.95   American Lung Association Bulletin. American Lung Association, 1740 Broadway, New York, N.Y. 10019. Monthly
(except July, February). 1914 to date.

4.96   Cancer Nursing, An International Journal for Cancer Care.
Cancer Nursing, 14 East 60th Street, Suite 1101, New York,
N.Y. 10022. Bimonthly. 1978 to date.

4.97   Cardiovascular Nursing. American Heart Association, Inc.,
7320 Greenville Avenue, Dallas, Tex. 75231. Bimonthly.
1965 to date.

4.98   Critical Care Quarterly. Aspen Systems Corporation, 20010
Century Boulevard, Germantown, Md. 20767. Quarterly.
1978 to date.

4.99   Current Perspectives in Oncologic Nursing. C.V. Mosby
Co., 11830 Westline Industrial Drive, St. Louis, Mo. 63141.
Biannually. 1976 to date. Cloth.

4.100   Diabetes Care. American Diabetes Association, Inc., 600
Fifth Avenue, New York, N.Y. 10020. Bimonthly.
1978 to date.

4.101 Diabetes Forecast. American Diabetes Association, Inc.,
       600 Fifth Avenue, New York, N.Y. 10020. Bimonthly.
       1948 to date.

4.102 Heart and Lung: Journal of Critical Care. C.V. Mosby Co.,
       11830 Westline Industrial Drive, St. Louis, Mo. 63141 (For
       the American Association of Critical Care Nurses).
       Bimonthly. 1972 to date.

4.103 Journal of Neurosurgical Nursing. American Association of
       Neurosurgical Nurses, 27 West Ridgeview Street, Chicago,
       Ill. 60185. (Distributed by Williams & Wilkins Co., 428
       E. Preston Street, Baltimore, Md. 21202.) Quarterly.
       1969 to date.

4.104 ONA Journal; Orthopedic Nurses' Association Journal.
       Charles B. Slack, Inc., 6900 Grove Road, Thorofare, N.J.
       08086. Monthly. 1974 to date.

5

The Natural Sciences and Nursing

One of the major bases for nursing practice is the natural sciences. This chapter focuses on anatomy, physiology, and biochemistry; chemistry, physics, and toxicology; immunology; mathematics and statistics; nutrition; pathology and pathophysiology; and pharmacology. Some books emphasize nursing; some are medical references. The chapter ends with a list of selected periodicals useful for nursing.

GENERAL

5.1   Elhart, Dorothy; Firsich, Sharon C.; Gragg, Shirley H.; et al. Scientific Principles in Nursing, 8th ed. St. Louis: Mosby, 1978.

> 689 pp. Paper. Index. Additional readings.
> For beginning students of nursing as they learn to apply the nursing process and acquire knowledge basic to quality nursing care. Presents material that underlies basic cognitive and psychomotor nursing skills in depth. Unit 1: Introduction; Unit 2: Preparing to Meet the Patient's Needs; Unit 3: Planning the Patient's Nursing Care; Unit 4: Nursing Interventions to Support Adaptation; Unit 5: Administration of Medications and Therapeutic Agents; Unit 6: Common Situations That Threaten Adaptation; and, Unit 7: Common Medical-Surgical Conditions. Chapter summaries, learning activities, and appendixes are included.

5.2   Nordmark, Madelyn T.; Rohweder, Anne W. Scientific
       Foundations of Nursing, 3d ed. Philadelphia: Lippincott,
       1975.
           426 pp. Paper. Index.
           For use by nursing students as they learn to relate the
           basic sciences to nursing and for nurse educators as
           they facilitate student learning. Part I: Orientation;
           Part II: The Biologic and Physical Sciences and Re-
           lated Nursing Care; Part III: Psychosocial Principles
           and Nursing Application; Part IV: A Guide to Use for
           Nursing Educators. Includes content from anatomy,
           physiology, pathology, microbiology, physics, chem-
           istry, psychology, and sociology. Written in outline
           form. Each chapter contains a section on selected
           principles followed by a section on nursing that gives
           examples of how the sciences are used.

ANATOMY, PHYSIOLOGY, AND BIOCHEMISTRY

5.3   Anthony, Catherine P.; Thibodeau, Gary A. Textbook of
       Anatomy and Physiology, 10th ed. St. Louis: Mosby, 1979.
           731 pp. Cloth. Index. Supplementary readings.
           Glossary.
           A classic text for nursing students. Up-to-date, clear,
           concise, this text is written for college level introduc-
           tory courses in human anatomy and physiology. Has
           charts, diagrams, illustrations. New material for this
           edition includes sections on basic chemistry, transpor-
           tation, immune system, and articulations in the skele-
           tal system.

5.4   Guyton, Arthur C. Function of the Human Body, 4th ed.
       Philadelphia: Saunders, 1974.
           473 pp. Cloth. Index. References.
           A textbook whose eight sections cover human physiology
           and the cell; the blood cells and immunity; the heart and
           the cardiovascular system; body fluids and the urinary
           system; oxygen and respiration; the nerves and
           muscles; the gastrointestinal system and metabolism;

and endocrinology and the reproductive system. Covers the basics in the field of human physiology and the function of the human body. Fifth edition (1979) not available for annotation.

5.5   Guyton, Arthur C. Textbook of Medical Physiology, 5th ed. Philadelphia: Saunders, 1976.
   1194 pp. Cloth. Index. References.
   Written for medical students, this text presents "an integrated study of the body's functional systems." (p. v) Covers the basic physiology useful for various other health professionals including nursing. Uses two print sizes. The smaller type adds additional information that is not required to understand the bulk of the text. Sixth edition due 1980.

5.6   Metheny, Norma M.; Snively, W. D., Jr. Nurses' Handbook of Fluid Balance, 3d ed. Philadelphia: Lippincott, 1979.
   406 pp. Paper. Index. Bibliography.
   A thorough revision that includes the latest scientific knowledge and also considers the newer roles of nurses involved in caring for patients with body fluid disturbances. Discusses the fundamentals of cellular and extracellular fluids and electrolytes; transport mechanisms; homeostasis; disturbances of balance and treatment; and nursing's role in prevention, observation, and treatment. Includes specific clinical applications.

5.7   White, Abraham; Handler, Philip; Smith, Emil L.; et al.; eds. Principles of Biochemistry, 6th ed. New York: McGraw-Hill, 1978.
   1492 pp. Cloth. Index. References.
   A medical text that looks at the principles of the mammalian, and principally human, biochemistry. Topic areas: major constituents of cells, catalysts, metabolism, body fluids and specialized tissues, biochemistry of the endocrine glands, and nutrition.

5.8   Wilson, Marion E.; Mizer, Helen E.; Morello, Josephine A.
       Microbiology in Patient Care, 3d ed. New York: Macmillan,
       1979.
           669 pp. Cloth. Index. Additional readings.
           Written for students in the health field who utilize the
           concepts and principles of microbiology in clinical
           practice. Part I is Basic Principles of Microbiology;
           Part II is Microbial Diseases and Their Epidemiology.

CHEMISTRY, PHYSICS, AND TOXICOLOGY

5.9   Diem, K.; Lentner, C., eds. Scientific Tables, 7th ed.
       [Documenta Geigy.] Basel, Switzerland and Ardsley, N.Y.:
       Ciba-Geigy, Ltd., 1970.
           809 pp. Cloth. Index. Bibliography.
           Designed "to provide doctors and biologists with basic
           data in a concise form and thus spare them much
           searching in the literature." (publisher's foreword)
           Gives information concerning mathematics and statis-
           tics, physics, physical chemistry, biochemistry, nu-
           trition, composition and functions of the body, body
           fluids, body measurements, hormones. Includes In-
           ternational Biological Standards and Reference Prepara-
           tions and charts for testing vision.

5.10   Gosselin, Robert E.; Hodge, Harold C.; Smith, Roger P.;
       et al. Clinical Toxicology of Commercial Products, Acute
       Poisoning, 4th ed. Baltimore: Williams & Wilkins, 1976.
           1780 pp. (approx.) Cloth. Indexes by ingredients,
           therapeutics, trade name.
           Intended to help the physician in dealing effectively
           with acute poisoning. Seven sections are included in
           this massive work: First Aid and General Emergency
           Treatment; Ingredients Index; Therapeutics Index; Sup-
           portive Treatment; Trade Name Index; General Formu-
           lations; and Manufacturers' Names and Addresses.
           Each section has color-coded pages to assure easy and
           quick access.

5.11 Hawley, Gessner G. The Condensed Chemical Dictionary,
       8th ed.   New York: Van Nostrand Reinhold Co., 1971.
          971 pp. Cloth. Bibliography. Index.
          "Gives compact, accurate summaries of pertinent
          facts about many thousands of chemicals and chemical
          phenomena." (p. ix)

5.12 Loomis, Ted A. Essentials of Toxicology, 3d ed. Phila-
       delphia: Lea & Febiger, 1978.
          245 pp. Cloth. Index. References.
          An introductory text that presents general principles
          along with specific examples of the harmful effects of
          chemicals on biologic tissues. Discusses harmful ef-
          fects, factors that modify such effects, antidotes, and
          toxicologic testing methods.

5.13 Sunshine, Irving; Seligson, David; eds. CRC Handbook.
       CRC Series in Clinical Laboratory Science; Section B:
       Toxicology, Vol. 1. West Palm Beach: CRC Press, 1978.
          414 pp. Cloth. Index. Bibliography.
          Part of a multisection handbook series sponsored by
          the Chemical Rubber Company. Reviews and explains
          basic principles of toxicology and includes current
          relevant data on many therapeutic agents.

5.14 Weast, Robert C., ed. CRC Handbook of Chemistry and
       Physics; A Ready-Reference Book of Chemical and Physical
       Data, 59th ed. West Palm Beach: CRC Press, 1978.
          2488 pp. Cloth. Index.
          This reference book contains mathematical tables and
          information on organic and inorganic compounds.

5.15 Windholz, Martha, ed. The Merck Index; An Encyclopedia of
       Chemicals and Drugs, 9th ed. Rahway: Merck and Co., 1976.
          1313 pp. Cloth. Indexes.
          A "comprehensive, interdisciplinary encyclopedia of
          chemicals, drugs, and biological substances." (p. v)
          For the health professional this book provides a source
          of "succinct information on the use, principal pharma-
          cological action, and toxicity of these substances." (p. v)

IMMUNOLOGY

5.16 Barber, Hugh R. K. Immunobiology for the Clinician. New
York: Wiley, 1977.
310 pp. Cloth. Index. References. Bibliography.
Glossary.
Brings the basics of immunology together in a readable
format that is concise and useful as a framework in
clinical practice. Discusses these topics among others:
antigens, antibodies, B and T cells, hypersensitivity,
autoimmune diseases, aging and cancer, immunosup-
pression, tests, and the future of immunology. Includes chapter summaries.

5.17 Bellanti, Joseph A. Immunology, Basic Processes.
Philadelphia: Saunders, 1979.
287 pp. Paper. Index. Bibliography.
This text focuses on the principles, mechanisms, and
clinical applications of immunology at a level appropriate for undergraduate, predoctoral, nursing, and
medical technology students.

5.18 Blake, Patricia J.; Perez, Rosanne C. Applied Immunological Concepts. New York: Appleton-Century-Crofts,
1978.
159 pp. Paper. Index. Suggested readings.
Describes current immunological concepts in terms of
their application to health promotion and maintenance.
Employs a developmental framework. Includes normal
and altered structures and functions. The implications
for nursing conclude the book. This is one of the first
attempts to describe and make usable important information from immunology that has relevance for nursing.

MATHEMATICS AND STATISTICS

5.19 Beyer, William H., ed. Handbook of Tables for Probability
and Statistics, 2d ed. West Palm Beach: CRC Press, 1968.
642 pp. Cloth. Index.
A substantial collection of useful, relatively standard
statistical tables.

5.20 Brown, Meta. Basic Drug Calculations. St. Louis: Mosby, 1979.
>   189 pp. Paper.
>   A workbook for the health professional student on basic math, including metric and apothecaries' systems related to giving medications. Sectional quizzes as well as a comprehensive quiz are included.

5.21 Dunn, Olive J. Basic Statistics: A Primer for the Biomedical Sciences, 2d ed. New York: Wiley, 1977.
>   218 pp. Cloth. Index.
>   A text for a one-semester course in the basics of statistics useful to physicians, nurses, public health workers, and persons involved in research projects. One year of high school algebra is sufficient to understand the text. Covers both descriptive and inferential statistics. Includes exercises and tables.

5.22 Hart, Laura K. The Arithmetic of Dosages and Solutions: A Programmed Presentation, 4th ed. St. Louis: Mosby, 1977.
>   74 pp. Paper.
>   A programmed text dealing with the metric system, calculation of fractional dosages, the apothecaries' system, conversion of approximate equivalents, household measures, solutions from pure drugs and stock solutions, and calculation of infants' and children's dosages. Each chapter or unit has review and practice problems with answers.

5.23 Klecka, William R.; Nie, Norman H.; Hull, C. Hadlai. SPSS Primer; Statistical Package for the Social Sciences Primer. New York: McGraw-Hill, 1975.
>   134 pp. Paper. Index. References.
>   A brief introduction to the SPSS computer system. Includes introductory information on computers, statistical analysis of data, components of the SPSS system, and the like.

5.24 Knapp, Rebecca Grant. Basic Statistics for Nurses. New York: Wiley, 1978.

308 pp. Paper. Index. Bibliographies.
An introductory text for nursing or allied health personnel in beginning statistics or research methodology
courses. Uses examples from actual research studies
in nursing, either published or ongoing. Chapters
cover a basic description of statistics, inferential
statistics, and computer applications. Includes appendixes of statistical tests. Each chapter has an
overview, objectives, exercises, summary of concepts. Solutions to exercises are included in the appendix as well.

5.25 Loether, Herman J.; McTavish, Donald G. Descriptive Statistics for Sociologists: An Introduction. Boston: Allyn and
Bacon, 1974.
388 pp. Paper. Subject and name indexes. References.
Sections treat descriptive statistics in detail. For a
beginning course of sociological statistics. Boxed summaries of main points are very helpful. Each chapter
has questions and problems. A companion volume discusses Inferential Statistics for Sociologists.

5.26 Martinson, Ida M.; Kepner, G. R. Mathematics for Health
Professionals. New York: Springer Publishing Co., 1977.
253 pp. Paper.
A practical book for students in the health field that
presents general math concepts related to the biological
sciences. For those without much prior mathematical
background. Includes a review of basic algebra, expo-
nents, logarithms, functions, linear power, and graphing.

5.27 Nie, Norman H.; Hull, C. Hadlai; Jenkins, Jean G.; et al.
SPSS; Statistical Package for the Social Sciences, 2d ed.
New York: McGraw-Hill, 1975.
675 pp. Paper. Name and subject indexes.
References.
A manual for use with the SPSS system of computer
programs for statistical analysis of social science
data. SPSS is being used in nearly 600 installations.
Includes an introduction and then specific information

as to the preparation of cards, production of statistical data, other versions of SPSS, etc.

5.28 Sackheim, George I; Robins, Lewis. Programmed Mathematics for Nurses, 4th ed. New York: Macmillan, 1979.
280 pp. Paper.
A programmed text with three major sections: Units
and Measurements, Preparation of Solutions, and
Miscellaneous Medications and Procedures. Each unit
has several practice tests. Chapters cover important
practices in current use.

5.29 Saxton, Dolores F.; Ercolano, Norma H.; Walter, John F.
Programmed Instruction in Arithmetic, Dosages, and Solutions, 4th ed. St. Louis: Mosby, 1977.
64 pp. Paper.
Clarifies the math used to prepare and give medications safely. Uses actual patient situations as examples. Deals with   1) Basic Concepts; 2) Systems of
Measurement; 3) Math Involved in Computing Dosage
of Medications or Preparing Solutions. Includes tests
for self-study. Appendixes cover symbols, abbreviations, and tables of equivalents.

NUTRITION

5.30 Altschule, Mark D. Nutritional Factors in General Medicine.
Springfield, Ill.: Thomas, 1978.
184 pp. Cloth. Index. References.
Contains nutritional information for use by physicians
with their patients. Major sections cover organic
macronutrients, inorganic macronutrients, trace elements, vitamins, and miscellaneous topics.

5.31 Briggs, George M.; Calloway, Doris Howes. Bogert's
Nutrition and Physical Fitness, 10th ed. Philadelphia:
Saunders, 1979.
682 pp. Cloth. Index. Bibliography.
A college text focusing on foods and nutrition for both
majors in nutrition and nonmajors. Major parts examine   nutrients, food intake, and nutrition. In-

cludes appendixes. Ninth edition by L. J. Bogert with
Briggs and Calloway.

5.32 Burton, Benjamin T. Human Nutrition, 3d ed. New York:
McGraw-Hill, H. J. Heinz Co., 1976.
    530 pp. Cloth. Index.
    A key nutrition reference book whose object is "to pre-
    sent concise, up-to-date and accepted information."
    (p. xii) The book has general information on foods and
    their components, normal nutrition throughout the life
    span, and nutritional aspects of disease states. The
    last part deals with emergencies, toxicology, and other
    added topics. An appendix includes composition and
    nutritive value of foods, and tables of food composition.

5.33 Church, Charles Frederick; Church, Helen Nichols. Food
Values of Portions Commonly Used, 12th ed., revised.
Philadelphia: Lippincott, 1975.
    197 pp. Paper (spiral bound). Index. Bibliography.
    Formerly by A. D. Bowes and C. F. Church. De-
    signed "to supply authoritative data on the nutritional
    values of foods in a form for quick and easy refer-
    ence." (Preface to the first edition) Includes infor-
    mation on nutrients, Recommended Daily Allowances,
    diets, body weights. The major part of the book con-
    tains tables for common food portions, including gram
    weights, calories, cholesterol and fat, amino acids,
    minerals, and vitamins. Thirteenth edition due 1980.

5.34 Haynes, R. Brian; Taylor, D. Wayne; Sackett, David L.
Compliance in Health Care. Baltimore: The Johns Hopkins
Press, 1979.
    516 pp. Cloth. Index. Annotated bibliography.
    References.
    This book consists of materials from a workshop/sym-
    posium on compliance with therapeutic regimens held
    in 1977. Describes the knowledge of compliance as it
    has advanced through multidisciplinary research efforts.
    It looks at problems related to compliance: measure-
    ment, determinants, strategies to improve, providers,
    and research. Contains useful reference materials.

5.35 Howard, Rosanne B.; Herbold, Nancie H. Nutrition in Clinical Care. New York: McGraw-Hill, 1978.
    642 pp. Cloth. Index. References.
    Discusses the principles of nutrition, food and the human environment, and the consequences of disease. Diagrams, tables, illustrations, and case presentations enhance this book. For the student who will be integrating nutritional concepts and theory into the health care delivery system.

5.36 Iowa Hospitals and Clinics. Recent Advances in Therapeutic Diets, 3d ed. Ames: Iowa State University Press, 1979.
    232 pp. Paper. Index. Bibliography.
    A diet manual developed for use by health professionals that includes sections on normal nutrition, hospital diets, diets modified in specific ways (minerals, calories, carbohydrates, protein, etc.), test diets, and parenteral feeding.

5.37 Katch, Frank I.; McArdle, William D. Nutrition, Weight Control, and Exercise. Boston: Houghton Mifflin, 1977.
    365 pp. Paper. Index. References.
    Contains " the most relevant, up-to-date information pertaining to nutrition, weight control, and exercise." (p. xiv) A text for courses at the university level, non-credit courses, and in the professional preparation of exercise specialists. Part I: Nutrition and Energy for Exercise; Part II: Body Composition and Weight Control; Part III: The Ventilatory and Cardiovascular Systems; Part IV: Physiological Conditioning.

5.38 Scarpa, Ioannis S.; Kiefer, Helen Chilton. Sourcebook on Food and Nutrition. Chicago: Marquis Academic Media, 1978.
    498 pp. Cloth. Index. References.
    Provides in one volume a wide variety of well-documented information on nutritional subjects. Section headings: Introduction; The Nutrients; Dietary Allowances and Labelling; Nutrition and the Life Cycle; Dieting and Weight Control; Special Diets; Nutrition and Health Problems; Food Additives, Carcinogens,

and Food-Drug Interactions; Perspectives on World
Food Production; Organizations and Agencies Interested in Food and Nutrition.

5.39 Williams, Sue R. Nutrition and Diet Therapy, 3d ed.
St. Louis: Mosby, 1977.
> 723 pp. Cloth. Index. References.
> A well-known text for health professionals, especially
> the nurse. Four major sections are: Foundations of
> Nutrition, Applied Nutrition in Community Health, Nu-
> trition in the Health Care Specialty, and Nutrition in
> Clinical Care. Includes appendixes.

PATHOLOGY AND PATHOPHYSIOLOGY

5.40 Boyd, William; Sheldon, Huntington. An Introduction to the
Study of Disease, 7th ed. Philadelphia: Lea & Febiger, 1977.
> 584 pp. Cloth. Index. Bibliography.
> "A survey of disease organized in a traditional manner
> and written for the assistants of the physician known as
> the paramedical personnel." (p. vii) Uses pictures,
> diagrams, charts but discussion of topics is brief.

5.41 Garb, Solomon. Laboratory Tests in Common Use, 6th ed.
New York: Springer Publishing, 1976.
> 247 pp. Cloth. Index. References.
> Part 1 looks at tests according to the type of specimen
> involved, urine, blood, etc. Part 2 contains tables of
> tests according to body organ, system, infection,
> poisoning. Includes tables of drugs and mixtures that
> interfere with tests.

5.42 Henry, John Bernard. Todd-Sanford-Davidsohn Clinical
Diagnosis and Management by Laboratory Methods, 16th ed.
Philadelphia: Saunders, 1979.
> 2107 pp. Cloth. Index. Bibliography.
> For clinical pathologists, medical technologists, medi-
> cal students, internists, and family physicians. This
> book provides a reference for the identification of

appropriate measures and their timing as well as interpretation of findings and the relevant pathophysiology used in the diagnosis and management of disease.

5.43 Netter, Frank H. Ciba Collection of Medical Illustrations.
Summit, N.J.: CIBA Pharmaceutical Co., 1953-79.
7 folios. Cloth. Index. References.
This collection by the well-known medical illustrator/
physician includes the nervous system; reproductive
system; digestive system; endocrine system; heart;
kidney, ureters, urinary bladder; and respiratory system.

5.44 Price, Sylvia A.; Wilson, Lorraine M.; eds. Pathophysiology: Clinical Concepts of Disease Processes. New York:
McGraw-Hill, 1978.
848 pp. Cloth. Index. Bibliography.
A well-illustrated text for health professionals, using
a self-instructional format, that focuses on the disruptions of physiology, anatomy, biochemistry that are
disease. Each chapter begins with objectives and ends
with questions. Chapter contributors include both physicians and nurses. Discusses the mechanisms of
disease and specific body systems. Examines concepts pertinent to understanding the basis of disease,
its symptoms and treatment.

5.45 Robbins, Stanley L. Pathologic Basis of Disease. Philadelphia: Saunders, 1974.
1595 pp. Cloth. Index. References.
For students of disease, this text covers the normal
cell, cell injury and death, neoplasia, genetic disorders, systemic diseases, infectious diseases, diseases of aging, the heart, the various body systems
and their diseases, and the like. Chapters include a
brief outline at the beginning. Second edition (1979)
not available for annotation.

5.46 Walter, John B. An Introduction to the Principles of Disease.
Philadelphia: Saunders, 1977.

739 pp. Cloth. Index. Selected references.
A text written for the medical student which can also
be used by other health professionals to increase their
knowledge in the area of diagnosis and treatment.
Part 1 covers the general principles of disease and
conditions of the body as a whole. Part 2 looks at diseases of individual organs. Review questions are included.

5.47 Widmann, Frances K. Clinical Interpretation of Laboratory
Tests, 8th ed. Philadelphia: Davis, 1979.
656 pp. Paper. Index. References.
Formerly Goodale's Clinical Interpretation of Laboratory Tests. For primary care providers as they select
procedures and evaluate the results. The focus is on
pathophysiology rather than on lab procedures. The
book is organized into sections on hematology, immunology, chemistry, microbiology, endocrine system,
and other tests.

PHARMACOLOGY

5.48 American Pharmaceutical Association. Evaluation of Drug
Interactions, 2d ed. Prepared with the cooperation and assistance of the American Dental Association, the American
Podiatry Association, the American Society of Hospital Pharmacists, the Food and Drug Administration, and the National
Library of Medicine. Washington, D.C.: American Pharmaceutical Association, the National Professional Society of
Pharmacists, 1976.
520 pp. Paper. Index. References.
Provides assessments of drug interaction information
after review by a panel of experts. Drugs are indexed
by nonproprietary names, drug trade names, and
"classlike" categories. Information on each drug is
arranged in alphabetical order. Included is a summary
of the interaction, use of the drug with related drugs,
pharmacological mechanisms, clinical data recommendations for dealing with the interaction, references,

and a list of nonproprietary and trade names. A separate section includes other information on interactions
relating to drug absorption, drug metabolism, drug
distribution. A third section gives pharmacological
aspects of drug interactions by therapeutic class (acid-
base balance, antihistamine, antitussive, muscle re-
laxant, therapy, etc.). The fourth section includes
tables on laboratory tests and clinical values.

5.49 Asperheim, Mary K.; Eisenhauer, Laurel A. The Pharmacologic Basis of Patient Care, 3d ed. Philadelphia: Saunders,
1977.
   565 pp. Cloth. Index. Bibliography.
   Gives the background on pharmacology and drug therapy and then groups drugs by category (e.g., topical
   anti-infectives, drugs that affect the skin and mucous
   membrane, etc.). For each drug, provides a general
   description, toxicity, dose, among other things. The
   end of each chapter contains a guide for nursing assessment and questions for review and discussion. This edition has a revised chapter on drug abuse and dependence.

5.50 Barofsky, Ivan, ed. Medication Compliance: A Behavioral
Management Approach. Thorofare, N.J.: Slack, 1977.
   221 pp. Cloth. References.
   A series of papers on behavioral management procedures available to help patients with their treatment
   regimens. Stresses the contribution of the patient to
   his own care. Part 1 specifies the problem, Part 2
   discusses the factors that determine compliance, and
   Part 3 focuses on intervention techniques that can be
   used to increase compliance. Includes the role of the
   physician, nurse, pharmacist as well as educational
   approaches.

5.51 Bergersen, Betty S.; Goth, Andres. Pharmacology in
Nursing, 14th ed. St. Louis: Mosby, 1979.
   779 pp. Cloth. Index. References. Glossary.
   A classic text for the practicing nurse and the nursing
   student that provides essential knowledge for therapy.
   Includes a section on toxicology.

5.52 Bergersen, Betty S.; Sakalys, Jurate A. Review of Pharmacology in Nursing, 2d ed. St. Louis: Mosby, 1978.
>303 pp. Paper. Index. References.
>Asks questions about the basic and most essential information concerning the major classifications of drugs. The answers are phrased to increase the reader's understanding of the drug's action and application to the clinical setting. Contents include chapters on the more traditional drug categories: those that affect the central nervous system, cardiovascular drugs, hormones, etc.

5.53 del Bueno, Dorothy J. Case Studies in Pharmacology. Boston: Little, Brown, 1976.
>170 pp. Paper. Index. References.
>Uses selected case studies as the framework for examining the actions, uses, and nursing implications of specific pharmacologic agents. Primarily for the graduate nurse's continuing education.

5.54 Gahart, Betty L. Intravenous Medications: A Handbook for Nurses and Other Allied Health Personnel, 2d ed. St. Louis: Mosby, 1977.
>236 pp. Paper. Index.
>Contains information needed to give intravenous medications correctly and safely. Useful for students but most useful as a reference in the areas where such medications are given. Concise and well organized, it includes only information related to the intravenous use of drugs. Each entry includes generic and trade names, usual dose, dilution, rate of administration, actions, indications and uses, precautions, contraindications, incompatibilities, side effects, and antidotes.

5.55 Goodman, Louis S.; Gilman, Alfred, eds. The Pharmacologic Basis of Therapeutics, 5th ed. New York: Macmillan, 1975.
>1704 pp. Cloth. Index. Bibliography.
>A classic medical text that correlates pharmacology

and the medical sciences, focusing on the actions and use of drugs in therapeutic intervention in clinical situations. Discusses all major categories of drugs. Sixth edition due 1980.

5.56 Govoni, Laura E.; Hayes, Janice E. Drugs and Nursing Implications, 3d ed. New York: Appleton-Century-Crofts, 1978.

> 818 pp. Paper. Index. Bibliography.
> Drugs are arranged alphabetically by generic name. Information for each entry includes actions and uses, absorption and rate, contraindications and precautions, adverse reactions, route and dosage, and the nursing implications. This edition continues to use prototypes as major sources of information about drug groups. New features include "drug interactions, drug-induced interferences with clinical tests, and pediatric drug dosages." (p. vii) A useful monograph for students and nurses in practice.

5.57 Griffith, H. Winter. Drug Information for Patients. Philadelphia: Saunders, 1978.

> 450 pp. (approx.). Cloth.
> A convenient source of information and instructions for patients about prescription drugs. Includes reproducible masters for about 500 drugs (those most frequently prescribed in the United States). To be used in addition to one-to-one dialogue. Each sheet includes instructions, precautions, possible side effects, effects on activities of daily living, storage, refills, and what to do about overdosage.

5.58 Hansten, Philip D. Drug Interactions: Clinical Significance of Drug-Drug Interactions and Drug Effects on Clinical Laboratory Results, 4th ed. Philadelphia: Lea & Febiger, 1979.

> 552 pp. Paper. Index. References.
> Major sections in this very useful resource are Drug-Drug Interactions (including drug-food interactions) and Drug Effects on Clinical Laboratory Test Results. Entries are arranged by drug or drug class and the

clinical significance of the interaction is indicated by
type face. Discusses the mechanisms of drug interaction, relevant patient factors, and factors relating to
drug administration.

5.59 Irons, Patricia Duggan. Psychotropic Drugs and Nursing
Intervention. New York: McGraw-Hill, 1978.
154 pp. Paper. Index. Bibliography.
Provides comprehensive information about psychotropic drugs that includes actions, use, contraindications, dosage, side effects, nursing actions, and drug
interactions. Especially for nurse practitioners and
nursing students in mental health. Topics include
drugs used in psychotic disorders, anxiety states, de-
pressive disorders, childhood psychiatric disorders,
drug abuse, and alcoholism.

5.60 Johns, Marjorie P. Drug Therapy and Nursing Care. New
York: Macmillan, 1979.
694 pp. Cloth. Index. Bibliography.
A text that focuses on "the effects of drugs on physio-
logic process, drug therapy, and nursing interven-
tion." (p. viii) Unit 1: General Aspects of Drug Ther-
apy; Unit 2: Drugs Used to Maintain Hemodynamic
Equilibrium; Unit 3: Drugs Used to Maintain Cellular
Reproduction and the Integrity of Tissues; Unit 4:
Drugs Used to Maintain Gas Exchange and Removal of
Toxicants and Wastes; Unit 5: Drugs Used to Maintain
Rest, Activity, and Emotional Equilibrium; and Unit 6:
Drugs Used to Maintain Nutritional Balance. Focuses
on drug therapy without including extensive discussions
on non-pharmacologic therapy of specific disease conditions. Includes common drugs currently in use. In-
dicates nursing interventions. Includes physiologic
and pathophysiologic considerations.

5.61 Johns, Marjorie P., Brogan, Anne M.; Lynch, M. Marcia;
et al. Case Studies in Drug Therapy: Physiologic Correlations and Nursing Intervention. New York: Macmillan, 1979.
275 pp. Paper. References.

A workbook for use with Johns' book Drug Therapy and Nursing Care. Selected patient situations in various settings give students an opportunity to apply their knowledge of pharmacology. Following each situation, study questions focus on pathophysiologic correlations, nursing interventions, and drug correlations. Can be used with other standard pharmacology texts. An answer key is provided.

5.62 Loebl, Suzanne; Spratto, George; Wit, Andrew; with comprehensive nursing implications by Estelle Heckheimer. The Nurse's Drug Handbook. New York: Wiley, 1977.
803 pp. Cloth. Index. Bibliography. Glossary.
A comprehensive reference text, divided into two parts. Part 1 gives general information about drugs including Safety Precautions for Preparation and Storage of Medications, and Drug Interactions: General Considerations. Part 2 takes types of drugs (anti-infectives, drugs affecting the central nervous system, etc.) and gives classification, dosage, administration, contraindications, reactions, nursing implications, etc., where applicable. Book is well highlighted with bold-face type, tables, etc. Second edition due 1980.

5.63 Physicians' Desk Reference, 34th ed. Oradell: Medical Economics, 1980.
2047 pp. Cloth.
An annual publication with supplements that contains the latest information on about 2,500 products. Product information (white section), diagnostic information (green section), product classification index (blue section), and the generic and chemical name index (yellow section) provide sources of helpful information for physicians and nurses. The information is compiled from the drug manufacturers' package inserts that meet FDA requirements. Includes a section on toxicology and a list of poison control centers.

5.64 Ralston, Susan E.; Hale, Marion E. Review and Application of Clinical Pharmacology. Philadelphia: Lippincott, 1977.

260 pp. Paper. Index. References.
A supplementary book to be used with pharmacology
texts in nursing courses that integrate pharmacology,
for review by new graduates, and for preparation for a
return to practice by other nurses. Each chapter has
a section for review and application. Answers to questions are included. Major drug categories are the central focus.

5.65 Smith, Dorothy L. Medication Guide for Patient Counseling.
Philadelphia: Lea & Febiger, 1977.
442 pp. Paper. Bibliography. Index.
Contains reproducible drug instruction sheets for distribution to patients, arranged alphabetically by generic
name. A comprehensive set of drug instructions for
use by all health professionals. The importance of explanations is stressed in helping the patient become an
active reliable partner in his drug therapy. Uses layman's language. Includes diagrams and other illustrations when appropriate. Useful for teaching and for
reference at home.

5.66 Swonger, Alvin K. Nursing Pharmacology: A Systems Approach to Drug Therapy and Nursing Practice. Boston:
Little, Brown, 1978.
329 pp. Paper. Index. References.
For nursing students as they learn the basics of pharmacology. Prototypes of the major drug categories
are stressed, but includes other drugs so that the book
can serve as a useful reference. The five sections are:
An Introduction to Pharmacology in Nursing, the Regulatory Systems of the Body, Systems Regulating the Internal Environment, Systems That Interface with the
External Environment, and Other Topics in Pharmacology. To be used with other drug references.

INDEXES

5.67 Biological Abstracts, References, Abstracts, and Indexes to
the World's Life Sciences Research Literature. BioSciences

Information Service of Biological Abstracts, 2100 Arch
Street, Philadelphia, Pa. 19103. Semimonthly. 1926 to
date.

5. 68 Chemical Abstracts. Chemical Abstracts Service (for the
American Chemical Society), Box 3012, Columbus, O. 43210.
Weekly with annual cumulations. 1907 to date.
Indexes and abstracts in English new chemical information published in more than 50 languages. Covers
over 14,000 journals, patents issued in 26 countries,
books, conference proceedings, government reports,
and dissertations.

5. 69 Current Contents/Life Sciences. Institute for Scientific Information, 325 Chestnut Street, Philadelphia, Pa. 19106.
Weekly. 1958 to date.

5. 70 Science Citation Index. Institute for Scientific Information,
325 Chestnut Street, Philadelphia, Pa. 19106. Six issues
annually. 1961 to date.
A unique approach to the indexing of over 2,600 journals from over 100 scientific fields. Based on the
premise that a bibliography can be compiled by noting
those current articles that cite (or refer to) an earlier
published paper of known relevancy. Includes a Per-
muterm Subject Index (by key word).

PERIODICALS

5. 71 American Dietetic Association Journal. American Dietetic
Association, 430 North Michigan Avenue, Chicago, Ill.
60611. Monthly. 1925 to date.

5. 72 Drug Intelligence & Clinical Pharmacy; An Interdisciplinary
Drug Journal for Physicians, Pharmacists and Nurses.
Drug Intelligence & Clinical Pharmacy, Inc., 1806 24th
Street N.W., Washington, D.C. 20008. Monthly. 1967 to
date.

5. 73 Drugs of Choice. C.V. Mosby Co., 11830 Westline Industrial Drive, St. Louis, Mo. 63141. Biannually. 1958 to
date.

5. 74 FDA Drug Bulletin. U.S. Food and Drug Administration,
5600 Fisheries Lane, Rockville, Md. 20852. Bimonthly.
1971 to date.

5. 75 Hospital Formulary. Harcourt Brace Jovanovich Health
Care Publications, 4015 W. 65th Street, Minneapolis, Minn.
55435. Monthly. 1966 to date.

5. 76 Nutrition Today. Nutrition Today, Inc., 101 Ridgely Avenue,
Box 465, Annapolis, Md. 21404. Bimonthly. 1966 to date.

6

The Behavioral Sciences and Nursing

In this chapter we have grouped psychology texts for nurses, general psychology texts and resources, and other useful books on topics of psychological significance. In addition, communication materials, including those on nurse-patient relations, are enumerated. Books on anthropology and sociology of relevance to nurses close the subject listings. As usual, periodicals are listed in alphabetical order at the end of the chapter.

PSYCHOLOGY

Nursing Texts

6.1 Auger, Jeanine R. Behavioral Systems and Nursing. [Scientific Foundations of Nursing Practice Series.] Englewood Cliffs: Prentice-Hall, 1976.
> 212 pp. Cloth. Index. Bibliography.
> One of a series of monographs that offers a new approach to the subject matter underlying nursing practice. The book presents the model of nursing developed by Dorothy E. Johnson and adopts the behavioral systems approach as an orderly way to understand complex behavior. It examines systems theory, the behavior system, the function of behavior, the influence of the external environment on behavior, regulators of behavior, and behavior and nursing assessment

and gives samples of behavioral assessment in the clinical setting.

6.2   Berni, Rosemarian; Fordyce, Wilbert. Behavior Modification and the Nursing Process, 2d ed. St. Louis: Mosby,
1977.
 160 pp. Paper. References.
 Discusses behavioral methods and their application by
nurses and other health care professionals in medical
settings. The focus is on behavioral analysis and the
procedures and principles to follow in approaching
problems. Chapters 1-4 deal with behavioral analysis,
Chapters 5-9 cover behavioral reinforcement, and
Chapters 10-14 look at ethical issues and the future.

6.3   Bowden, Charles L.; Burstein, Alvin G. Psychosocial Basis
of Medical Practice: An Introduction to Human Behavior, 2d
ed. Baltimore: Williams & Wilkins, 1979.
 231 pp. Paper. Index. References.
 A concise text for undergraduates preparing for careers
in the health field that focuses on psychosocial variables
and relationship skills. Major section headings are
Working with Patients; The Life Cycle: Adaptation and
Change; Physician, Heal Thyself.

6.4   Brown, Martha Montgomery; Fowler, Grace R. Psycho-
dynamic Nursing: A Biosocial Orientation, 4th ed. Phila-
delphia: Saunders, 1971.
 358 pp. Cloth. Index. Bibliographies.
 Five parts deal with   1) Low-Visibility Functions in
Nursing (general points on psychiatric patients),
2) High-Visibility Nursing Functions in the Care of
Psychiatric Patients, 3) The Psychiatric Patient and
His Socio-Environmental Milieu, 4) Psychiatric-Mental
Health Nursing in Community Settings, and 5) The
Teaching-Learning Milieu for Psychosocial Nursing.
Each chapter has a bibliography and suggestions for
further reading which include both books and articles.
The appendix contains a code for nurse-patient inter-
action.

6.5   Burnside, Irene Mortenson; Ebersole, Priscilla; Monea,
       Helen Elena, eds. Psychosocial Caring Throughout the Life
       Span. New York: McGraw-Hill, 1979.
              655 pp. Cloth. Name and subject indexes. References
              and other resources (including organizations and films).
              The three parts of this book address the life span:
              1) Infancy through Adolescence; 2) Young Adulthood,
              Middle Age, and Preretirement; and 3) Young Old Age
              Through Old Age. The authors, all master's degree
              nurses, emphasize the aging process. They also em-
              phasize the normal rather than the pathological growth
              and development associated with each phase.

6.6   Carlson, Carolyn E.; Blackwell, Betty, eds. Behavioral
       Concepts and Nursing Intervention, 2d ed. Philadelphia:
       Lippincott, 1978.
              298 pp. Paper. References.
              Includes concepts common to most nursing curricula
              and research. This edition focuses on substantive
              rather than process concepts. Several new ones have
              been added and many from the previous edition have
              been expanded or changed to reflect changes in nursing.
              The major sections are   1) Fundamental Concepts in
              Illness and Disability; 2) Responses to Changes in
              Health Status: Concepts with Negative Connotations;
              3) Responses to Changes in Health Status: Concepts
              with Positive Connotations; 4) Example of Applying
              Concepts from a Theory to Nursing: Transactional
              Analysis Concepts. The concepts included are body
              image, stigma, shame, loss, trust, hope, privacy,
              and others.

6.7   Francis, Gloria M.; Munjas, Barbara A. Manual of Social-
       psychologic Assessment. New York: Appleton-Century-
       Crofts, 1976.
              209 pp. Paper. Index. References.
              Presents a systematic method of assessing the social
              and psychologic aspects of clients. Written for health
              professionals, it includes an assessment form. The
              introduction covers the assessment process. The next

chapters look at sociologic and psychologic aspects
separately. The last chapter discusses the assessment
form in detail.

6.8   Jasmin, Sylvia; Trygstad, Louise N. Behavioral Concepts
and the Nursing Process. St. Louis: Mosby, 1979.
193 pp. Paper. Index. References.
Chapters discuss The Nursing Person, Nursing Process,
Nurse-Patient Relationships, Stress, Separation, De-
pendency, Depression, Aggression, and Ambivalence
and Conflict. Chapters include summaries and study
questions. Has clinical examples with steps of the
nursing process used in analyzing and planning intervention.

6.9   Loomis, Maxine E.; Horsley, Jo Anne. Interpersonal
Change: A Behavioral Approach to Nursing Practice. New
York: McGraw-Hill, 1974.
182 pp. Paper. Index. References.
This text is designed to be a practical guide for nurses
interested in the clinical application of operant learning theory. The model presented differs from other
models since it deals with the individual's behavior
both in the hospital and at home. Chapters discuss
operant conditioning, techniques for modifying behavior, treatments.

6.10   Roberts, Sharon L. Behavioral Concepts and Nursing
Throughout the Life Span. Englewood Cliffs: Prentice-Hall,
1978.
301 pp. Cloth. Author and subject indexes.
Bibliography.
A useful text for undergraduate and graduate students
as well as practitioners. Discusses vital concepts for
all practice settings as applied to all ages. Concepts include anxiety, stress, loss, hopelessness, and
others. Uses a systems model to discuss major behaviors of hospitalized patients and the application of
the concepts to nursing.

6.11 Schwartz, Lawrence H.; Schwartz, Jane Linker. The Psycho-
dynamics of Patient Care: A Life Cycle Approach for Nursing
and Related Health Fields. Englewood Cliffs: Prentice-
Hall, 1972.
>422 pp. Cloth. Index. References. Glossary.
>Written by a psychiatrist and a nurse, this book dis-
>cusses psychoanalytic psychology in general and the
>application of many of its tenets to nursing. After be-
>ginning chapters on the nurse–patient relationship and
>psychoanalytic concepts, the book goes through the en-
>tire life cycle, from infancy to old age and death and
>dying.

6.12 Simons, Richard C.; Pardes, Herbert, eds. Understanding
Human Behavior in Health and Illness. Baltimore: Williams
& Wilkins, 1977.
>718 pp. Cloth. Author and subject indexes.
>References.
>Written for medical students, this book includes the
>study of human behavior, the behavioral sciences as
>related to medicine, and the clinical aspects of human
>behavior. Discusses normal development, the life
>cycle, mind–body relationships, psychopathology.
>Part 1) Human Behavior and the Physician; Part 2)
>Childhood and Adolescence: The Years of Growth and
>Development; Part 3) Adulthood: The Years of Maturity
>and the Completion of the Life Cycle; Part 4) Psychol-
>ogy of Medical Illness; Part 5) Normal Development
>and Psychopathology: The Continuum Between Health
>and Illness; and Part 6) Medical Education and the
>Teaching of Human Behavior.

General

6.13 Eysenck, H. J.; Arnold, W.; Meili, R., eds. Encyclopedia
of Psychology. 3 vols. New York: Herder and Herder, 1972.
>3 volumes. Cloth. Bibliography.
>An alphabetic listing which includes brief dictionary-

style definitions as well as lengthier articles that deal
with important terms and concepts. All entries are
signed and many include bibliographies for further
reading. Designed for both the professional psychologist and other interested persons.

6.14 Neel, Ann. Theories of Psychology: A Handbook, rev. and
enl. Cambridge, Mass.: Schenkman, 1977.
699 pp. Cloth. Index. Bibliography.
Deals with matured theories and this edition adds behavior modification, Piaget, and mini-theories of cognition, motivation, learning, and behavior. Contents
include reference points for organizing psychological
theory, nature of theory, chronological treatment of a
number of theories, and current theoretical developments. Enables the reader to trace relationships,
origins, and ramifications of an idea.

6.15 Wolman, Benjamin B., comp. and ed., with Gerhard Adler
et al. Dictionary of Behavioral Science. New York: Van
Nostrand Reinhold, 1973.
478 pp. Cloth.
An alphabetical arrangement that spans the fields of
psychology, psychiatry and related areas. Entries are
brief and concise and include concepts, proper names,
tests, disease states, etc. Appendixes include the
American Psychiatric Association's Classification of
Mental Disorders and Ethical Standards of Psychologists.

Other

6.16 Brown, Marie S. Normal Development of Body Image.
[Nursing Concept Modules.] New York: Wiley, 1977.
106 pp. Paper. Bibliography.
Uses a format of pretest, learning objectives, directions, activities, progress checks, post-test. Employs
an integrated, conceptual approach. After an introduction, discusses body image development from birth to

old age. For use in self-instruction or for class or
seminar.

6.17 Coelho, George V.; Hamburg, David A.; Adams, John E.,
eds. Coping and Adaptation. New York: Basic Books, 1974.
454 pp. Cloth. References.
Deals with the subject in five major sections: Social
Interaction and Motivation in Adaptive Behavior; Coping
Tasks and Strategies in the Development of Compe-
tence; Coping with Real-Life Crises; Assessment of
Coping Functions; Coping and Adaptation.

6.18 Garfield, Charles A., ed. Stress and Survival: The Emotional Realities of Life-Threatening Illness. St. Louis:
Mosby, 1979.
388 pp. Cloth. Index. Suggested readings.
An anthology for nurses, physicians, mental health professionals and volunteers, the clergy, and family members who face the emotional situations of life-threatening illness. This book focuses on the capacity of persons to live under protracted crisis situations, gives
insights into the importance of emotional support in
such situations, and suggests optional ways of providing that support.

6.19 Jersild, Arthur T.; Brook, Judith S.; Brook, David W. The
Psychology of Adolescence, 3d ed. New York: Macmillan,
1978.
616 pp. Cloth. Author and subject indexes.
Bibliography.
Focuses on the period in which the person makes the
transition from childhood to adulthood. Covers adolescence, physical development, emotional development, social development, vocation, and the future.
This edition is updated to reflect changes in attitudes
and social forces that influence youth. This book
should be useful to health practitioners who care for
adolescent clients.

6.20 Lynch, James J. The Broken Heart: The Medical Conse-
      quences of Loneliness. New York: Basic Books, 1977.
          271 pp. Cloth. Index. Bibliography.
          A monograph whose purpose is to "document the fact
          that reflected in our hearts there is a biological basis
          for our need to form loving human relationships."
          (p. xiii) Social isolation, lack of human companion-
          ship, death or absence of parents in early childhood,
          sudden loss of love, and chronic human loneliness are
          significant contributors to premature deaths.

6.21 Moustakas, Clark E. Turning Points. Englewood Cliffs:
      Prentice-Hall, 1977.
          120 pp. Cloth. References.
          The author examines his roots (childhood, adolescence,
          and adulthood) and the significant forces in his life as a
          teacher, therapist, and a person by which he came to
          understand those conditions which foster healthy growth
          and those which interfere. He calls such events "be-
          ginnings" and "turning points." Describes seven situa-
          tions that precipitate acute identity experience. In-
          cluded are crises related to illness, peak experiences,
          sudden loss of important relationships, and others.

6.22 Selye, Hans. Stress in Health and Disease. Boston:
      Butterworths, 1976.
          1256 pp. Cloth. Author and subject indexes.
          Bibliographies.
          A "classified collection of concise abstracts" on the
          physiology and pathology of stress covering, primarily,
          the years from 1956. Small print sections are concise,
          impersonal abstracts; critical reviews by the author of
          highlights in the literature are in large print. Includes
          seven sections: History and General Outline of the
          Stress Concept; Stressors and Conditioning Agents;
          Characteristic Manifestations of Stress; Diseases of
          Adaptation; Treatment; Theories; and Various Other Re-
          lated Topics. A very useful reference in the field of
          stress.

6.23 Selye, Hans. The Stress of Life, rev. ed. New York:
McGraw-Hill, 1976.
     515 pp. Cloth. Index. Annotated references.
Glossary.
The author describes this book "as a simplified sum-
mary of contemporary views on the scientific bases of
the entire stress concept as it applies to any field."
(p. xi) Books are entitled   The Discovery of Stress,
The Dissection of Stress, The Diseases of Adaptation,
Sketch for a Unified Theory, and Implications and Ap-
plications.

6.24 Selye, Hans. Stress Without Distress. Philadelphia:
Lippincott, 1974.
     171 pp. Cloth. Index. Bibliography. Glossary.
This small book discusses and updates Selye's creed,
the philosophy of gratitude, introduced in The Stress
of Life. This philosophy is based on his laboratory
experiments which are explained in nontechnical
terms. Chapters include   The Stress of Life, Motivation, What Is the Aim of Life?, To Earn Your Neigh-
bor's Love.

6.25 Stevenson, Joanne S. Issues and Crises During Middlescence.
New York: Appleton-Century-Crofts, 1977.
     230 pp. Paper. Index. References. Suggested
readings.
A text for college students with special emphasis on
situations and problems of interest to nurses and
others. Three parts cover   1) Historical and Conceptual Bases of Adult Life Phases; 2) Significant Issues
During the Middle Years; and 3) The Crises of Adult
Life Phases Including the Impact of Illness. Describes
the developmental tasks and discusses the theoretical
bases, which include a systems approach and role
theory. Covers such topics as work, family, community participation, and development of maturity. The
last section examines both maturational and situational
crises. Very useful to those studying the life span.

6.26 Vaillant, George E. Adaptation to Life. Boston: Little,
Brown, 1977.
>396 pp. Cloth. Index. Bibliography. References.
The report of a grant study begun in 1937 on adult development. The study focused on mental health, styles
of adaptation, and consequences of adaptation. The in-
vestigators studied those who were well and did well in
both their physical and psychological aspects.

6.27 Weiss, Robert S. Loneliness: The Experience of Emotional
and Social Isolation. Cambridge: The MIT Press, 1973.
>236 pp. Cloth. Bibliography.
In this study of loneliness, Weiss discusses what loneliness is, who is lonely, and what the responses to
loneliness are.

COMMUNICATION

6.28 Blondis, Marion Nesbitt; Jackson, Barbara E. Nonverbal
Communication With Patients: Back to the Human Touch.
New York: Wiley, 1977.
>110 pp. Paper. Index. Bibliography.
This book on nonverbal communication stresses the
necessity for human understanding in nursing care
along with competence in nursing skills. Chapters
discuss nonverbal communication, nurse-patient nonverbal communication, nonverbal communication in
pediatrics, geriatrics, death, crisis intervention, and
the like. Includes brief accounts of actual patient care
situations.

6.29 Clark, Carolyn C. Assertive Skills for Nurses. Wakefield:
Contemporary Publishing, 1978.
>236 pp. Paper. Bibliography.
A workbook for self-study or for use in a course
(basic, graduate, or continuing education). Uses a
modular approach with pre- and post-tests, focus for
learning, information to read, learning activities,
problems to solve, and an evaluation. Modules look

at assertive, aggressive, and acquiescent behavior;
factors that support or deter them; and strategies that
are useful in being assertive and responding to asser-
tiveness.

6.30   Clark, Carolyn C. The Nurse As Group Leader. [Springer
Series on the Teaching of Nursing, 3.] New York: Springer
Publishing, 1977.
179 pp. Paper. Index. Bibliography. Glossary.
For nursing students and/or graduate nurses in a
variety of settings. This text is designed for a basic
course in group dynamics and is broad enough to cover
the wide range of group situations in which nurses work.
After an introduction, chapters discuss group process,
group problems, group dynamics, group leadership,
etc. Simulated exercises end each chapter.

6.31   Collins, Mattie. Communication in Health Care: Understanding and Implementing Effective Human Relationships.
St. Louis: Mosby, 1977.
261 pp. Paper. Index. References.
Bibliography.
The purpose of this text is "to assist in the transfer
of theoretical concepts concerning human relationships
to the reality of people care." (p. vii) Two parts deal
with (1) Concepts Related to Communication and (2) Decision Making in Communication: Exercises in Interpersonal Relations. The last part presents actual
patient problem situations with discussion.

6.32   Enelow, Allen J.; Swisher, Scott N. Interviewing and
Patient Care, 2d ed. New York: Oxford University Press,
1979.
255 pp. Cloth. Index. References.
A text for medical and other health professional students on a topic that is fundamental to successful
clinician-client relationships. Includes basic interviewing as well as how to interview children and families. Discusses the use of the problem-oriented
method of recording data.

6.33   Epstein, Charlotte. Effective Interaction in Contemporary
       Nursing. Englewood Cliffs: Prentice-Hall, 1974.
           174 pp. Cloth.
           A mix of didactic and case situations dealing with
           problems in nursing, nurse-patient relations, the
           nurse and her environment, the nurse as a health pro-
           fessional, and the nurse and aging and death.

6.34   Hames, Carolyn Cooper; Joseph, Dayle Hunt, eds. Basic
       Concepts of Helping: A Wholistic Approach. New York:
       Appleton-Century-Crofts, 1980.
           272 pp. Paper. Index. References. Selected
           readings.
           Designed to acquaint the reader with the role and re-
           sponsibilities of a professional helper. Each chapter be-
           gins with behavioral objectives and ends with reminders
           and individual and group activities. Chapters are
           Adaptation, Culture, Threat, Problem Management,
           Helping, Communication, Therapeutic Communication
           Skills, Barriers to Effective Communication, Learn-
           ing, and Group Dynamics.

6.35   Hein, Eleanor C. Communication in Nursing Practice,
       2d ed. Boston: Little, Brown, 1980.
           311 pp. Paper. Index. Bibliography.
           Presents a systematic view of communication through
           a therapeutic communication model. Within this frame-
           work, discusses messages, channels of communication,
           evaluation of communication, and interviewing.

6.36   Herman, Sonya J. Becoming Assertive: A Guide for Nurses.
       New York: Van Nostrand, 1978.
           189 pp. Paper. Index. Bibliography.
           Written as a self-help book for nursing students in in-
           troductory community or psychiatric nursing courses
           as well as for others. Improvement of communica-
           tion skills, self-development, and increasing personal
           and professional effectiveness are goals. Major topics
           include the place of assertiveness training in nursing,
           how to become assertive, barriers to becoming

assertive, and others. One appendix contains scripts
for behaving assertively and another is a statement of
ethics in assertive behavior training.

6.37 Johnson, Margaret Anne. Developing the Art of Understanding, 2d ed. New York: Springer Publishing, 1972.
299 pp. Paper. Index. Suggested readings.
Chapters deal with emotional reactions to illness, pain,
death, surgery, and childbirth. Has a chapter on understanding and examples of questions or projects for
further discussion.

6.38 Lewis, Garland K. Nurse-Patient Communication, 3d ed.
[Foundations of Nursing Series.] Dubuque: Wm. C. Brown,
1978.
104 pp. Paper. Index. Bibliographies.
Examines both verbal and nonverbal communication
and how it affects nurse-patient interaction. Discusses
language, perceptions, feelings, nurse-patient communication, patient's communication, etc.

6.39 Litwack, Lawrence; Litwack, Janice M.; Ballou, Mary B.
Health Counseling. New York: Appleton-Century-Crofts,
1980.
304 pp. Cloth. Index. References. Selected
readings.
Includes both theory and practice of health counseling.
Has learning exercises and activities at the end of
each chapter.

6.40 Mercer, Lianne S.; O'Conner, Patricia. Fundamental
Skills in the Nurse-Patient Relationship: A Programmed
Text, 2d ed. Philadelphia: Saunders, 1974.
216 pp. Paper. Glossary.
An eight- to ten-hour instructional unit which is not designed to be comprehensive, but rather to give a student
some of the basics, including practical examples of
nurse-patient communication. Uses a programmed format with questions and correct answers given. Useful
appendixes include examples of charts and forms and
material for criterion testing.

6.41 O'Brien, Maureen J. Communications and Relationships in
      Nursing, 2d ed. St. Louis: Mosby, 1978.
         245 pp. Paper. Index. Bibliography.
         For nurses and nursing students, this book looks at
         both oral and written communication. The latter, how-
         ever, does not include writing for publication. Exam-
         ples of communication interaction help to clarify the
         content.

6.42 Pluckhan, Margaret L. Human Communication: The Matrix
      of Nursing. New York: McGraw-Hill, 1978.
         196 pp. Paper. Index. Bibliographies.
         Two parts deal with communication in general (defini-
         tion, models, interpersonal relations, problems in
         communication, and the like) and communication in
         nursing (the process of nursing, nurse-patient rela-
         tions, the nurse as teacher and/or learner, change,
         etc.).

6.43 Purtilo, Ruth. Health Professional/Patient Interaction, 2d
      ed. Philadelphia: Saunders, 1978.
         286 pp. Paper. Index. References.
         Written for the health professional whose minimum
         preparation includes studies in the liberal arts, basic
         science, and a particular health profession. Discusses
         those methods of interactions with patients that most
         increase the effectiveness of the professional. Im-
         proved interaction with other health care providers as
         well as the patient is the goal.

6.44 Sierra-Franco, Miriam Hoglund. Therapeutic Communica-
      tion in Nursing. New York: McGraw-Hill, 1978.
         402 pp. Paper. Selected references.
         A programmed text designed primarily for the begin-
         ning student in a health profession. Covers communi-
         cation from an overview and a discussion of the fac-
         tors which affect it to a look at techniques, timing,
         and clues. Each chapter includes objectives. Chap-
         ters are arranged by frames and the student progresses
         systematically through the book by answering correctly

the multiple-choice questions at the end of each frame.
Includes exercises and discussion topics for each
chapter.

6.45 Smith, Voncile M.; Bass, Thelma A. Communication for
Health Professionals. Philadelphia: Lippincott, 1979.
238 pp. Paper. Index. References.
Written for health professional students, this book
looks at communication in general, then at the application of relevant factors in the improvement of communication skills. Chapters have objectives, summaries, and exercises.

6.46 Sundeen, Sandra J.; Stuart, Gail Wiscarz; Rankin, Elizabeth
DeSalvo; et al. Nurse-Client Interaction: Implementing the
Nursing Process. St. Louis: Mosby, 1976.
200 pp. Paper. Index. References. Suggested
readings.
Stresses holistic nursing care. The chapters address
growth, development, the nurse-patient relationship,
the nursing process, and nursing interventions. Each
chapter includes study questions.

ANTHROPOLOGY

6.47 Bauwens, Eleanor E. The Anthropology of Health. St.
Louis: Mosby, 1978.
218 pp. Paper. Index. References.
A collection of original papers by different authors
which introduces the reader to areas of medical anthropology. Main sections explore culture and its relationship to medicine, food habits in different cultures,
and aging and dying in anthropological perspective. Includes case studies for understanding and discussion.

6.48 Branch, Marie Foster; Paxton, Phyllis Perry, eds. Providing Safe Nursing Care for Ethnic People of Color. New York:
Appleton-Century-Crofts, 1976.
272 pp. Paper. Index. References.

A group of "ethnic nurses of color" have designed this
book as a means of providing cultural perspective for
nursing, to show approaches to nursing the person of
color, and to present curriculum models for use in
nursing education. Parts include Introduction; Cultural Health Traditions: Implications for Nursing
Care; Curricula Supplements. Includes case studies
with discussion.

6.49 Brink, Pamela J., ed. Transcultural Nursing: A Book of
Readings. Englewood Cliffs: Prentice-Hall, 1976.
289 pp. Paper. References.
Blends anthropology and nursing in order to raise the
cultural consciousness of the reader. Discusses cultural differences in relation to child rearing, language,
value system, personality, and research methods.

6.50 Brownlee, Ann T. Community, Culture, and Care: Cross-
Cultural Guide for Health Workers. St. Louis: Mosby, 1978.
297 pp. Paper. Index. Bibliography.
Provides a practical guide for health workers and students. It includes material from many sources that is
useful in learning about one's own culture and the sur-
rounding culture. Sections are organized by what to
find, why, and how. Part 1: General Information
examines general community information and methods
of gathering it. Part 2: Community Systems and Their
Relation to the Health Program includes communication, language, the family, politics, economics, education, and religion. Part 3: The Health Systems of
the Community discusses health practices and beliefs,
health care systems and relationships. Should be helpful to those planning research in this subject area.

6.51 Leininger, Madeleine. Nursing and Anthropology: Two
Worlds to Blend. New York: Wiley, 1970.
181 pp. Cloth. Index. Footnotes. Suggested
readings.
Dr. Leininger, an R.N. who is also a Ph.D., believes

the study of anthropology in nursing will lead to a better
understanding between people and, thus, to better patient care. Chapters explore the nature of anthropology, the nature of nursing, anthropology's potential
contribution to nursing, American values, cultural values and differences and their impact on patient care,
health institutions from a sociocultural perspective,
and the like. Includes a discussion of case studies
within some chapters.

6.52 Leininger, Madeleine. Transcultural Nursing: Concepts,
Theories, and Practices. New York: Wiley, 1978.
    532 pp. Cloth. Index. Bibliography. References.
    ". . . a substantive, comprehensive, and scholarly
    book on the new field of transcultural nursing. The
    ultimate goal is to help nurses to incorporate cultural
    concepts, theories, and research findings into nursing
    care practices and into nursing education." (p. ix)
    Four parts: theory, research, and trends in transcul-
    tural nursing; culture and transcultural nursing; actual
    transcultural models in the United States and in other
    areas of the world; and curricula in nursing schools
    dealing with culture and transcultural nursing. Sequel
    to Nursing and Anthropology: Two Worlds to Blend.

6.53 Spector, Rachel E. Cultural Diversity in Health and Illness.
New York: Appleton-Century-Crofts, 1979.
    324 pp. Paper. Index. Bibliographies.
    References.
    The author, a nurse educator, has written this book to
    help health care providers interact effectively with
    people from varying cultural backgrounds. Units are
    entitled: Provider Self-Awareness; Issues of Delivery
    and Acceptance of Health Care: A Barrier and a
    Bridge; and Traditional Views of Health and Illness.
    Explores the question, "Is health care a right?" from
    both sides. Focuses on the Asian, Black, Hispanic,
    and Native American (Indian) communities. Includes
    contributions by Manuel Spector and Irving Kenneth
    Zola.

SOCIOLOGY AND SOCIAL WORK

6.54 Bracht, Neil F. Social Work in Health Care: A Guide to
Professional Practice. New York: Haworth Press, 1978.
     346 pp. Cloth. Index. Bibliography.
     Includes material by Neil Bracht, a social worker and
     educator, and 25 contributors. A comprehensive, up-
     to-date guide to professional social work practice in
     the health field. Discusses social work and health
     care delivery, social and behavioral aspects of health
     and illness, social work in hospitals, nursing homes,
     primary care, and prevention programs, consultation
     and teaching, community health services, research,
     and administration and accountability in social work
     programs.

6.55 Davis, Alan; Horobin, Gordon; eds. Medical Encounters:
The Experience of Illness and Treatment. New York: St.
Martin's Press, 1977.
     223 pp. Cloth. References.
     A collection of essays by sociologists and anthropolo-
     gists on the subject of illness and patienthood. An
     interesting perspective by trained observers.

6.56 Davis, Fred. Illness, Interaction, and the Self. [Wadsworth
Series in Analytical Ethnography.] Belmont, Ca.: Wadsworth, 1972.
     155 pp. Paper. Index. Footnotes.
     A collection of eight papers (seven published earlier)
     by a medical sociologist. Papers are divided into two
     sections: the first deals with nursing students and their
     growth into their profession, the second with the im-
     pact of illness in theory and in actuality.

6.57 Jaco, E. Gartly, ed. Patients, Physicians, and Illness; A
Sourcebook in Behavioral Science and Health, 3d ed. New
York: The Free Press, 1979.
     479 pp. Cloth. Name and subject indexes. References.
     An anthology that focuses on the behavioral sciences
     and health. Sections cover Society, Illness, and the

Use of Health Services; Health and Illness Behavior;
Societal Coping with Disease and Injury; and Society
and the Organization of Health Systems. Contributors
include   Renée C. Fox, Barney G. Glaser, John H.
Knowles, Theodor J. Litman, Hans A. Mauksch,
David Mechanic, and Talcott Parsons.

6.58 Kosa, John; Zola, Irving K.; eds. Poverty and Health: A
Sociological Analysis, rev. ed. Cambridge: Harvard University Press, 1975.
456 pp. Cloth. Index. Footnotes.
A series of essays that help document the relationship
between poverty and poor health. They include topics
such as social aspects of illness, social differences of
physical health, the nature of poverty, and rehabilitation.

6.59 Milio, Nancy. The Care of Health in Communities: Access
for Outcasts. New York: Macmillan, 1975.
402 pp. Paper. Index. References.
Chapters discuss rich versus poor nations; distribution, organization, and payment for health care; access to health training; decision making and reshap-
ing health care directions. Includes information on
health care in other countries. Appendixes include
statistical facts, some international data.

6.60 Skipper, James K.; Leonard, Robert C., eds. Social Interaction and Patient Care. Philadelphia: Lippincott, 1965.
399 pp. Paper. Index. Footnotes. References.
A collection of papers by doctors, nurses, sociologists, psychiatrists, psychologists, anthropologists,
and patients, which stress the role of the social and
behavioral sciences in patient care. Five sections are
included: Social and Psychological Aspects of the
Nurse's Role; The Importance of Communication; The
Patient's View of His Situation; The Structural and
Cultural Context of Patient Care; and Doctor, Nurse,
and Patient: Role and Status Relationships.

6.61   Storlie, Frances.   Nursing and the Social Conscience.   New
York: Appleton-Century-Crofts, 1970.
      222 pp. Paper. Footnotes. References.
      A thought-provoking book "for the young, the inquisi-
      tive, the impudent, the student of nursing or student
      of life, who seeks from history and provocation some
      light to help guide her for the present." (p. x) The
      author urges nursing to move out of the institution and
      into caring more for the sick in society in general.
      Chapters include Nursing Is Not for the Sick Alone;
      Nursing Organizations; The Migrant Poor; The Ghetto
      Poor; The Aged Poor, etc. Appendixes include a
      sample letter to be used in writing to nursing associa-
      tions, information on regulations in migrant camps in
      some states, etc.

6.62   Twaddle, Andrew C.; Hessler, Richard M.   A Sociology of
Health. St. Louis: Mosby, 1977.
      349 pp. Paper. Subject and author indexes.
      References.
      The major sections are 1. Toward a Sociology of
      Health; 2. Disease and the Sick Person; 3. The Heal-
      ing Occupations; 4. The Organization of Health Ser-
      vices; and 5. Some Urgent Issues. Considers medi-
      cine and health from a sociological perspective. Dis-
      cusses relevant research. Useful for students in the
      health professions.

INDEXES

6.63   *Psychological Abstracts.   American Psychological Association, 1200 17th Street N.W., Washington, D.C. 20036.
Monthly with semiannual cumulations. 1927 to date.

6.64   Social Sciences Index: An Author and Subject Index to Periodicals in the Fields of Anthropology, Area Studies, Eco-

---

*See Chapter 16 for more detailed explanation of this index.

nomics, Environmental Science, Geography, Law and
Criminology, Medical Sciences, Political Science, Psychol-
ogy, Public Administration, Sociology and Related Subjects.
Quarterly. H.W. Wilson Company, 950 University Avenue,
Bronx, N.Y. 10452. 1974 to date.

6.65 Sociological Abstracts. Sociological Abstracts, Inc., Box
22206, San Diego, Ca. 92122. Bimonthly. 1952 to date.

PERIODICALS

6.66 American Journal of Psychology. University of Illinois
Press, 54 E. Gregory, Champaign, Ill. 61801. Quarterly.
1887 to date.

6.67 American Journal of Sociology. University of Chicago
Press, 5801 S. Ellis Ave., Chicago, Ill. 60637. Bimonthly.
1895 to date.

6.68 American Sociological Review. American Sociological
Association, 1722 N. Street N.W., Washington, D.C. 20036.
Bimonthly. 1936 to date.

6.69 Journal of Clinical Psychology. Clinical Psychology Publishing Co., Inc., 4 Conant Square, Brandon, Vt.
05733. Quarterly. 1945 to date.

6.70 Journal of Educational Psychology. American Psychological
Association, 1200 17th Street N.W., Washington, D.C.
20036. Bimonthly. 1910 to date.

6.71 Journal of Psychology: The General Field of Psychology.
Journal Press, 2 Commercial Street, Provincetown, Mass.
02657. Bimonthly. 1936 to date.

6.72 Psychological Review. American Psychological Association,
1200 17th Street N.W., Washington, D.C. 20036. Bimonthly.
1894 to date.

7
Mental Health and Psychiatric Nursing

Psychiatric-mental health nursing focuses on both illness and prevention and includes books relevant to both inpatient and community settings. The organization of this chapter is similar to previous ones, that is, nursing texts first, in general and specific categories, followed by medical books. A listing of relevant nursing and medical periodicals concludes the chapter.

NURSING

General

7.1   Aguilera, Donna Conant. Review of Psychiatric Nursing. St. Louis: Mosby, 1977.
         159 pp. Paper. Index. References. Glossary.
         An overview of material on mental health nursing designed to give background and a review, and to encourage the nurse to look for further information. Chapters cover mental health, ego, patients with maladaptive behaviors, patients with behavior problems, patients who can't care for themselves, psychiatric units, ethics, treatment of psychiatric emergencies, crisis intervention, etc.

7.2   Backer, Barbara A.; Dubbert, Patricia M.; Eisenman,
Elaine J. P. Psychiatric/Mental Health Nursing: Contemporary Readings. New York: Van Nostrand, 1978.
499 pp. Paper. References.
An anthology that includes specific views and approaches to nursing intervention in order to help students move from the theoretical and general to the
specific client situation. Looks at assessment and
interventions with families, groups, and individuals;
change; and issues in psychiatric nursing.

7.3   Bailey, David S.; Dreyer, Sharon O. Therapeutic Approaches to the Care of the Mentally Ill. Philadelphia:
Davis, 1977.
278 pp. Paper. Index. Annotated bibliography.
A text for the mental health worker on concepts, techniques, and procedures used with the mentally ill in
prevention, treatment, and rehabilitation. Post-tests
follow each chapter. Topics include theoretic considerations, treatment and therapy, approaches
to inappropriate behavior, and specific types of
patient groups. A rather traditional approach
to psychiatric nursing.

7.4   Burgess, Ann Wolbert; Lazare, Aaron. Community Mental
Health: Target Populations. Englewood Cliffs: Prentice-
Hall, 1976.
276 pp. Cloth. Index. References.
This book focuses upon community populations that
have often been ignored in the past using a conceptual
approach useful to solve their mental health problems.
Written for the interdisciplinary health care team
which sees members of these target groups (the infer-
tile couple, alcoholics, abusers of drugs, victims of
violence, and the prostitute).

7.5   Burgess, Ann Wolbert; Lazare, Aaron. Psychiatric Nursing in the Hospital and the Community, 2d ed. Englewood
Cliffs: Prentice-Hall, 1976.
520 pp. Cloth. Index. Bibliography.

The focus is on the student and the practitioner in the
psychiatric setting (hospital and community) but the
concepts are applicable to all nursing. Emphasizes
the human dimension of patients and students. It includes material necessary for interdisciplinary collaboration (clinical syndromes) and for meeting the
increasing responsibilities of the psychiatric nurse who
often is the primary caretaker.

7.6   Carter, Frances Monet. Psychosocial Nursing, Theory
and Practice in Hospital and Community Mental Health,
2d ed. New York: Macmillan, 1976.
       538 pp. Cloth. Index. References. Suggested
       readings.
       A good psychiatric nursing sourcebook that uses intra-
       psychic, developmental life cycle, and sociocultural
       approaches. Chapter topics include loss, aggression,
       suicide, and the psychotic child. A history of psy-
       chiatric nursing has been added to this edition. Ap-
       pendixes cover development, diagnostic nomenclature,
       and drugs used for mind alteration.

7.7   Dreyer, Sharon; Bailey, David; Doucet, Will. Guide to
Nursing Management of Psychiatric Patients, 2d ed.
St. Louis: Mosby, 1979.
       247 pp. Paper. Bibliography.
       A workbook for use in psychiatric nursing courses.
       The book has three major parts: General Theoretical
       Considerations, Nursing Management of Psychiatric
       Patients, and Special Problems. Each chapter has a
       defined objective, overview, questions, and a post-
       test. This edition has a clinical evaluation tool for
       use with students.

7.8   Dunlap, Lois Craft, ed. Mental Health Concepts Applied to
Nursing. New York: Wiley, 1978.
       232 pp. Paper. Index. Bibliography.
       Consists of readings (prepared for this book) on the
       application of mental health concepts to nursing in

hospital settings, community, and in specialty areas.
A sourcebook for diploma and associate degree registered nurses returning to school and for basic nursing
students. Emphasizes the importance of psychiatric-
mental health concepts in nonpsychiatric settings, and
examines the creative work of innovative clinicials.
Includes chapters on spiritual needs of the patient,
legal rights, art and poetry therapy, understanding
suicide, family-focused intervention, hospice nursing,
the emotional aspects of cancer, and others.

7.9   Grace, Helen K.; Layton, Janice; Camilleri, Dorothy.
Mental Health Nursing: A Socio-Psychological Approach.
Dubuque: Wm. C. Brown, 1977.
542 pp. Cloth. Index. Bibliography. Glossary.
Divided into two major sections, A Socio-Psychological View of Behavior, and Interventions. Written for
traditional and innovative curricular patterns, it provides a bridge between the traditional past and the
evolving future psychiatric nursing as it is trans-
formed into mental health nursing. Includes not only
the illness model but also social roles, networks of
groups, and both hospital and community settings.
Not limited to one specialty group. Contains chapter
summaries and learning activity plans.

7.10   Haber, Judith; Leach, Anita M.; Schudy, Sylvia M.; et al.,
eds. Comprehensive Psychiatric Nursing. New York:
McGraw-Hill, 1978.
752 pp. Cloth. Index. Bibliography. Glossary.
Written to assist the basic nursing student to utilize
primary, secondary, and tertiary prevention in the
delivery of mental health care. A resource for practitioners and educators that "utilizes psychiatric
mental health nursing principles to formulate an integrated approach to client care across the life span
and in a variety of settings." (p. xiii) The first chapter develops a conceptual framework, reviews historical and sociocultural factors, and provides a theoretical base. Of special interest is the chapter, Nursing

Management of the Family System Without Manifest
Psychiatric Disorders, in which concepts are applied
to clients outside the psychiatric setting. The last
chapter looks at the future and discusses research,
legislation, education, and private practice. Learning objectives are included for each chapter.

7.11 Irving, Susan. Basic Psychiatric Nursing, 2d ed. Philadelphia: Saunders, 1978.
361 pp. Paper. Index. References. Glossary.
A psychiatric nursing text which covers human needs,
communication, growth and development, adjustment,
stress, nurse/patient relations, etc. Includes case
examples with discussion. Appendixes include useful
information on psychoactive drugs.

7.12 Joel, Lucille A.; Collins, Doris I. Psychiatric Nursing:
Theory and Application. New York: McGraw-Hill, 1978.
421 pp. Cloth. Index. Bibliography. Suggested
readings.
Proposes that nursing move away from the medical
model and use developmental theory as a base for
practice in both content and process. For use by
nursing students in one-to-one, group, family, and
crisis nursing intervention. The goal is to help the
patient assume or resume self-care in relation to
positive behaviors. Major sections: Psychiatric
Nursing: A Scientific Theory; One-to-One Relationship; Working with Groups of Patients; The Patient as
a Member of the Family; The Patient in Crisis; and
Conclusion: The Community as Patient.

7.13 Longo, Dianne C.; Williams, Reg Arthur; eds. Clinical
Practice in Psychosocial Nursing: Assessment and Intervention. New York: Appleton-Century-Crofts, 1978.
382 pp. Paper. Index. References.
The authors discuss complex, abstract, and difficult
to apply concepts. They operationalize the principles
of psychosocial nursing and integrate physical health
and physiological variables. For use with other basic

psychiatric nursing texts. Especially helpful for integrated baccalaureate curricula. Topics include,
among others, life change, adaptation and illness,
sexuality, group process, dysfunction in the family
system, and social networks.

7.14 Manfreda, Marguerite Lucy; Krampitz, Sydney Diane.
Psychiatric Nursing, 10th ed. Philadelphia: Davis, 1977.
525 pp. Cloth. Index. Suggested readings. Glossary.
Begins with the National Association for Mental
Health's Facts About Mental Illness and Mental Illness Can Be Prevented, along with the ANA's Standards of Psychiatric and Mental Health Nursing Practice. The six units address mental illness, psychiatric nursing, behavior, therapies for mental illness,
and nursing care of psychiatric patients. An appendix
includes the diagnostic nomenclature for mental disorders.

7.15 Mereness, Dorothy A.; Taylor, Cecelia Monat. Essentials
of Psychiatric Nursing, 10th ed. St. Louis: Mosby,
1978.
592 pp. Cloth. Index. Suggested sources of additional information. Glossary.
Presents a concise, comprehensive look at psychiatric nursing. Sections address mental health and
mental illness, communication, therapeutic interventions, various types of inappropriate behaviors, crisis
intervention, the law and psychiatric nursing, etc.

7.16 Morgan, Arthur James; Johnston, Mabyl K. Mental Health
& Mental Illness, 2d ed. Philadelphia: Lippincott, 1976.
301 pp. Paper. Index. References. Glossary.
An introductory text for nursing students, students in
social work or psychology, or for health professionals
working in this area. Each chapter includes behavioral
objectives. Chapters are grouped into six units covering human behavior; development of personality; mental illness—history, categories, etc.; specific types of
disorders; developmental disabilities; and interventions.

7.17 Robinson, Lisa. Psychiatric Nursing as a Human Experi-
      ence, 2d ed. Philadelphia: Saunders, 1977.
          459 pp. Cloth. Index. References. Annotated sug-
          gested readings. Glossary.
          For nursing students—with a focus on the student who
          develops self-awareness and the patient who is helped
          by the therapeutic nurse-patient relationship. Pro-
          poses an eclectic theoretical basis from major fields
          of psychiatric thought. Uses patient case materials
          to illustrate the ideas being presented. Discusses
          various settings for psychiatric nursing and includes
          individual, family, and group approaches. A useful
          text for an integrated curriculum.

7.18 Stuart, Gail Wiscarz; Sundeen, Sandra J. Principles and
      Practice of Psychiatric Nursing. St. Louis: Mosby, 1979.
          636 pp. Cloth. Index. References. Glossary.
          This text uses the nursing process as a framework.
          Part 1 looks at the principles of nursing; Part 2 looks
          at the practice of psychiatric nursing as well as cur-
          rent treatment modalities. Describes the most used
          models of psychiatric care, groups, and family ther-
          apy among other topics. Includes chapter summaries.

7.19 Topalis, Mary; Aguilera, Donna Conant. Psychiatric Nurs-
      ing, 7th ed. St. Louis: Mosby, 1978.
          445 pp. Cloth. Index. References. Additional read-
          ings. Glossary.
          Succinct and comprehensive treatment of personality
          and behavior, nursing and the nurse-patient relation-
          ship, patients with dysfunctional behavior problems,
          patients with organic behavior difficulties, patients
          with alcohol or drug abuse problems, and children's
          behaviors and problems. Appendixes include the
          ANA's Standards of Psychiatric-Mental Health Nurs-
          ing Practice.

7.20 Wilson, Holly Skodol; Kneisl, Carol Ren. Psychiatric Nurs-
      ing. Menlo Park, Ca.: Addison-Wesley, 1979.
          855 pp. Cloth. Index. Bibliography. Glossary.

An inclusive basic text intended for psychiatric nursing courses, that is organized by concepts and designed to fit with most nursing curricula. Also available with this book are a teacher's manual and a workbook of tools and heuristics. Organized into five
parts: Theoretical Bases for Psychiatric Nursing;
The Processes of Psychiatric Nursing Practice; Life
Theories for Psychiatric Nursing; Intervention Modes;
and the Social, Political, and Economic Context of
Practice. Chapters include a brief outline, learning
objectives, and a summary. Appendixes cover ￼Draft
of Axes I and II of DSM—III Classification; ANA Standards of Psychiatric-Mental Health Nursing Practice;
a form for mental health assessment with rating information, a listing of mental health organizations, etc.

Specialized

7.21 Burkhalter, Pamela K. Nursing Care of the Alcoholic and
Drug Abuser. New York: McGraw-Hill, 1975.
    297 pp. Paper. Index. References.
    Primarily for the nursing student or practitioner, this
    book provides clear and succinct information on the
    alcoholic and the drug abuse patient and on the rehabili-
    tation and nursing care of these patients.

7.22 Deloughery, Grace W.; Gebbie, Kristine M.; Neuman,
Betty M. Consultation and Community Organization in Com-
munity Mental Health Nursing. Baltimore: Williams &
Wilkins, 1971.
    219 pp. Paper. Index. Bibliography.
    The stated purpose is "to provide a theoretical frame-
    work for consultation and community organization in
    community mental health nursing." (p. vii) Written
    for graduate and post-graduate students and nurses in
    community mental health settings. Major sections

cover history, mental health consultation, community organizations and programs, and the future.

7.23 Doona, Mary Ellen. Travelbee's Intervention in Psychiatric Nursing, 2d ed. Philadelphia: Davis, 1979.
280 pp. Cloth. Index. Bibliographies.
"The purpose of this text is to assist nurses in caring for mentally ill persons." (p. v) Chapters define and discuss psychiatric nursing, anxiety, the psychiatric nursing process, the nurse-patient relationship, one-to-one relationships, and the supervisory process. First edition by Joyce Travelbee.

7.24 Fagin, Claire M. Family-Centered Nursing in Community Psychiatry; Treatment in the Home. Philadelphia: Davis, 1970.
190 pp. Cloth. Index. Bibliography.
Contains the conceptual framework developed for two courses in the master's program in psychiatric-mental health nursing at New York University. The chapters are papers by students describing their participation in the clinical experience with a theoretical discussion by the appropriate instructor. Should be useful for students of nursing and for other disciplines studying family therapy.

7.25 Glaser, Frederick B.; Greenberg, Stephanie W.; Barrett, Morris. A Systems Approach to Alcohol Treatment. Toronto: Addiction Research Foundation, 1978.
303 pp. Paper. References.
The report of a study done in 1973 of the treatment of alcoholism in Pennsylvania. The authors found no systematic, coordinated treatment program or plan. Section 1 contains general and introductory material; Section 2 presents the data gathered in the survey of treatment programs; Section 3 discusses other intervention efforts. A final section contains conclusions and recommendations.

7.26 Goldman, Elaine, ed. Community Mental Health Nursing:
      The Practitioner's Point of View. New York: Appleton-
      Century-Crofts, 1972.
           268 pp. Cloth. Annotated bibliography.
           Reports on a conference on the nature and signifi-
           cance of the nurse's role in community mental health
           programs. Part 1: Current Innovations in Commu-
           nity Mental Health Nursing Practice; Part 2: Theoreti-
           cal Considerations; and Part 3: The Conference Model.
           Conference was sponsored by the ANA's Psychiatric
           Mental Health Division on Nursing Practice (New
           York, 1970).

7.27 Hall, Joanne E.; Weaver, Barbara R., eds. Nursing of
      Families in Crisis. Philadelphia: Lippincott, 1974.
           264 pp. Paper. Index. Bibliography.
           Uses crisis theory as a conceptual approach to the
           nursing of families. After the introduction, the con-
           tributions of various nurses look at maturational and
           situational crises. The examples come from various
           clinical settings. Very useful for nursing students
           and faculty, especially in integrated baccalaureate
           programs.

7.28 Hankoff, L. D.; Einsidler, Bernice, eds. Suicide: Theory
      and Clinical Aspects. Littleton, Mass.: PSG Publishing,
      1979.
           464 pp. Cloth. Index. References.
           Presents current knowledge from many areas about
           the phenomena of suicidal behaviors. After an his-
           torical introduction, major sections are Contempo-
           rary Value Systems; Biology of Suicide; The Suicidal
           Person; Specific Risk Subgroups; Management and Pre-
           vention; and Conclusion: The Dialectics of Suicide.

7.29 Hatton, Corrine Loing; Valente, Sharon McBride; Rink,
      Alice. Suicide: Assessment and Intervention. New York:
      Appleton-Century-Crofts, 1977.
           220 pp. Paper. Index. References.
           For caregivers (physicians, social workers, nurses,

teachers, psychologists, clergy, police) this book
covers the history of suicide, the theoretical
basis of suicide, assessment of suicidal risk, intervention in suicide, survivors of suicide, clinical examples, prevention of suicide and the like. Chapters
include a discussion of issues or questions.

7.30 Johnson, Suzanne Hall, ed. High-Risk Parenting: Nursing
Assessment and Strategies for the Family at Risk. Philadelphia: Lippincott, 1979.
    424 pp. Paper. Index. References. Additional
    readings.
    High-risk children and high-risk parents are the sub-
    ject of this monograph that discusses related family
    difficulties and nursing interventions. The contribu-
    tors use an holistic approach, identify problems com-
    mon to a number of situations, and write for the nurse
    in any setting or in any specialty. Includes a variety
    of tools used to assess child development.

7.31 Leininger, Madeleine M., ed. Contemporary Issues in
Mental Health Nursing. Boston: Little, Brown, 1973.
    196 pp. Cloth. Index. References.
    "Reflects the scholarly thinking of [seven] nurse-
    scientists whose education and work has consistently
    focused on theoretical, practical, and research issues
    of importance to psychiatric nursing." (p. ix) Covers
    futuristic ideas, critical issues, and research possi-
    bilities. Includes sociological, anthropological, physio-
    logical, clinical practice, historical, educational, and
    humanistic issues.

7.32 Loomis, Maxine E. Group Process for Nurses. St. Louis:
Mosby, 1979.
    170 pp. Paper. Index. References.
    This book's purpose is to give nurses assessment,
    intervention, and evaluation tools in order to use the
    small group medium to advantage. Four parts cover
    the uses of small groups and the advantages and dis-
    advantages; the development and structure of the small

group so as to provide help for the client; the small group process; and, finally, results and outcomes that can be brought about by small groups.

7.33 Marram, Gwen D. The Group Approach in Nursing Practice, 2d ed. St. Louis: Mosby, 1978.
247 pp. Paper. Index. References.
The author's goal is to increase understanding of groups and the group process by nurses in general and by those in psychiatric-mental health nursing in particular. She uses an eclectic theoretical orientation and points out the advantages and disadvantages of this approach. The second edition has more clinical examples and recognizes the expanding role of the nurse in conducting groups independently.

7.34 O'Connor, Andrea B., comp. Psychotherapeutic Nursing Practice. [Contemporary Nursing Series.] New York: The American Journal of Nursing Co., 1977.
331 pp. Paper. References.
This collection of articles explores the application of therapeutic techniques in both psychiatric and physical illness. The articles originally were published in the American Journal of Nursing Company's periodicals.

7.35 Robinson, Lisa. Liaison Nursing: Psychological Approach to Patient Care: Philadelphia: Davis, 1974.
238 pp. Cloth. Index. Bibliographies. Glossary.
Liaison nursing refers to the care given by a nurse trained in psychiatry to patients in the hospital setting who have other physical problems. The liaison nurse can be called the "clinical specialist, psychiatric nurse clinician, or psychiatric nurse coordinator." (p. ix) This discussion of liaison nursing examines the logistics of liaison nursing, actual types of patients, and ways to deal with these patients.

7.36 Robinson, Lisa. Psychological Aspects of the Care of Hospitalized Patients, 3d ed. Philadelphia: Davis, 1976.
108 pp. Paper. Index. Bibliographies. Glossary.

Designed to aid nurses in communicating better with
patients, this brief book attempts to bridge the gap between detachment and too much personal involvement
on the part of the nurse. Chapters address specific
problems (surgery, depression, fear, etc.) and the
nurse's role in these situations.

7.37 Satir, Virginia. Peoplemaking. Palo Alto: Science and
      Behavior Books, 1972.
              304 pp. Paper.
              This book on family process is written by an expert in
              family therapy. She believes that all ingredients in a
              family that count (for example, individual self-worth,
              communication, and rules) are changeable and cor-
              rectable. The book contains exercises that a family
              can use to increase self-awareness, communication
              within the family, and to revise family styles.

7.38 Saxton, Dolores F.; Haring, Phyllis W. Care of Patients
      With Emotional Problems, 3d ed. St. Louis: Mosby, 1979.
              132 pp. Paper. Index. Bibliography. Glossary.
              Designed to help nursing students identify and meet
              patients' emotional needs. Four parts explore devel-
              opment of emotions, illness and emotions, types of
              emotional disorders in patients, and basic psychiatric
              nursing roles and types of patients. Provides study
              questions after each chapter.

7.39 Simmons, Janet A. The Nurse-Client Relationship in Mental
      Health Nursing: Workbook Guides to Understanding and Man-
      agement, 2d ed. Philadelphia: Saunders, 1976.
              248 pp. Paper. Bibliography.
              A workbook for the nurse who is establishing a thera-
              peutic relationship with persons under emotional stress.
              Consists of chapters containing several pages of didac-
              tic information followed by questions and exercises for
              the nurse to work through. Can be used with an instruc-
              tor or alone. Chapters are arranged in four parts:
              observing and collecting data, theory of the nurse-
              client relationship, implementing the plan of care, and
              evaluating the progress of the plan.

7.40 Smoyak, Shirley, ed. The Psychiatric Nurse as a Family
Therapist. New York: Wiley, 1975.
>251 pp. Paper. Index. Bibliographies.
>For the psychiatric nurse, to enable her to view the
>patient within the framework of the family of which he
>is a part. An outgrowth of a course taught at Rutgers
>College of Nursing and Graduate School. Original
>papers are grouped into six parts: the therapist, in-
>creasing frames of reference, covert communication,
>scapegoating and labeling, children, and problems in
>families. Very practical with many examples.

MEDICAL

General

7.41 Arieti, Silvano, chief ed. American Handbook of Psychiatry,
2d ed. New York: Basic Books, 1974-1975.
>6 vols. Cloth. Name and subject indexes. Bibliographies.
>The six volumes of this monumental work cover: The
>Foundations of Psychiatry, edited by Silvano Arieti;
>Child and Adolescent Psychiatry, Socio-Cultural and
>Community Psychiatry, edited by Gerald Caplan; Adult
>Clinical Psychiatry, edited by Silvano Arieti and
>Eugene B. Brody; Organic Disorders and Psychoso-
>matic Medicine, edited by Morton F. Reiser; Treat-
>ment, edited by Daniel X. Freedman and Jarl E.
>Dyrud; and New Psychiatric Frontiers, edited by
>David A. Hamburg and H. Keith Brodie.

7.42 Hill, Oscar, ed. Modern Trends in Psychosomatic Medicine 3. London: Butterworths, 1976.
>520 pp. Cloth. Index. References.
>Discusses data on the impact of psychosocial function
>and the genesis of bodily disease. Selected topics in-
>clude: an overview; research in animals; pheromones;
>noise; biofeedback techniques; life events and illness;
>chronic hypertension; bronchial asthma; essential
>hypertension; coronary artery disease; anorexia
>nervosa; death and obesity.

7.43 Kolb, Lawrence C. Modern Clinical Psychiatry, 9th ed.
      Philadelphia: Saunders, 1977.
             910 pp. Cloth. Index. Bibliography.
             A text for nursing and medical students as they study
             the areas related to psychiatry. This book first pre-
             sents the evolution of psychiatric thought, and its base
             of biologic and psychosocial concepts and assessment
             skills. The next part presents specific personality
             dysfunctions (according to American Psychiatric Asso-
             ciation classification). The last chapters discuss mod-
             ern approaches, including social and community psy-
             chiatry, drug therapy, shock, and physical therapy.
             The last chapter focuses on law in relation to psychi-
             atry. Case materials are presented as part of a
             totally medical approach.

7.44 Lipp, Martin R. Respectful Treatment: The Human Side of
      Medical Care. Hagerstown: Harper & Row, 1977.
             232 pp. Paper. Index. Bibliography.
             A most unusual handbook in practical psychiatry for
             non-psychiatrists. Very helpful for faculty and prac-
             titioners moving into integrated educational programs
             or primary care practice settings, as well as for
             graduate students. It presumes considerable knowl-
             edge of psychiatric-mental health nursing. Chapters
             include Psychosocial Conditions Disguised as Physi-
             cal Illness; Medical Conditions in Psychiatric Dis-
             guise; Emotional Aspects of Major Disease Categories;
             The Family: Whose Patient Is This?; Consultation and
             Referral: Calling for Help; and others.

Specialized

7.45 Aguilera, Donna C.; Messick, Janice M. Crisis Interven-
      tion: Theory and Methodology, 3d ed. St. Louis: Mosby,
      1978.
             190 pp. Paper. Index. References. Additional
             readings.
             A text for health professionals that blends the history,

theory, and practical methods of crisis resolution.
Topics include how crisis intervention differs from
psychotherapeutic techniques, the use of group therapy
concepts, importance of sociocultural factors, the
problem-solving approach, situational crises, and
maturational crises. In the last two sections, case
material is used to clarify the theoretical material.

7.46 DeRosis, Helen. Working With Patients: Introductory
Guidelines for Psychotherapists. New York: Agathon
Press, 1977.
>194 pp. Cloth. Index.
Documents the numerous problems that face the beginning psychotherapist and discusses the human approaches that help solve these problems as one works
with patients. Topics include limiting preconceptions
and assumptions, misconceptions, positive assets of
patients, and intuitive insights of the beginning therapist. Written for beginners and supervisors.

7.47 Freeman, Arthur M., III; Sack, Robert L.; Berger, Philip A.,
eds. Psychiatry for the Primary Care Physician. Baltimore:
Williams & Wilkins, 1979.
>422 pp. Paper. Index. References.
Written for physicians and others in primary care and
for students preparing for such practice. Chapter
topics include   the place of psychiatry in primary
care, physical illness, surgery, aging, family crises,
obesity, chronic pain, alcoholism, drug abuse, and
sexual dysfunction. Also describes major psychiatric
syndromes and, in the last chapters, discusses therapeutic techniques.

7.48 Goldfried, Marvin R.; Davison, Gerald C. Clinical Behavior Therapy. New York: Holt, Rinehart and Winston,
1976.
>301 pp. Cloth. Index. References. Bibliography.
For clinical psychologists, psychiatrists, social workers, counselors, teachers, peer counselors, and
paraprofessionals. The authors discuss their use of

behavior therapy in their roles as teachers, researchers, practitioners, and clinical supervisors. Presents a broad picture that speaks to concerns of behavior therapy, how it fits, how it can approach client
problems. A reasoned, rational, "pro" position. Includes selected clinical problems. Patient-therapist
conversation with the therapist's thoughts in italics
is helpful.

7.49 Gottesfeld, Harry. The Critical Issues of Community Mental Health. [Community Mental Health Series.] New York:
Behavioral Publications, 1972.
    296 pp. Cloth. Bibliography.
    Report of an empirical study on the philosophic issues
    underlying community mental health. The issues are
    discussed from both sides of the controversy by dis-
    tinguished leaders in the psychiatric-mental health
    field. Topics are Community Context, Radicalism,
    Traditional Psychotherapy, Prevention, Extending the
    Definition of Mental Health, and Role Diffusion.

7.50 Haley, Jay. Problem-Solving Therapy: New Strategies for
Effective Family Therapy. [Jossey-Bass Behavioral Science
Series.] San Francisco: Jossey-Bass, 1977.
    275 pp. Cloth. Index. Footnotes.
    For therapists and teachers of therapists, presents an
    approach that focuses on solving the client's problems
    within the framework of the family. Emphasizes the
    social context of human problems and describes ways
    of intervening to solve these problems. Of special in-
    terest is the discussion of "labeling" and the therapist
    as part of the problem.

7.51 Hoff, Lee A. People in Crisis: Understanding and Helping.
Menlo Park, Ca.: Addison-Wesley, 1978.
    336 pp. Paper. Index. References.
    This book focuses on crisis intervention, interventions
    in specific cases, and comprehensive services for
    crisis intervention. Many case examples and vignettes
    add clarity. The book is written for the professional

who works directly with people in crisis, the health
educator, and the general reader, since the author
believes that crisis intervention is not the special
domain of any one group.

7.52 Kreitman, Norman, ed. Parasuicide. New York: Wiley,
1977.
      193 pp. Cloth. Index. References.
      Describes a series of empirical studies on attempted
      suicide. Parasuicide is defined as a nonfatal act in
      which the individual deliberately causes self-injury or
      ingests a substance in excess of any prescribed or
      generally recognized therapeutic dosage. It is not
      just failed suicide. Chapters cover epidemiology,
      sociocultural aspects, psychological studies, recog-
      nition and prevention of parasuicide.

7.53 Labov, William; Fanshel, David. Therapeutic Discourse:
Psychotherapy as Conversation. New York: Academic
Press, 1977.
      392 pp. Cloth. Author and subject indexes.
      References.
      The investigators, psychotherapists, examine linguis-
      tic forms of patient and therapist interaction. Five
      episodes are analyzed and the rules of discourse,
      paralinguistic cues, propositions, interactional terms,
      and utterances are indexed. Includes directions for
      microanalysis of conversation considering historical
      and factual content.

7.54 Minuchin, Salvador; Rosman, Bernice L.; Baker, Lester.
Psychosomatic Families: Anorexia Nervosa in Context.
Cambridge: Harvard University Press, 1978.
      351 pp. Cloth. Index. Bibliography.
      Written by a psychiatrist, a pediatrician, and a psy-
      chologist after ten years of research on the influences
      of the family in psychosomatic syndromes in children.
      Four case studies show models of therapeutic inter-
      vention.

7.55 Morse, Stephen J.; Watson, Robert I., Jr.; eds. Psycho-
therapies: A Comparative Casebook. New York: Holt,
Rinehart and Winston, 1977.
>   421 pp. Cloth. Subject and author indexes.
>   Bibliography.
>   Describes the differences and similarities of therapeu-
>   tic process in different schools of psychotherapy.
>   Each major section contains an introduction, histori-
>   cal and technical overview, and a case presentation
>   (what the therapist did and why). Case contributions
>   are by Freud, Franz Alexander, Erik Erikson, Carl
>   Rogers, Eric Berne, and John Wolpe, among others.
>   For graduate students and advanced practitioners.

7.56 Parad, Howard J., ed. Crisis Intervention: Selected
Readings. New York: Family Service Association of
America, 1965.
>   368 pp. Paper. Index. Footnotes.
>   Presents a range of theoretical formulations of crisis
>   theory. The book uses "psychoanalytic personality
>   theory in combination with selected social science con-
>   cepts to extend and enrich the concept of person-
>   situation configuration as the unit of attention in psy-
>   chosocial treatment." (p. xi) Part 1: Theoretical
>   Explorations; Part 2: Common Maturational and Situa-
>   tional Crises; Part 3: Clinical Applications; Part 4:
>   The Measurement of Crisis Phenomena. Contains 29
>   papers, most of which are reprinted, by professionals
>   in social work, community health services, psychiatry,
>   and sociology-anthropology.

7.57 Van Hoose, William H.; Kottler, Jeffrey A. Ethical and
Legal Issues in Counseling and Psychotherapy. [Jossey-
Bass Behavioral Science Series.] San Francisco: Jossey-
Bass, 1977.
>   224 pp. Cloth. Index. References. Annotated
>   bibliography.
>   Considers ethical principles and decision-making in
>   therapy and the legal constraints within which thera-
>   pists work. Presents illustrative ethical situations

and dilemmas including several landmark cases. The authors believe ethics has received far too little attention and they document practices that cause difficulties for the therapist and criticism and ridicule for the profession. They describe the influence of laws, court decisions, and regulations.

7.58 West, Norman D. Psychiatry in Primary Care Medicine. Chicago: Year Book, 1979.
>   266 pp. Cloth. Index. References.
>   Written for primary care physicians to help them "recognize primary or secondary psychiatric symptoms in their patients." (p. vii) Other personnel in primary care, including nurses, will find this a useful resource. Chapter topics include general concepts; specific psychiatric diagnostic categories; alcohol, drug, and sexual problems; and testing, consultation, and community resources. Brief case histories are included in each chapter.

PERIODICALS

Nursing

7.59 Current Perspectives in Psychiatric Nursing. C.V. Mosby Co., 11830 Westline Industrial Drive, St. Louis, Mo. 63141. Annually. 1976 to date.

7.60 Issues in Mental Health Nursing. Health Professions Publising Group, McGraw-Hill Book Co., 1221 Avenue of the Americas, New York, New York 10020. Quarterly. 1978 to date.

7.61 Journal of Psychiatric Nursing and Mental Health Services. Charles B. Slack, Inc., 6900 Grove Road, Thorofare, New Jersey 08086. Monthly. 1963 to date.

7.62 Perspectives in Psychiatric Care. Nursing Publications, Inc., Box 218, Hillsdale, New Jersey 07642. Quarterly. 1963 to date.

Medical

7.63   American Journal of Psychiatry.   American Psychiatric
Association, 1700 18th Street, N.W., Washington, D.C.
20009.   Monthly.   1844 to date.

7.64   Archives of General Psychiatry.   American Medical Association, 535 N. Dearborn Street, Chicago, Illinois 60610.
Monthly.   1959 to date.

7.65   Community Mental Health Journal.   Human Sciences Press,
72 Fifth Avenue, New York, New York 10011.   Quarterly.
1965 to date.

7.66   Hospital and Community Psychiatry.   American Psychiatric
Association, 1700 18th Street, N.W., Washington, D.C.
20009.   Monthly.   1950 to date.

7.67   International Journal of Group Psychotherapy.   International
Universities Press, Inc. (for the American Group Psycho-
therapy Association), 315 Fifth Avenue, New York, New
York 10016.   Quarterly.   1951 to date.

7.68   Journal of Clinical Psychiatry.   Physicians Postgraduate
Press, Box 38293, Memphis, Tennessee 38138 (Cosponsors:
Eastern Psychiatric Association and Titus Harris Society).
Monthly.   1940 to date.   Formerly Diseases of the Nervous
System.

7.69   Journal of Nervous and Mental Diseases; An International
Journal of Neuropsychiatry.   Williams & Wilkins Co.,
428 E. Preston Street, Baltimore, Maryland 21202.
Monthly.   1874 to date.

7.70   MH (Mental Hygiene).   National Association for Mental
Health, 1800 N. Kent Street, Rosslyn, Virginia 22209.
Quarterly.   1917 to date.

7. 71 Menninger Clinic Bulletin. Menninger Foundation, Box 829,
Topeka, Kansas 66601. Bimonthly. 1936 to date.

7. 72 Psychiatry; Journal for the Study of Interpersonal Processes.
William Alanson White Psychiatric Foundation, Inc. , 1610
New Hampshire Avenue, N.W. , Washington, D.C. 20009.
Quarterly. 1938 to date.

8
Community Health

In this chapter, we have first grouped books on community health nursing and on community health in general. Next, books are grouped by frequent concerns of nonhospitalized clients of varying ages, including death and dying, gerontology and geriatrics, human sexuality, marriage and the family, occupational health, primary care, resources for consumers, and school health. At the end of the chapter, periodicals in the various subject areas are listed alphabetically.

COMMUNITY HEALTH NURSING

8.1   Archer, Sarah Ellen; Fleshman, Ruth P. Community Health Nursing: Patterns and Practice, 2d ed. North Scituate, Mass.: Duxbury Press, 1979.
>   647 pp. Cloth. Index. Bibliography.
>   A sourcebook for the nursing student and community nurse that addresses the complexity, variability, and continuity of nursing in the community. Includes a conceptual frame of reference and tools for community nursing as well as examples of community nurses at work.

8.2   Braden, Carrie Jo; Herban, Nancy L. Community Health: A Systems Approach. New York: Appleton-Century-Crofts, 1976.

178 pp. Paper. Index. References. Recommended
readings. Glossary.
Provides a systems approach to the study of the community. Section 1 gives background about general
systems theory and presents a theoretical model of
the community. Section 2 explores assessment, planning and implementation, and evaluation in decision-
making in community health. Section 3 contains a
look toward the future. Appendixes include a chronol-
ogy of medical care in the United States.

8.3   Clark, Carolyn Chambers. Mental Health Aspects of Community Health Nursing. New York: McGraw-Hill, 1978.
275 pp. Paper. Index. References.
This book is designed more for the community health
nurse working with people who have a physical com-
plaint than for the nurse working with the psychiatric
client. Part 1, Theory and Concepts, discusses the
nurse/client relationship; Part 2, Observation and Communication Guides, provides frameworks for the assessment of mental health status. A review question section is included after each chapter in the first two parts;
answers are at the end of the book. Part 3, Case Con-
sultations and Discussions, gives cases with discussion
afterward to help in the application of concepts discussed in the earlier sections. Part 4, Case Studies
for Practice, includes case presentations with study
questions listed after them. Part 5, Simulated Situations for Practice, includes situations for group role
playing with discussion questions after each situation.

8.4   Fromer, Margot Joan. Community Health Care and the
Nursing Process. St. Louis: Mosby, 1979.
467 pp. Cloth. Index. Bibliographies.
Discusses developments in community health nursing
rather than telling how to function in this setting.
Uses the holistic approach to development which recognizes the need for the community nurse to know about
family therapy, epidemiology, community planning,
etc. Chapters deal with the health care system, the

community health providers, ethics in health care,
the community and the nurse, epidemiology, crises,
the nursing process in community nursing, keeping
records, school and industrial nursing. Includes some
case examples.

8.5   Hall, Joanne E.; Weaver, Barbara R., eds. Distributive
Nursing Practice: A Systems Approach to Community
Health. Philadelphia: Lippincott, 1977.
     536 pp. Cloth. Index. Bibliography.
     A text for students that focuses on the nursing of popu-
lations at risk. Those enrolled in community, public
health, or distributive nursing courses should find it
useful. Uses a general systems approach as a conceptual framework for examining practice, education,
and settings and clients. Part 1: Introduction; Part
2: Conceptual Foundations of Practice; Part 3: Strategies and Tactics of Nursing Intervention; Part 4: Preparation of Distributive Nursing Practice; Part 5: Distributive Nursing Arenas.

8.6   Hymovich, Debra P.; Barnard, Martha Underwood, eds.
Family Health Care, 2d ed. New York: McGraw-Hill,
1979.
     2 vols. Paper. Index. References.
     The first edition (1973) has grown to this two-volume
second edition. Volume 1: General Perspectives, has
three parts: Introductory Considerations (information
on family development, parenthood, family crisis,
family nursing, etc.); Factors Affecting the Family
(law, economics, culture, urban life, nutrition,
mothers with careers, etc.); Approaches to Assessment and Intervention (family assessment, family
counseling, genetic counseling, sexuality, etc.). The
two parts of Volume 2: Developmental and Situational
Crises, cover Expanding and Contracting Families (family planning, expectant families, adolescence, adoption,
etc.) and Situational Crises (birth defects, the terminally ill child, child abuse, alcoholism). Both volumes
contain original papers by numerous contributors.

8.7   Knafl, Kathleen Astin; Grace, Helen K.   Families Across
the Life Cycle: Studies for Nursing. Boston: Little,
Brown, 1978.
>   380 pp. Paper. Index. References.
>   With twenty contributing authors, this book combines
>   theoretical considerations and research findings.
>   Part 1: Theoretical and Methodological Underpinnings;
>   Part 2: Family Beginnings: Premarital Relationships;
>   Part 3: Family Beginnings: Marital Interaction; Part
>   4: The Expanding Family; Part 5: The Child Rearing
>   and Child Launching Family; Part 6: The Family and
>   the Nurse. Of special interest is the last chapter in
>   which problems and concerns of nurse researchers
>   are shared by the authors.

8.8   Leahy, Kathleen M.; Cobb, M. Marguerite; Jones, Mary C.
Community Health Nursing, 3d ed. New York: McGraw-
Hill, 1977.
>   432 pp. Cloth. Index. Bibliography.
>   For nursing students as they begin their involvement
>   in the community. Part 1 discusses entry into and
>   interaction with client systems in the community.
>   Part 2 contains a community study, case studies, and
>   case situations. The authors suggest that the material
>   included be supplemented by the use of lectures,
>   audiovisual material, experiential assignments, and
>   so forth.

8.9   Sobol, Evelyn G.; Robischon, Paulette. Family Nursing,
A Study Guide, 2d ed. St. Louis: Mosby, 1975.
>   182 pp. Paper. Suggested readings.
>   After an introduction to family nursing, provides case
>   studies on types of families, e.g., families that are
>   beginning, families with children of school age, fam-
>   ilies in the middle years, and older families. Includes
>   a description and other useful data for each family,
>   then poses questions and points for further study or
>   discussion. Good for illustrating the move from
>   theory to practice in family nursing.

8.10 Spradley, Barbara Walton, ed. Contemporary Community
      Nursing. Boston: Little, Brown, 1975.
            467 pp. Paper. Index. References.
            A collection of articles, chiefly reprinted from other
            sources, that illustrates the scope of community nurs-
            ing. Eight sections discuss Community Nursing; The
            Community Nurse Role and Settings; The Expanded
            Nurse Role and Team Relationships; The Cultural
            Dimension of Community Nursing; The Nursing Pro-
            cess; Communication; The Family in Community Nurs-
            ing; and Community Assessment and Health Planning.
            Includes introductions before each section and before
            each article.

8.11 Tinkham, Catherine W.; Voorhies, Eleanor F. Community
      Health Nursing: Evolution and Process, 2d ed. New York:
      Appleton-Century-Crofts, 1977.
            299 pp. Cloth. Index. References. Bibliographies.
            Chapters take an historical look at community health
            nursing, a current look at community health nursing
            (including information on families and the nurse's in-
            teraction with the family unit) and, finally, a look at
            the future of community health nursing. Appendixes
            include forms for data collection on families and sur-
            veys by community nurses.

8.12 Warner, Anne R., ed. Innovations in Community Health
      Nursing: Health Care Delivery in Shortage Areas. St.
      Louis: Mosby, 1978.
            235 pp. Paper. References.
            The 22 registered nurses that contributed to this book
            give a new perspective on the delivery of health care
            to shortage areas, especially inner cities and rural
            areas. For use as a supplemental text in community
            health nursing courses, it can also be used by nurses
            who are contemplating changing their practice and for
            recruiting persons into nursing. Describes creative,
            innovative ways to meet the health need in inner city
            clinics, rural health centers, outreach programs,
            mobile health units, and others.

COMMUNITY HEALTH

8.13 Anderson, C. L.; Morton, Richard F.; Green, Lawrence W.
      Community Health, 3d ed. St. Louis: Mosby, 1978.
           374 pp. Cloth. Index. References.
           The focus in this book is on the coordination and inte-
           gration of health care activities with the needs, goals,
           and resources of the community. Major sections are:
           Overview; Promoting Community Health; Preventing
           Disorders and Disabilities; Environmental Health; and
           Health Services. Useful for all health professionals.
           Each chapter has questions and exercises.

8.14 Hanlon, John J.; Pickett, George E. Public Health; Admin-
      istration and Practice, 7th ed. St. Louis: Mosby, 1979.
           787 pp. Cloth. Index. References.
           A classic text that discusses the beginnings of public
           health as well as the socioeconomic, legal, and man-
           agement aspects of public health. Also included are
           topics related to health and development, behavior,
           and environment.

8.15 Lopata, Helena Z., consulting ed. Family Factbook.
      Chicago: Marquis Academic Media, 1978.
           676 pp. Cloth. Index. References.
           Materials in areas related to the family are found in
           six sections: Family (General); Adults; Children;
           Health; Work and Income; Housing. The family in the
           United States is the focus. The text and statistics in-
           cluded should be a useful reference for many profes-
           sionals who work with families.

8.16 MacMahon, Brian; Pugh, Thomas F. Epidemiology;
      Principles and Methods. Boston: Little, Brown, 1970.
           376 pp. Cloth. Index. References.
           A textbook that introduces epidemiologic principles
           and methods as they relate to chronic disease. Topics
           include classification, measurement, data sources,
           and various methods of study.

8.17 Peterson, Donald R.; Thomas, David B. Fundamentals of
Epidemiology: An Instruction Manual. Lexington, D.C.
Heath, 1978.
>   97 pp. Paper. Index. Footnotes.
>   A self-instruction manual by two physicians with pub-
>   lic health degrees. An introduction is followed by a
>   discussion of disease rates, disease incidence, epi-
>   demics, prevalence of disease, epidemiology, statis-
>   tics, etc. Includes specific problems with answers as
>   well as sample exam questions with answers.

8.18 Pratt, Lois. Family Structure and Effective Health Behavior: The Energized Family. Boston: Houghton Mifflin,
1976.
>   230 pp. Paper. Index. References.
>   Explores the contemporary family in chapters that
>   cover health care and the family, the medical care
>   system, the family structure, social action, and the
>   like. The author stresses the need for the "energized"
>   family. "The energized concept refers to the unleash-
>   ing of people's potential so that they may develop them-
>   selves to their fullest capacities." (p. xi) Much of the
>   author's data are based on a field study from a grant
>   from the U.S. Public Health Service and the appendix
>   includes information on this study.

8.19 Wilner, Daniel M.; Walkley, Rosabelle Price; O'Neill,
Edward J. Introduction to Public Health, 7th ed. New
York: Macmillan, 1978.
>   533 pp. Cloth. Index. References. Additional
>   readings.
>   Provides an overview of the health field for students
>   in all the health professions. Topics include health
>   care organization, financing, the work force, mental
>   health care, environmental health, and consumer pro-
>   tection, organized into the following sections: The
>   Framework of Public Health; Medical Care, Mental
>   Health, and Environmental Health; Health and Disease
>   of Population Groups; and Selected Public Health Sup-
>   portive Services. An instructor's manual is available.
>   First five editions by H. S. Mustard.

8.20 Wing, Kenneth R. The Law and the Public's Health. [Issues
      and Problems in Health Care.] St. Louis: Mosby, 1976.
          167 pp. Paper. References.
          Written for students and professionals, this book looks
          at public health law. Focuses on general principles of
          law in discussing nine topics relevant to understanding
          the law and the public's health: law and the legal sys-
          tem; governmental authority in the public's health;
          limits to government's authority; individual rights;
          governmental benefits by statutes; malpractice;
          patient's rights; governmental control of health insti-
          tutions; and public obligations of non-profit hospitals.

DEATH AND DYING

8.21 Barton, David, ed. Dying and Death: A Clinical Guide for
      Caregivers. Baltimore: Williams & Wilkins, 1977.
          238 pp. Paper. Index. References.
          ". . . multifaceted and multidisciplinary information
          that provides the caretaker with insights into the psy-
          chology and pathos of dying, allowing him to formulate
          his own approach to the problem." (p. vii) The book
          is written for physicians, clergy, pastoral counselors,
          students, and others working with or interested in the
          process of caring for the dying and their families.
          Part 1 is entitled An Approach to Caring for Dying
          Persons. Part 2: Perspectives, contains contributions
          by philosophers, a clergyman, a pediatrician, a geri-
          atric specialist, a nurse, and two dying patients.

8.22 Castles, Mary Reardon; Murray, Ruth Beckmann. Dying in
      an Institution: Nurse/Patient Perspectives. New York:
      Appleton-Century-Crofts, 1979.
          356 pp. Paper. Index. References.
          Written for all nurses who care for dying patients.
          This report of a research study looks at attitudes,
          patients' perceptions, nurses' perceptions, the insti-
          tution within which care is given, and strategies of
          care. The appendixes include information on ethical

statements; legal aspects, hospices, families and
death, and death and rituals.

8.23   Dealing with Death and Dying, 2d ed. [Nursing '77 Skillbook
Series.] Jenkintown, Pa.: Intermed Communications, 1976.
189 pp. Cloth. Index.
Approaches the practical problems of thanatology with
specific guidelines to help make the nurse's role in
caring for the dying patient clearer. Specifically,
focuses on how to deal with the feelings and fears of
all involved. Skill checks are included as examples of
situations as well as to check progress through the
book. Major units cover Dealing with the Patient,
the Family, Yourself, the Staff, and Some Personal
Views (of patients and others). An especially helpful
chapter focuses on children's needs. The last chapter
reports a survey of nurses' responses to caring for
dying patients.

8.24   Earle, Ann M.; Argondizzo, Nina T.; Kutscher, Austin H.;
eds. The Nurse as Caregiver for the Terminal Patient and
His Family. New York: Columbia University Press, 1976.
252 pp. Cloth. Index. Bibliography.
A collection of papers on death and the nursing relationship in dying situations. This volume was encour-
aged by the Foundation of Thanatology and includes
chapters on The Nurse as Crisis Intervener; The
Deadborn Infant: Supportive Care for Patients; Coping
with Staff Grief; Female Chauvinism in Nursing; Teaching to Individual Differences; etc. Appendix includes a
course outline from the University of Washington
School of Nursing, Seattle, by Jeanne Quint Benoliel
and a bibliography by the same author.

8.25   Epstein, Charlotte. Nursing the Dying Patient: Learning
Processes for Interaction. Reston: Reston Publishing, 1975.
210 pp. Cloth. Index. Bibliography.
Intended for both students and teachers. Seven sections cover self-awareness, the stages of death, the
"trajectories" of dying, death at different stages of

life, silence and death, observation in order to identify effective and ineffective behaviors, and helping the
professional deal with death. Includes exercises to
assist nurses to confront the conflict inherent in the
commitment to life-saving goals and the presence of
dying patients.

8.26 Feifel, Herman. New Meanings of Death. New York:
McGraw-Hill, 1977.
      367 pp. Cloth. Name and subject indexes.
      References.
      This book consists of contributions by a variety of
      health professionals and others, including laypersons,
      and is an update of The Meaning of Death (1959). Pro-
      vides "the reader with clinical and empirical findings,
      horizons, and strategies pertinent to professional
      practice, existing conceptual frameworks, and public
      policy in the areas of dying, death, and bereavement."
      (pp. xiii-xiv) Contributors include Jeanne Benoliel,
      Charles Garfield, Orville Kelly, Cicely Saunders, and
      Avery Weisman.

8.27 Garfield, Charles A., ed. Psychosocial Care of the Dying
Patient. New York: McGraw-Hill, 1978.
      430 pp. Cloth. Subject and author indexes.
      References.
      An anthology meant to inspire as well as to inform.
      Contributors include a chaplain, physician, psychia-
      trist, patient, volunteer, school teacher, family mem-
      ber, and social worker. The aim is to assist the phy-
      sician and allied health professional to identify the
      emotional needs of the dying patient and his family and
      to suggest helpful ways to provide the needed support.
      It also recognizes the professional's need for support.
      Chapters look at terminal care, life-threatening ill-
      ness, doctor-patient relationships, helping with
      psychological needs, counseling and the family.

8.28 Hollingsworth, Charles E.; Pasnau, Robert O. The Family in Mourning: A Guide for Health Professionals. [Seminars

in Psychiatry.] New York: Grune & Stratton, 1977.
    213 pp. Cloth. Index. Bibliography.
    Part 1 discusses a family coping with their lethal
    stress from the standpoint of the members of the
    health team. Five other parts cover Informing Fam-
    ilies of Death; Observations on Mourning; Helping the
    Family in Mourning; Helping the Helpers: The Role
    of Liaison Psychiatry; and Conclusion. The focus is
    on the living.

8.29 Horan, Dennis J.; Mall, David, eds. Death, Dying, and
    Euthanasia. Washington: University Publications of
    America, 1977.
    821 pp. Cloth. References.
    Contains essays relevant to the major issues addressed
    in this volume. These issues are 1) Death: When
    Does It Occur and How Do We Define It?; 2) Death as
    a Treatment of Choice; 3) Involuntary Euthanasia of
    the Defective Newborn; 4) Euthanasia: Ethical, Reli-
    gious, and Moral Aspects; 5) Euthanasia: The Legal
    Aspects of "Mercy Killing"; 6) How Should Medicine
    and Society Treat the Dying?; 7) Legalized Euthanasia:
    Social Attitudes and Governmental Policies; and 8) Sui-
    cide and the Patient's Right to Reject Medical Treat-
    ment.

8.30 Kastenbaum, Robert J. Death, Society, and Human Ex-
    perience. St. Louis: Mosby, 1977.
    328 pp. Paper. Index. References. Suggested
    readings.
    For the student in a course or the individual exploring
    death, society, and the human experience. Topics in-
    clude death-related phenomena and the interpenetra-
    tion of death into life.

8.31 Ladd, John, ed. Ethical Issues Relating to Life and Death.
    New York: Oxford University Press, 1979.
    214 pp. Cloth. Index. Bibliography.
    A series of essays by six philosophers and one physi-
    cian on ethical issues related to euthanasia. The

essays represent varying points of view relating to
this controversial subject and are designed to increase
the public's understanding.

8.32 McMullin, Ernan, ed. Death and Decision. [AAAS Selected
Symposia, no. 18.] Boulder: Westview Press, American
Association for the Advancement of Science, 1978.
154 pp. Cloth. Footnotes.
This book focuses on the "kind of decision the voluntary termination of life represents." (p. v) Discusses
the moral, medical, legal, and economic issues associated with death and dying that face health professionals. Chapters include 1) Definitions of Death: Where
to Draw the Lines and Why; 2) What Is the Function of
Medicine; 3) Psychosocial Factors in Coping with Dying; 4) The Right to Die Garrulously; 5) Euthanasia:
The Right to Die and the Obligation to Care; 6) Allowing to Die, Killing for Mercy, and Suicide; 7) Demands
for Life and Requests for Death: The Judicial Dilemma.

8.33 Miller, Albert Jay; Acri, Michael James. Death: A Bibliographic Guide. Metuchen, N.J.: The Scarecrow Press, 1977.
420 pp. Cloth. Author and subject indexes.
A research tool for scholars, professional people, and
laymen that covers material from ancient times to the
present. Included are articles, books, letters, edi-
torials, pamphlets, and media information. Some
entries are annotated. Major headings are General
Works, Education, Humanities, Medical Profession
and Nursing, Religion and Theology, Science, Social
Sciences, and Audiovisual Media.

8.34 Rossman, Parker. Hospice; Creating New Models of Care
for the Terminally Ill. New York: Association Press, 1977.
238 pp. Cloth. References.
Part of the movement to make death humane, the hospice is seen as a place outside of the religious institution which is dedicated to the care of incurable patients.
This volume offers a carefully designed regimen and
environment sensitive to the dying person's needs and

rights—family, pain relief, personal and family counseling, attractive surroundings. Includes a description of New Haven Branford Hospice, the first to be
established in the United States. For those interested
in establishing special units for the care of dying cancer patients.

8.35 Russell, O. Ruth. Freedom to Die: Moral and Legal Aspects of Euthanasia, rev. ed. New York: Human Sciences
Press, 1977.
    413 pp. Cloth. Index. Bibliography.
    Discusses the many aspects of euthanasia and the
    necessary safeguards to make it a basic human right.
    Three parts cover Changing Attitudes Toward Death
    and Dying; Historical Review of Thought and Action on
    Euthanasia; Legislation of Euthanasia: Arguments and
    Proposals. Appendix includes The Hippocratic Oath,
    information on legislative proposals, the definition of
    death, and the like. Includes cases of individuals who
    have acted to end hopeless suffering or who have advo-
    cated the right to refuse treatment.

8.36 Shibles, Warren. Death: An Interdisciplinary Analysis.
Whitewater, Wisc.: The Language Press, 1974.
    558 pp. Cloth. Index. Bibliography.
    An excellent resource that examines death from many
    perspectives. Includes information from Greek and
    Roman writings through the ages to modern times.
    Presents humanistic, psychological, and sociological
    approaches. Death in art, in various cultures, from
    the child's view, and the funeral industry are a few of
    the many topics.

8.37 Stoddard, Sandol. The Hospice Movement: A Better Way of
Caring for the Dying. New York: Stein and Day, 1978.
    266 pp. Cloth. Index. Bibliography.
    An exploration of the hospice movement that inter-
    twines historical background and modern development
    with the author's experiences at St. Christopher's Hos-
    pice, at the first hospice in the United States in New

Haven, Connecticut, and involvement in establishing
a hospice.

8.38 Wilcox, Sandra Galdieri; Sutton, Marilyn. Understanding
Death and Dying: An Interdisciplinary Approach. Port
Washington: Alfred Publishing, 1977.
>   474 pp. Paper. Index. Bibliography.
>   A text for an introductory course in thanatology that
>   consists of readings from many fields: philosophy,
>   ethics, psychology, sociology, gerontology, medicine,
>   nursing, anthropology, literature, and law. Includes
>   selections from fiction and non-fiction, prose and
>   poetry, essays and research reports. Each of the five
>   sections contains an encounter, readings, questions,
>   projects, structured exercises, and further readings.
>   The major headings are The Definition and Meaning
>   of Death; The Experience of Dying; Grief, Mourning,
>   and Social Functions; Death and the Child; and Choices
>   and Decisions in Death.

8.39 Worden, J. William; Proctor, William. PDA* Personal
Death Awareness. Englewood Cliffs: Prentice-Hall, 1976.
>   196 pp. Cloth. Index. References.
>   Contains informative tests and exercises to help de-
>   termine how aware one is of one's death. For the gen-
>   eral audience, the book includes material the author
>   (Worden) uses to teach death awareness to medical
>   students. The five major sections are Waking Up to
>   Yourself, The Death of Fear, Freedom from Futility,
>   Changing Your Life Span, and Free at Last. Points
>   out that thinking about death gives one freedom and
>   the opportunity to make choices not only about dying
>   but also about living.

GERONTOLOGY AND GERIATRICS

8.40 Aker, J. Brooke; Walsh, Arthur C.; Beam, James R.
Mental Capacity: Medical and Legal Aspects of the Aging.
Colorado Springs: Shepard's, 1977.

372 pp. Cloth. Index. References.
This work draws together published materials in the
medical literature on mental capacity in aging. It is
designed to help both the medical and legal professions.
Part 1 includes an overview of the brain, theories of
aging, and certain legal matters. Part 2 discusses
causes of organic brain damage with aging. Parts
3-5 describe sy' ms of brain damage, diagnosis,
and treatment. Part 6 contains a series of questions
that might be asked of treating physicians and expert
witnesses. The format includes a listing of legal
cases and lends itself to use as a ready reference.

8.41   Atchley, Robert C.; Seltzer, Mildred M., eds. The Sociology of Aging: Selected Readings. Belmont: Wadsworth,
1976.
291 pp. Paper. References.
A set of readings on some important sociological
ideas about aging in selected areas that are theoreti-
cally and practically relevant. Chapters include
Age Grading and the Life Course; Individual Aging and
Social Evolution: Methodological Issues; Socialization; the Family; Economics; Politics; and Aging and
Social Stratification.

8.42   Botwinick, Jack. Aging and Behavior: A Comprehensive
Integration of Research Findings, 2d ed., updated and exp.
New York: Springer Publishing, 1978.
404 pp. Cloth. Index. References.
For anyone interested in aging and behavior. The
book is a comprehensive study of the literature on the
psychology of aging. Topics include factors in longev-
ity, survival, sexuality, rigidity, intelligence, learning and memory, among others.

8.43   Brickner, Philip W. Home Health Care for the Aged: How
to Help Older People Stay in Their Own Homes and Out of
Institutions. New York: Appleton-Century-Crofts, 1978.
306 pp. Cloth. Index. References.
After describing the home-bound aged, the author

discusses the development and implementation of a
home health care program for the aged. Considers
goals, methods of organization, functions of involved
health professionals, financial aspects, and life support services. Uses case materials to illustrate the
concepts and positions presented.

8.44 Brocklehurst, J. C., ed. Textbook of Geriatric Medicine
and Gerontology, 2d ed. Edinburgh: Churchill, Livingstone,
1978.
>   838 pp. Cloth. Index. References.
>   A "reference to all aspects of aging and medicine
>   in old age." (Preface) Based on research and current
>   practice, this text considers the biological, psycho-
>   logical, and social aspects of aging.

8.45 Brody, Elaine M. Long-Term Care of Older People; A
Practical Guide. [Gerontology Series.] New York: Human
Sciences Press, 1977.
>   402 pp. Cloth. Index. Bibliography.
>   This book is concerned with those older people who
>   find themselves in congregate facilities of an institu-
>   tional nature. Focuses on the social aspects of caring
>   for clients and their families and the role of social
>   work in improving services to such clients.

8.46 Burnside, Irene Mortenson, ed. Nursing and the Aged.
New York: McGraw-Hill, 1976.
>   654 pp. Cloth. Subject and name indexes.
>   References.
>   An important contribution to the nursing literature
>   focusing on aging. Written for nurses, nursing stu-
>   dents, and others, this book presents a multidisci-
>   plinary, comprehensive approach that covers both
>   psychosocial and physiologic aspects. The major
>   parts of the book are Aging and Nursing; the Normal
>   Aging Process; Deviations of the Aging Process:
>   Geropsychiatry; Deviations of the Aging Process:
>   Pathophysiology; the Nursing Process; Social Forces
>   and Aging; Implications for Nursing; Research in

Aging; and Epilogue. An instructor's manual, Teaching Gerontological Nursing: A Multimedia Approach by Helen Monea, is available. Second edition due 1981.

8.47 Burnside, Irene Mortenson, ed. Working With the Elderly: Group Process and Techniques. North Scituate, Mass.: Duxbury Press, 1978.
421 pp. Paper. Index. Bibliography.
For students and practitioners. Contains four sections: Introduction to Group Work, Theoretical Concepts Applicable to Group Work, The Practice of Group Work with the Elderly, and The Future of Group Work with the Aged. Contributors are nurses, social workers, administrators, teachers, family therapists, among others. At the end of each chapter, there are exercises to help the student solve special problems encountered in group work with older people. Includes suggestions for curricular changes that would promote group approaches to experiential learning.

8.48 Busse, Ewald W.; Pfeiffer, Eric, eds. Behavior and Adaptation in Late Life, 2d ed. Boston: Little, Brown, 1977.
382 pp. Paper. Index. References.
Contains much basic, interdisciplinary information relating to how people grow old. Chapters cover Theories of Aging; Sociological Aspects of Aging; Economics of Retirement; Living Arrangements and Housing of Old People; Sexual Behavior in Old Age; Intelligence and Cognition in the Aged; Organic Brain Syndromes; Nursing of Older People; Training in Geropsychiatry; The Aged and Public Policy, etc. Includes much information from investigations and studies done at the Duke University Center for the Study of Aging and Human Development.

8.49 Butler, Robert N.; Lewis, Myrna I. Aging and Mental Health: Positive Psychosocial Approaches, 2d ed. St. Louis: Mosby, 1977.

365 pp. Paper. Author and subject indexes.
References. Glossary.
Written by a physician and a social worker, this text
is useful for all health professionals involved with
aging clients and in particular those involved in mental health care. Part 1: The Nature and Problems of
Old Age; Part 2: Evaluation, Treatment, and Prevention. Includes appendixes which have sources of relevant literature, organizations, government programs,
and training programs.

8.50 Eliopoulos, Charlotte. Gerontological Nursing. New York:
Harper & Row, 1979.
384 pp. Cloth. Index. Bibliography.
This text provides an introduction to nursing the aged
client using a theoretical approach, emphasizing the
normal process of aging, and clarifying features of
age-related illness. Also includes special topics
like self care, sexuality, pharmacology, and dying.
A chapter on services for the aged is especially
helpful.

8.51 Epstein, Charlotte. Learning to Care for the Aged.
Reston, Va.: Reston Publishing, 1977.
219 pp. Paper. Index. Bibliography.
Contains "material that will facilitate continued development of awareness, sensitivity, and skill—especially in their relationships with old people." (p. xi) Odd-
numbered chapters contain background material, research findings, opinions of those in the field of aging,
and experiences of people involved in their personal
lives with aged relatives and friends. Even-numbered
chapters contain exercises with cases and analyses,
guided discussion plans, checklists, and values clarification.

8.52 Good, Shirley R.; Rodgers, Susan S. Analysis for Action;
Nursing Care of the Elderly. Englewood Cliffs: Prentice-
Hall, 1980.
208 pp. Paper. References.

Uses a series of case studies with specific study guide
questions to help nursing students examine the problems of aging clients. Problems included are those
met frequently: physical disability, poverty, dependence, death, and isolation. Discusses physical,
psychosocial, and cultural problems.

8.53 Gunter, Laurie M.; Estes, Carmen A. Education for
Gerontic Nursing. [Springer Series on the Teaching of Nursing, vol. 5.] New York: Springer Publishing, 1979.
    212 pp. Paper. Index. Bibliography.
    Outlines the field of nursing education, practice, and
    research related to the elderly. Describes levels of
    practice and curricular implications. Includes guide-
    lines and resources for registered nurses at the vary-
    ing levels—generic, masters, and doctoral programs.

8.54 Gunter, Laurie M.; Ryan, Joanne E. Self-Assessment of
Current Knowledge in Geriatric Nursing; 1,311 Multiple
Choice Questions and Referenced Answers. [Self-Assess-
ment Books.] Flushing: Medical Examination, 1976.
    216 pp. Paper (spiral bound). References.
    For practicing nurses, instructors, and students to
    use for review and assessment of knowledge in geri-
    atric nursing. Multiple choice questions cover the
    aging process; human development; mental health and
    the aging; nutrition and the aging; clinical aspects of
    aging; medical-surgical problems; rehabilitation; and
    the arthritic patient, etc. Answers are given as well
    as references to pertinent literature.

8.55 Kart, Cary S.; Metress, Eileen S.; Metress, James F.
Aging and Health: Biologic and Social Perspectives.
Menlo Park, Ca.: Addison-Wesley, 1978.
    341 pp. Cloth. References. Glossary.
    A text that introduces the health professional and other
    students to both the physical and social concerns of the
    aging person. Emphasizes health maintenance. Writ-
    ten by three professors in the fields of sociology,
    health education, and anthropology.

8.56 Lewis, Clara. Nutritional Considerations for the Elderly.
Philadelphia: Davis, 1978.
> 48 pp. Paper. Index. Bibliography.
> A programmed instruction booklet that covers param-
> eters of the nutritional status of the elderly, psycho-
> social deterrents to good nutrition, and useful com-
> munity services. Has review questions and a post-test.

8.57 Pearson, Linda Buck; Kotthoff, Mary Ernestine. Geriatric
Clinical Protocols. Philadelphia: Lippincott, 1979.
> 590 pp. Paper. Index. References.
> This text meets the need for protocols for the common
> clinical problems of elderly clients. The protocols
> for presenting complaints and chronic problems in-
> clude: overview, problem list, historic descriptors,
> physical exam components, worksheet rationale,
> assessment, plan, and bibliography. Topics include
> falls and hip injuries, hearing problems, peripheral
> edema, constipation, hypertension, and others.

8.58 Rossman, Isadore, ed. Clinical Geriatrics, 2d ed.
Philadelphia: Lippincott, 1979.
> 704 pp. Cloth. Index. References.
> A medical text for the clinician involved in geriatrics.
> Six parts cover Aging Changes; The Aged Patient—
> General Principles; The Aged Patient and the Clinical
> Specialties; Musculoskeletal Problems in the Aged
> Patient; Psychiatric and Behavioral Considerations in
> the Aged Patient; and Special Topics in Geriatrics.

8.59 Saxon, Sue V.; Etten, Mary Jean. Physical Change and
Aging; A Guide for the Helping Professions. New York:
Tiresias Press, 1978.
> 192 pp. Cloth. Index. Bibliography.
> A concise text for nurses, social workers, psycholo-
> gists, clergy, counselors, and others who need to
> understand the physical aspects of aging and their im-
> plications for behavior. Part 1 discusses aging in gen-
> eral; Part 2 discusses each organ system in detail; and
> Part 3 discusses special topics: homeostasis,

nutrition, exercise, and others. The appendixes contain safety hints and agencies that offer information on aging.

8.60 Schultz, Phyllis R. Primary Health Care to the Elderly:
An Evaluation of Two Health Manpower Patterns. Denver:
Medical Care and Research Foundation, 1977.
109 pp. Paper. Bibliography.
This report discusses a research project that examined whether the primary health care of elderly clients in private practice was more effective by an adult health nurse practitioner and physician team than by the physician alone. The study concluded that the physician-only pattern was cost effective for the clients who could come to the clinic, while the physician-nurse team pattern was more cost effective if the client was homebound or in a nursing home.

8.61 Seltzer, Mildred M.; Corbett, Sherry L.; Atchley, Robert C.;
eds. Social Problems of the Aging: Readings. [Lifetime
Series in Aging.] Belmont, Ca.: Wadsworth, 1978.
345 pp. Paper. Index. References. Further readings. Glossary.
A book of readings that focuses on the descriptive and statistical information needed for a more accurate picture of the needs and problems of the aged. Part 1: Ageism, Age Prejudice, and Age Discrimination; Part 2: Role Change; Part 3: Social Problems Within Social Institutions; Part 4: Multiple Jeopardy; Part 5: Solutions: Current and Future; and Epilogue: A Glance into the Future.

8.62 Troll, Lillian E.; Israel, Joan; Israel, Kenneth, eds.
Looking Ahead: A Woman's Guide to the Problems and Joys
of Growing Older. Englewood Cliffs: Prentice-Hall, 1977.
216 pp. Cloth. Index. References.
Combines the approaches of gerontology and the feminist movement to raise the consciousness of the reader. Examines changing viewpoints about the older woman. Sections include The Body, New Worlds, Differences, Help, and Power.

8.63 Yurick, Ann Gera; Robb, Susanne S.; Spier, Barbara
      Elliott; et al. The Aged Person and the Nursing Process.
      New York: Appleton-Century-Crofts, 1980.
            576 pp. Cloth. References. Recommended readings.
            Glossary.
            A textbook for nursing students who work with the el-
            derly. Part 1 provides information necessary to un-
            derstand the elderly within the context of American
            society and the health care system. Part 2 applies
            the nursing process to major areas of the aged per-
            son: developmental tasks, cognition, sensory ex-
            periences, nutrition and elimination, activity, and
            bodily protection. The last chapter deals with medica-
            tions. Appendixes include gerontologic course outline,
            organizations, print and audiovisual resources.

8.64 Zarit, Steven H., ed. Readings in Aging and Death: Con-
      temporary Perspectives, 1977-78 ed. [Contemporary
      Perspectives Reader Series.] New York: Harper & Row, 1977.
            307 pp. Paper. Bibliography.
            This book explores the process of development in
            later years and its impact on people. From differing
            perspectives, addresses major issues in geron-
            tology: social problems, love and family relation-
            ships, culture, and death. Includes an annotated table
            of contents. The readings are all since 1963, most
            from 1968-77. They are from professional journals
            and books as well as from books, magazines, and
            newspapers for the general reader.

HUMAN SEXUALITY

8.65 Green, Richard, ed. Human Sexuality; A Health Practi-
      tioner's Text, 2d ed. Baltimore: Williams & Wilkins, 1979.
            295 pp. Paper. Index. References.
            A text developed for medical and other health profes-
            sion students. Major sections are: General Issues in
            Medical Sex Education, General Health and Patient Is-
            sues in Human Sexuality, and Specific Medical Topics
            and Sexuality.

8.66 Heslinga, K.; Schellen, A.M.C.M.; Verkuyl, A. Not Made
      of Stone: The Sexual Problems of Handicapped People.
      Springfield, Ill.: Thomas, 1974.
           208 pp. Paper. Bibliography. Glossary.
           Discusses problems of a group frequently expected to
           have no sexual needs. Considers problems related to
           specific handicaps, contraceptive advice, and sex edu-
           cation. Illustrated. Translated from the Dutch.

8.67 Hogan, Rosemarie Mihelich. Human Sexuality: A Nursing
      Perspective. New York: Appleton-Century-Crofts, 1980.
           768 pp. Cloth. Index. References.
           Suggested readings.
           A comprehensive text for nurses. Examines biologic,
           psychologic, and sociocultural aspects of sexuality in
           health and illness. Implications for nursing care are
           presented in nursing process framework; teaching and
           counseling aspects are included.

8.68 Hubbard, Charles William. Family Planning Education, 2d
      ed. St. Louis: Mosby, 1977.
           241 pp. Paper. Index. References. Glossary.
           This text, written for students in the health profes-
           sions, provides information on contraception, abor-
           tion, sterilization, and venereal diseases. Includes
           family planning counseling information.

8.69 Kolodny, Robert C.; Masters, William H.; Johnson,
      Virginia E.; et al. Textbook of Human Sexuality for Nurses.
      Boston: Little, Brown, 1979.
           450 pp. Paper. Index. References.
           A text for nurses, specialist and nonspecialist, on
           matters of sexuality. After chapters on anatomy and
           physiology and development, the authors discuss the
           effects of illness, surgery, drug use, and aging on
           sexuality. Sexual dysfunction is included as a topic.

8.70 Oldershaw, K. Leslie. Contraception, Abortion, and
      Sterilization. Chicago: Year Book, 1975.

288 pp. Cloth. Index. References.
By a British physician, this book covers family planning, contraception, various contraceptive methods,
sterilization, abortion, and sexual problems and infertility.

8.71 Rudel, Harry W.; Kincl, Fred A.; Henzl, Milan R. Birth
Control, Contraception, and Abortion. New York:
Macmillan, 1973.
372 pp. Cloth. Indexes. References. Suggested
readings.
Chapters deal with family planning, intrauterine devices, abortion, the moral aspects of birth control,
etc. Appendixes list agencies concerned with conception control and the like. Each chapter begins with a
brief outline.

8.72 Woods, Nancy Fugate. Human Sexuality in Health and Illness, 2d ed. St. Louis: Mosby, 1979.
400 pp. Paper. Index. References.
Three units provide an holistic approach to human
sexuality, sexual health care, and sexuality in specific clinical situations (abortion, rape, chronic illness, paraplegia, etc.). Units include original papers
by the author and six other contributors. This edition
has been expanded and reorganized from the first edition. Most chapters include a summary, references,
media, references for clients.

MARRIAGE AND THE FAMILY

8.73 Dodson, Fitzhugh. How to Father. Edited by Jeanne Harris.
Los Angeles: Nash Publishing, 1974.
535 pp. Cloth. Index. Footnotes.
Written for fathers, this book begins with the child at
birth and progresses through the stages of development, especially the years from six to twenty-one.
Although written from the father's viewpoint, it is

useful to mothers as well. Includes a chapter on
divorce and remarriage. The appendixes provide
guides to toys and play equipment, children's books
and records, and a survival kit which suggests useful
books and other resources.

8.74 Duvall, Evelyn Millis. Marriage and Family Development,
5th ed. Philadelphia: Lippincott, 1977.
    559 pp. Cloth. Name and subject indexes.
    References. Glossary.
    A text that looks at marriage and family life today,
    taking into account the various patterns, potentials,
    settings, and stages of the family life cycle. Major
    sections are Generative Potentials in Human Sexual-
    ity; Societal Settings for Marriage and the Family;
    Development over the Life Cycle; Developing Families;
    The Second Half of Marriage; and For Better or for
    Worse. Prior editions entitled Family Development.

8.75 Gullick, Eugenia L.; Peed, Steven F., eds. The Health
Practitioner in Family Relationships: Sexual and Marital
Issues. Westport: Technomic Publishing Co., 1978.
    143 pp. Cloth. Author and subject index. References.
    Addresses the general considerations and basic issues
    in sexual dysfunction, intervention, and related issues.
    For the primary practitioner, family physician, and
    other health professionals who confront sexual and
    marital problems. It does not attempt to prepare a
    sex therapist or a marriage counselor.

8.76 Lantz, James E. Family and Marital Therapy: A Transac-
tional Approach. New York: Appleton-Century-Crofts, 1978.
    218 pp. Paper. Index. Bibliography.
    For the beginning practitioner, presents an introduc-
    tory view of family and marital therapy from the vary-
    ing helping professions. Should be used with experien-
    tial learning and supervision.

8.77 O'Neill, Onora; Ruddick, William, eds. Having Children:
Philosophical and Legal Reflections on Parenthood: Essays.

New York: Oxford University Press, Society for Philosophy
and Public Affairs, 1979.
    362 pp. Paper. Footnotes.
    The Society for Philosophy and Public Affairs is dedi-
    cated to philosophical analysis of issues of concern to
    the public. This collection of papers, largely re-
    printed from other sources, is organized around three
    parts: Becoming Parents; Caring for Children; and
    Growing Up and Apart. Includes contemporary papers
    as well as papers by such renowned political theorists
    as John Locke and Jean-Jacques Rousseau.

8.78 Ragan, Pauline K., ed. Aging Parents. Los Angeles:
      University of Southern California Press, Ethel Percy
      Andrus Gerontology Center, 1979.
          295 pp. Paper. Bibliography.
          This monograph addresses the middle generation,
          aging parents, and professionals, all of whom are
          concerned about relationships with aging parents. The
          contributors are psychologists, social workers, and
          sociologists. Major sections: Perspectives, The Fam-
          ily, Dependency and Interrelationship Issues, Implica-
          tions for Practice, and Challenge for the Future.

8.79 Salk, Lee. What Every Child Would Like Parents to Know
      About Divorce. New York: Harper & Row, 1978.
          149 pp. Cloth. Index.
          Written by a practicing psychologist, this book takes
          a common sense approach to divorce. Includes infor-
          mation on divorce, its effect on children, others in-
          volved in a divorce, custody, the law and divorce, and
          life after divorce. Includes questions and case ma-
          terial with discussion.

8.80 Stahmann, Robert F.; Hiebert, William J., eds. Klemer's
      Counseling in Marital and Sexual Problems; A Clinician's
      Handbook, 2d ed. Baltimore: Williams & Wilkins, 1977.
          375 pp. Paper. Index. Bibliography.
          Offers "sound, clinically tested suggestions for help-

ing patients who have very real and urgent marital and
sexual problems." (p. v) Has contributions from 25
persons who share information, ideas, and guidelines
for practicing marriage counselors. Discusses many
topics including: counseling the dissolving marriage,
parent-child relationships, resources for couple
growth and development, and premarital counseling.
Appendix includes information regarding the American
Association of Marriage and Family Counselors.
First edition by Richard H. Klemer.

OCCUPATIONAL HEALTH

8.81 Hutchison, Marilyn K., ed. A Guide to the Work-Relatedness
of Disease. DHEW (NIOSH) publication no. 77-123. Rockville,
Md.: National Institute for Occupational Safety and Health, 1976.
>115 pp. Paper. Bibliography. Glossary.
>A guide for those persons and agencies concerned with
>compensation for occupational disease. It includes a
>method for data collection and management in deter-
>mining whether a certain disease is work-related.
>Gives five examples (including noise and asbestos) and
>lists occupations with potential exposure to selected
>agents.

8.82 Lee, Jane A. The New Nurse in Industry: A Guide for the
Newly Employed Occupational Health Nurse. DHEW (NIOSH)
publication no. 78-143. Cincinnati: National Institute for
Occupational Safety and Health, Division of Technical Services, 1978.
>110 pp. Paper. Bibliographies.
>This brief publication is designed to provide nurses
>with a basic guide to the practice of occupational
>health nursing. Chapters give an introduction to oc-
>cupational health, a discussion of the field, qualifi-
>cations, education, experience, the work environ-
>ment, and pertinent legislation. Appendixes include
>organization listing, sample forms, and so on.

PRIMARY (AMBULATORY) CARE

8.83   Capell, Peter T.; Case, David B.   Ambulatory Care Manual
for Nurse Practitioners.   Philadelphia: Lippincott, 1976.
>   333 pp. Cloth. Index. References.
>   By two physicians, this is intended to be a reference
>   volume for nurses working in ambulatory care settings.
>   Chapters include General Evaluation of the Patient;
>   Review of Major Disease Mechanisms and Interpreta-
>   tion of Clinical Symptoms; Interpretation of Vital
>   Signs; Respiratory Illnesses; Gynecologic Problems;
>   Psychosocial Problems and Mental Illness; Dermatol-
>   ogy, etc. Includes case material with discussion.

8.84   Diekelmann, Nancy. Primary Health Care of the Well Adult.
New York: McGraw-Hill, 1977.
>   243 pp. Paper. Index. Bibliographies.
>   Focuses on health care of the well adult in young,
>   middle, and older stages of life. Discusses each
>   stage in general, and then considers nutrition, sexual-
>   ity, and special phases in each. Has "vignettes" of pa-
>   tient situations and suggests nursing actions. Includes
>   assessment information for preventive health care.

8.85   Gillies, Dee Ann; Alyn, Irene B.   Patient Assessment and
Management by the Nurse Practitioner. Philadelphia:
Saunders, 1976.
>   236 pp. Cloth. Index. Bibliographies.
>   For "the nurse who is giving primary care to chroni-
>   cally ill patients." (p. vi) Includes chapters on the
>   health interview, the physical examination, laboratory
>   tests, assessment, recording information, and plan-
>   ning patient care. In addition, has chapters discuss-
>   ing some specific patient care problems, e.g., hyper-
>   tension, diabetes, obesity, alcoholism, and others.
>   Includes Normal Laboratory Values of Clinical Impor-
>   tance by Rex B. Conn, M.D.

8.86   Goldsmith, Seth B. Ambulatory Care. Germantown, Md.:
Aspen Systems, 1977.

133 pp. Cloth. Index. Bibliography.
Looks at the administration and organization of insti-
tutionally based ambulatory care. Synthesizes the
major points and principles for review and discussion
by experienced health and hospital administrators.
Discusses group practice, hospital based ambulatory
care, and hospital based primary care.

8.87 Hudak, Carolyn M.; Hokanson, Nancy L.; Suzuki, Irene E.
Clinical Protocols: A Guide for Nurses and Physicians.
Philadelphia: Lippincott, 1976.
461 pp. Paper. Index. Bibliographies.
Includes guidelines for handling common problems of
patients both for teaching purposes and to insure a
standardized level of patient care. This book was developed largely by nurse practitioners in an ambulatory care setting of a major medical center. Four
units cover background on protocols; protocols for
self-limiting problems (nausea, chest pain, headache,
etc.); protocols for several chronic diseases (diabetes
mellitus, hypertension, etc.); and maintenance of
health. Protocols include worksheets, symptoms,
outline of pertinent data, and the like.

8.88 Jonas, Steven. Quality Control of Ambulatory Care: A Task
for Health Departments. [Springer Series on Health Care
and Society, vol. 1.] New York: Springer Publishing,
1977.
178 pp. Cloth. Index. References.
This monograph reports on a study of the New York
City Health Department and Suffolk County Ambulatory
Care Programs that examined the enforcement of standards of quality for health care in preparation for a
national health insurance program. Three governmental approaches to ambulatory care are considered:
1) inspection and regulation; 2) subsidy of local government efforts; and 3) contracts. The chapter on
health care quality measurement and control is especially interesting.

8.89 Leitch, Cynthia J.; Tinker, Richard V., eds. Primary
Care. Philadelphia: Davis, 1978.
589 pp. Cloth. Index. Bibliography.
Written for nurses and physicians engaged in the provision of primary care to help them recognize the
pathophysiology and psychology of health problems.
The Introduction looks at the family as a unit of
health care management, problem-oriented records,
and health maintenance and prevention. Part 2:
Evaluation and Management of Primary Care Problems; Part 3: Primary Health Care of the Child;
Part 4: Management of Medical Emergencies; Part 5:
Mental Health in Primary Care; and Part 6: Rehabilitation.

8.90 Murray, Ruth Beckmann; Zentner, Judith Proctor. Nursing
Assessment and Health Promotion Through the Life Span,
2d ed. Englewood Cliffs: Prentice-Hall, 1979.
448 pp. Cloth. Index. References.
Presents "knowledge of the highly complex normal and
well person." (p. ix) For use with Nursing Concepts
for Health Promotion (2.18, this volume). Views the
person and his family from birth to death from physiological, psychological, social, cultural, religious, and
moral perspectives.

8.91 Rakel, Robert E. Principles of Family Medicine. Philadelphia: Saunders, 1977.
536 pp. Cloth. Index. References.
Looks at the clinical medicine base for family medicine. It also focuses on the attitudes and behavioral
skills needed for effective application of the base by
students preparing for family medicine. Chapters
1 - 7 describe the content and practice of family medicine. Chapters 8 - 13 discuss the behavioral features
of family practice. Chapters 14 - 16 outline methods
to document and organize information, medical records,
and family charts.

8.92 Soper, Michael R. Guidelines for Chronic Care: A Team

Approach. Bowie: Robert J. Brady Company, 1977.
  215 pp. Paper. Suggested readings.
  By a physician, this book is designed to help the nurse
  in an ambulatory setting. The brief chapters contain
  information on and guidelines for the care of those with
  chronic disease such as diabetes, hypertension, arthritis, stress, etc. Includes a lengthy appendix with
  patient-oriented material on topics such as physical
  fitness, cholesterol, fatigue, etc. Also includes appendixes with questionnaires for patients, history taking information, and the like.

RESOURCES FOR CONSUMERS

8.93 Allen, Robert D.; Cartier, Marsha K., eds. The Mental
  Health Almanac. New York: Garland STPM Press, 1978.
     403 pp. Cloth. References.
     A source book in the field of mental health for the gen-
     eral public, students, and professionals. Provides a
     resource list and guide that can be read on three levels:
     Level 1 is a comprehensive view of what is taking place
     in major topics in the field; Level 2 is information of
     interest that can be found and then pursued in the li-
     brary; Level 3 is information that can be sought direct-
     ly from organizations, associations, etc., that are de-
     scribed. Major section headings are The Population,
     The Concern, and The Profession. The first refers to
     clients; the second includes topics such as health,
     therapy, rape, death, crises; the third looks at grad-
     uate programs, licensing, employment, and others.
     Each topic has an overview, lists of annotated books
     and articles, audiotapes, films and other sources.

8.94 American Public Health Association. Consumer Health
  Education: A Directory, 1976, rev. ed. DHEW publication
  no. (HRA) 77-607. Washington: Office of Health Resources
  Opportunity, 1976.
     49 pp. Paper. Index.
     Obtained from a survey of resources for health

education from the major voluntary U.S. health organizations. For each organization (arranged alphabetically by title) gives address, phone number, type
of organization, objectives of the organization, description of major health education activities, and
contract information. Lists approximately 48 organizations.

8.95 Biegel, Leonard. The Best Years Catalogue: A Source Book
for Older Americans Solving Problems and Living Fully.
New York: G.P. Putnam's Sons, 1978.
224 pp. Cloth. Index. Bibliography.
A source book designed for aging Americans. Chapters include the following topics: About Aging; Food;
Shelter; Health; Safety; Creative Leisure; Transportation and Travel; Money; Joining and Sharing; Communicating; and Rights and Legacies. The book is set in
large type.

8.96 Bloomfield, Harold H.; Kory, Robert B. The Holistic Way
to Health and Happiness: A New Approach to Complete Life-
time Wellness. New York: Simon and Schuster, 1978.
311 pp. Cloth. Index. Bibliography.
For the consumer, this book uses the holistic approach
to better health. Discusses good health, the principles
of good health (e.g., no smoking, moderate drinking,
etc.), health problems (overweight, depression, alcoholism, etc.), ways of solving health problems, etc.
Includes vignettes and appendixes.

8.97 Lazes, Peter M., ed. The Handbook of Health Education.
Germantown, Md.: Aspen Systems, 1979.
430 pp. Cloth. Index. Bibliography.
Describes efforts by individuals and communities to
improve their health. Suggests that health education
and disease prevention efforts may decrease the cost
of medical care services. Part 1, Where the Action
Is: Strategies and Settings for Implementing Consumer
Health Education Programs; Part 2, Action Tools
Needed for Change; Part 3, Legal and Consumer

Perspectives. Of special interest are discussions of
health education in schools and pre-schools and health
maintenance organizations and industry, as well as the
use of media and gaming and simulation, and self-help
guides for exercise and weight reduction. Helpful resources are found in the appendix.

8.98   National League for Nursing, Council of Home Health Agencies and Community Health Services. Directory of Home
Health Agencies Certified as Medicare Providers, 2d ed.
NLN publication no. 21-1648. New York: NLN, 1976.
88 pp. Paper.
Agencies certified by the Social Security Administration and the U.S. Department of Health, Education,
and Welfare are listed by state, giving the address
and category (private, official, etc.). Agencies accredited by the NLN are so designated.

8.99   Philbrook, Marilyn McLean. Medical Books for the Lay-
person: An Annotated Bibliography. Boston: Boston Public
Library, 1976.
113 pp. Paper. Index.
The reader may find sources on a particular illness,
the quality of the health system, or how to stay healthy.
Items included are from 1969 through mid-1975 and
are listed alphabetically by author. The table of contents has topic headings with an author listing. Topics
include nutrition, handicaps, medical ethics, hypertension, mental retardation, travel and health, etc.
A 46-page supplement was published in 1978 and includes books from mid-1975 through 1977.

8.100   Schmidt, Alice M. The Homemaker's Guide to Home
Nursing. Provo: Brigham Young University Press, 1976.
181 pp. Paper. Index. Bibliography.
A reference book for homemakers and other layper-
sons who need to know how to deal with illness, accident, or other emergencies. Includes tips on how to
prevent illness, treat illness, recognize illness, move
a patient, feed a patient, care for a patient, and

considerations in dealing with the aged or terminally
ill person. Has a section on first aid and the text is
highlighted for important points in each category,
e.g., cancer's seven danger signals.

8.101 Somers, Anne R., ed. Promoting Health: Consumer Edu-
cation and National Policy. Report of the Task Force on
Consumer Health Education. Germantown, Md.: Aspen
Systems, 1976.
    264 pp. Cloth. Index. Bibliography.
    Sponsored by the John E. Fogarty International Center
    for Advanced Study in the Health Sciences, the National
    Institutes of Health, and the American College of Pre-
    ventive Medicine. Discusses health information,
    health promotion, preventive health services, includ-
    ing occupational, social, and behavioral factors affect-
    ing and determining health. The section on health
    problems that can be prevented is especially interest-
    ing. Contains the task force's recommendations.

8.102 Stewart, Jane Emmert. Home Health Care. St. Louis:
Mosby, 1979.
    183 pp. Paper. Index. References. Glossary.
    By a nurse, this book is intended to serve as an intro-
    duction to the home health field. Chapters cover
    home health care in general; agencies concerned with
    home health care; services provided by home health
    care; financing of home health care; advantages of
    home health care; and current developments. Appen-
    dixes include a list of organizations.

8.103 Stolten, Jane Henry. Home Care: A Guide to Family Nursing. Boston: Little, Brown, 1975.
    400 pp. Cloth. Index.
    Written by a registered nurse, this book is designed
    for those who care for ill or older adults at home.
    Sections cover General Care (medicine, feeding, etc.);
    Care for Special Conditions (aged, death, stroke, etc.);

and Infant Care (pregnancy, feeding the infant, etc.).
Appendixes include definitions of specific types of
doctors, lists of helpful organizations, and the like.

SCHOOL HEALTH

8.104 Bryan, Doris S. School Nursing in Transition. St. Louis:
Mosby, 1973.
>204 pp. Cloth. Index. Footnotes. Selected readings.
>A comprehensive textbook covering the school nursing
>field. Chapters discuss the philosophy of school nurs-
>ing, the people in and the planning of school nursing
>programs, administration of school nursing programs,
>and new directions for change in school nursing. Each
>chapter includes a summary model.

8.105 Nader, Philip R., ed. Options for School Health: Meeting
Community Needs. Germantown, Md.: Aspen Systems,
1978.
>196 pp. Cloth. Index. References.
>This monograph, for school personnel and health care
>providers, reports on the National School Health Con-
>ference held in Galveston, Texas, in 1976. Maintains
>that there are roles for both groups in the education
>and the promotion of health of school children. Useful
>in developing a framework for school health in a com-
>munity. Includes actual examples, pre- and post-
>tests, with answers.

8.106 Willgoose, Carl E. Health Teaching in Secondary Schools,
2d ed. Philadelphia: Saunders, 1977.
>457 pp. Cloth. Index. Bibliography.
>Written for teachers of health education, this book is
>a resource for curriculum development, teaching
>strategies, and issues and trends in health education.
>The appendix includes objectives for major health
>topics in both junior and senior high schools.

PERIODICALS

8.107   *Aging. U.S. Administration on Aging, Office of Human Development, Department of Health, Education and Welfare,
Washington, D.C. 20201. 10 times annually. 1951 to date.

8.108   American Journal of Public Health. American Public Health
Association, 1015 18th Street N.W., Washington, D.C.
20036. Monthly. 1911 to date.

8.109   Current Literature in Family Planning. Planned Parenthood-
World Population. Katherine Dexter McCormick Library,
810 Seventh Avenue, New York, N.Y. 10019. Monthly.
1973 to date.

8.110   Current Literature on Aging. National Council on Aging,
1828 L Street N.W., Suite 504, Washington, D.C. 20036.
Quarterly. 1957 to date.

8.111   Current Practice in Family-Centered Community Nursing.
C.V. Mosby Co., 11830 Westline Industrial Drive, St. Louis,
Mo. 63141. Biannually. 1977 to date.

8.112   Current Practice in Gerontological Nursing. C.V. Mosby
Co., 11830 Westline Industrial Drive, St. Louis, Mo. 63141.
Annually. 1979 to date.

8.113   Family and Community Health, The Journal of Health Promotion and Maintenance. Aspen Systems Corporation,
20010 Century Boulevard, Germantown, Md. 20767.
Quarterly. 1978 to date.

8.114   Geriatrics: Devoted to Diseases and Processes of Aging.
Lancet Publications, Inc., 4015 West 65th Street,
Minneapolis, Minn. 55435. (For the American Geriatrics
Society.) Monthly. 1946 to date.

---

*Order from Superintendent of Documents, Washington, D.C. 20402.

8.115   Gerontologist. Gerontological Society, 1 Dupont Circle
        Number 520, Washington, D.C. 20036. Bimonthly.
        1961 to date.

8.116   Health Education Monographs. Charles B. Slack, Inc.,
        6900 Grove Road, Thorofare, N.J. 08086. Quarterly.
        1974 to date.

8.117   Health Values: Achieving High Level Wellness. Charles B.
        Slack, Inc., 6900 Grove Road, Thorofare, N.J. 08086.
        Bimonthly. 1977 to date.

8.118   Journal of Ambulatory Care Management. Aspen Systems
        Corporation, 20010 Century Boulevard, Germantown, Md.
        20767. Quarterly. 1978 to date.

8.119   Journal of Gerontological Nursing. Charles B. Slack, Inc.,
        6900 Grove Road, Thorofare, N.J. 08086. Bimonthly.
        1975 to date.

8.120   Journal of Gerontology. Gerontological Society, 1 Dupont
        Circle, Number 520, Washington, D.C. 20036. Bimonthly.
        1946 to date.

8.121   Medicolegal News. American Society of Law & Medicine,
        454 Brookline Avenue, Boston, Mass. 02215. Quarterly.
        1973 to date.

8.122   Milbank Memorial Fund Quarterly/Health and Society.
        Neale Watson Academic Publication, 156 Fifth Avenue,
        New York, N.Y. 10010. Quarterly. 1923 to date.

8.123   Nursing Homes. Heldret Publications, Inc., 4000 Albemarle
        St., N.W., Washington, D.C. 20016. (For the American
        College of Nursing Administrators.) Bimonthly. 1950 to date.

8.124   Occupational Health Nursing. Charles B. Slack, Inc., 6900
        Grove Road, Thorofare, N.J. 08086. (For the American Asso-
        ciation of Occupational Health Nurses, Inc.). Monthly. 1953
        to date.

8.125   Omega; Journal of Death and Dying. Baywood Publishing
Co., Inc., 120 Marine Street, Farmingdale, N.Y. 11735.
Quarterly. 1970 to date.

8.126   School Nurse. National Education Association, Department
of School Nurses, 1201 16th Street N.W., Washington,
D.C. 20036. Quarterly. 1969 to date.

8.127   School Nursing Monographs. American Alliance for Health,
Physical Education and Recreation, National Council for
School Nurses, 1201 16th Street N.W., Washington, D.C.
20036. Irregular. 1969 to date.

8.128   Sexuality and Disability; A Journal Devoted to the Study of
Sex in Physical and Mental Illness. Human Sciences Press,
72 Fifth Avenue, New York, N.Y. 10011. Quarterly. 1978
to date.

9

Women's Health

In this chapter, we enumerate some of the books which deal with the health of women. Books on gynecology and obstetrics are listed first, followed by books on special topics in women's health: the battered woman, breast cancer, breast feeding, feminism, home childbirth, middle years, midwifery, natural childbirth, nutrition, parent education, and psychology. Pertinent periodicals are listed at the completion of the chapter.

GYNECOLOGY

9.1 Beacham, Daniel Winston; Beacham, Woodward Davis. Synopsis of Gynecology, 9th ed. St. Louis: Mosby, 1977.
> 444 pp. Cloth. Index. References.
> A compact sourcebook by physicians for physicians. Covers anatomy and physiology, examination and diagnosis in gynecology, pelvic infections, infertility, medicolegal aspects, etc. Earlier editions by Harry Sturgeon Crossen and Robert James Crossen.

9.2 Benson, Ralph C. Handbook of Obstetrics and Gynecology, 6th ed. Los Altos: Lange, 1977.
> 772 pp. Paper. Index.
> A supplemental rather than primary text for the medical student, nurse practitioner, midwife, physician. A concise digest of material used in diagnosis and

treatment of obstetric-gynecologic problems. Topics range from anatomy and physiology of the female reproductive tract to home delivery, and from gynecologic history to gynecologic procedures. Also available in other languages.

9.3   Charles, David. Self-Assessment of Current Knowledge in Obstetrics and Gynecology, 1000 Multiple-Choice Questions and Referenced Answers, 2d ed. [Self-Assessment Books.] Flushing, N.Y.: Medical Examination, 1977.
203 pp. Paper (spiral bound). Bibliography.
Contains multiple-choice questions with an answer key in the back of the book. Citations are given to clarify references in the medical literature. By a physician for physicians.

9.4   Cowan, Belita. Women's Health Care: Resources, Writings, Bibliographies. Ann Arbor: Anshen, 1977.
52 pp. Paper.
Combines information and sources as well as how to do library research on the topic of women's health. Chapters include such topics as Your Rights as a Patient; Women and Drugs; Abortion; Women and Psychotherapy; Aging; Publications and Films; and Directory of Organizations.

9.5   Goodlin, Robert C. Handbook of Obstetrical and Gynecological Data. Los Altos: Geron-X, 1972.
526 pp. Paper. Index. References.
A handbook by a physician whose data "is in two broad classifications: an extensive section of gynecic laboratory and clinical data not found in textbooks and a brief section on diagnosis and therapy." (Preface)

9.6   Martin, Leonide L. Health Care of Women. Philadelphia: Lippincott, 1978.
391 pp. Cloth. Index. References.
For the nurse in the ambulatory setting who does not want to separate the female patient's physiological and psychosocial health care needs. Chapters cover

Health Maintenance for Women; Sexuality and Affec-
tional Relationships; Contraception; Menstrual Prob-
lems; Pregnancy; Labor, Delivery, and Postpartum;
Induced Abortion; Menopause; Vaginal Discharge and
Itching; Urinary Problems; Venereal Disease; Lower
Abdominal Pain; Breast Masses; Abnormal Pap Smears;
Nervousness and Fatigue; and Socialization of Women.

9.7   Novak, Edmund R.; Jones, Georgeanna Seegar; Jones,
Howard W., Jr. Novak's Textbook of Gynecology, 9th ed.
Baltimore: Williams & Wilkins, 1975.
    822 pp. Cloth. Index. References.
A standard medical text goes into Anatomy; Gyneco-
logical History; Examination and Operations; Menstru-
ation; Problems of the Vulva, Cervix, Uterus, etc.;
Family Planning; Sex Education; Gynecologic Clinical
Cytopathology, etc.

9.8   Romney, Seymour L., et al. Gynecology and Obstetrics:
The Health Care of Women. New York: McGraw-Hill, 1975.
    1163 pp. Cloth. Index. References.
A text for medical students and practicing physicians.
Goes into normal and diseased states and for specific
problems, often presents treatment, etiology, and the
like. An appendix includes information on the infertility
work-up, normal values, etc. Second edition due 1980.

9.9   Stewart, Felicia Hance; Guest, Felicia; Stewart, Gary K.;
et al. My Body, My Health: The Concerned Woman's Guide
to Gynecology. Clinician's Edition. New York: Wiley, 1979.
    566 pp. Cloth. Index. References.
Contains information the authors believe patients should
know. Also useful for the clinician who must undertake
the role of teacher, it is "a resource that approaches
health problems in a factual, balanced way." (p. x)
Opens with a section on patient education and informed
consent. The next chapters include discussions of
anatomy, physiology, contraception, abortion, common gynecologic problems, and sexual problems.

OBSTETRICS

Nursing

9.10 Anderson, Betty Ann; Camacho, Mercedes E.; Stark,
Jeanne. The Childbearing Family, 2d ed. New York:
McGraw-Hill, 1979.
> 2 vols. Paper. Index. Bibliography.
> This updated edition reflects new knowledge and the
> identification of clinical competencies in two pro-
> grammed texts: Vol. 1: Pregnancy and Family Health,
> and Vol. 2: Interruptions in Family Health During
> Pregnancy. Units in Volume 1 discuss the family, the
> nurse's role, human sexuality, maternal and fetal
> adaptations, pregnancy, the intrapartum period, and
> the postpartum period. Units in Volume 2 deal with
> interruptions in health during fetal growth and develop-
> ment, early and late pregnancy, intrapartum and post-
> partum, and the neonatal period.

9.11 Bethea, Doris C. Introductory Maternity Nursing, 3d ed.
Philadelphia: Lippincott, 1979.
> 365 pp. Paper. Index. References. Glossary.
> Includes chapters on maternity care, reproduction,
> pregnancy, development of the fetus, high risk factors
> in infants and families, labor, puerperium, the new-
> born, etc. Deals with both normal and abnormal situa-
> tions. Each chapter has detailed behavioral objectives
> at the beginning and a clinical case with questions at
> the end for review and discussion.

9.12 Bing, Elisabeth D. Moving Through Pregnancy: The Complete Exercise Guide for Today's Woman. Indianapolis:
Bobbs-Merrill, 1975.
> 143 pp. Cloth.
> A guide to exercises during and after pregnancy for
> the active woman. Profusely illustrated with tips on
> how to get out of bed in the morning comfortably, on
> getting dressed during pregnancy, for doing chores
> around the house with less strain on the pregnant

woman, etc. Includes exercise routines with illustrations and written instructions for both before birth and postpartum. For the lay person, but could be useful in the teaching of maternity patients.

9.13 Blair, Carole Lotito; Salerno, Elizabeth Meehan. The Expanding Family: Childbearing. Boston: Little, Brown, 1976.
     276 pp. Paper. Index. References. Related readings. Two main parts deal with the practice of nursing within the family and childbearing. Contains many examples and practical guides for applying the various theories discussed.

9.14 Bleier, Inge J. Workbook in Bedside Maternity Nursing, 2d ed. Philadelphia: Saunders, 1974.
     207 pp. Paper.
     A workbook not limited for use with a specific text and which itself contains some didactic information. "Tests medical knowledge and nursing skills and requires the use of the behavioral sciences and interpersonal relations." (p. iii) Presents questions (with space for answers) on topics such as anatomy of female reproduction, sex, the fetus, pregnancy, labor and delivery, contraception, etc. Has a final section containing multiple-choice review questions on the categories discussed.

9.15 Clark, Ann L., ed. Culture/Childbearing/Health Professionals. Philadelphia: Davis, 1978.
     190 pp. Cloth. Index. References.
     Looks specifically at the childbearing practices of a number of the cultures found in the United States. Each chapter focuses on one culture's response to children, control of conception, marriage, pregnancy, labor, puerperium, and neonatal care. After an opening chapter on culture, nine chapters by different contributors focus on the following: American Indian, Afro-American, Chinese American, Japanese American, Mexican American, Puerto Rican, Filipino American, American Samoan, and Vietnamese. Each

chapter begins with a short biographical sketch of the
contributor and includes some cultural data. The purpose of the book is to improve the health professional's
assessment skills in the cultural area.

9.16 Clark, Ann L.; Affonso, Dyanne D.; Harris, Thomas R.
Childbearing: A Nursing Perspective, 2d ed. Philadelphia:
Davis, 1979.
>   1052 pp. Cloth. Index. References. Bibliographies.
>   By two R.N.'s and a physician, this is an extensive
>   text divided into units. These units cover an intro-
>   duction to maternal-child health nursing; psychosocial
>   factors and concepts; culture; physiology and the pre-
>   natal, intrapartal, and postpartal periods; the newborn;
>   risks of childbearing; crises of childbearing; and legal
>   and other considerations. Includes brief outlines for
>   each chapter. Well illustrated.

9.17 Clausen, Joy Princeton; Flook, Margaret Hemp; Ford,
Boonie; et al. Maternity Nursing Today, 2d ed. New York:
McGraw-Hill, 1977.
>   883 pp. Cloth. Index. References. Bibliographies.
>   Glossary.
>   The five parts contain chapters by various contributors.
>   Topics include maternity nursing, childbearing and
>   childrearing, the nursing process in conjunction with
>   these activities, and, finally, problems in childbearing
>   and childrearing. Stresses new trends in maternity
>   nursing and includes chapters that deal with such things
>   as the single-parent family and communal living. An
>   appendix includes the ANA's Standards of Maternal and
>   Child Health Nursing Practice. Broader than many
>   maternity nursing texts.

9.18 Coffey, Lou; Reilly, Dorothy. Modules for Learning in
Nursing: Life Cycle and Maternity Care. Philadelphia:
Davis, 1975.
>   183 pp. Paper. Bibliographies.
>   This book is designed as a companion and sequel to the
>   authors' Modules for Independent-Individual Learning

in Nursing (2.5). The modules in this volume address
sexuality, pregnancy, nursing care during pregnancy,
stages of development (newborn through elderly adult),
etc. Includes self-study multiple-choice questions with
answers, lists of audiovisual software by format and
module number, audiovisual distributors with their
addresses, and a checklist for the student's maternity
experiences.

9.19 Dickason, Elizabeth J.; Schult, Martha O.; Morris, Elaine M.
Maternal and Infant Drugs and Nursing Intervention. New
York: McGraw-Hill, 1978.
367 pp. Paper. Index. Bibliography.
Discusses the problems associated with drug utilization
during pregnancy and lactation and during the perinatal
and neonatal periods. Presents current, accurate information relevant to administering drugs used in normal pregnancy and lactation, family planning, problem
pregnancies, labor and delivery, as well as drugs used
for the newborn and neonatal infant. Considers physiologic variables, such as altered maternal metabolism
and the stage of fetal development. Indicates nursing
implications and measures. There is good use of
charts throughout the book, and the appendix discusses
parenteral injections.

9.20 Disbrow, Mildred A.; Johnson, Nancy; Leitch, Janet, et al.
Maternity Nursing Case Studies, 53 Case Histories Related
to Maternal and Infant Care in 13 Families. [Case Study
Books.] Flushing, N.Y.: Medical Examination, 1976.
215 pp. Paper (spiral). Index. Bibliographies.
"Written primarily for undergraduate student nurses
and should serve as a supplement to textbooks, a study
guide for state board examinations and a handy reference for practicing professional nurses." (p. iii)
Presents data on actual cases with 13 families. Inter-
weaves case histories with multiple-choice questions
(with answers indicated and discussed). Bibliographies
are given after each family section. Uses a "family-
centered format" because "childbearing is, and should
be, a family affair." (p. iii)

9.21 Friesner, Arlyne; Raff, Beverly. Maternity Nursing, 2d ed.
      [Nursing Outline Series.] Flushing, N.Y.: Medical Exam-
      ination, 1977.
          219 pp. Paper. Index. Bibliography.
          Provides a concise, comprehensive review of maternity
          nursing for students and graduate nurses. Employs a
          compact, outline format. Useful as a supplement to a
          text on maternity nursing and as a handy reference and
          study guide for examinations. Topics include history
          and trends in maternal care; prenatal, intrapartal, and
          postnatal periods; and the newborn. Questions are
          included in each chapter.

9.22 Goerzen, Janice L.; Chinn, Peggy L. Review of Maternal
      and Child Nursing. St. Louis: Mosby, 1975.
          210 pp. Paper. Index. References. Suggested
          readings.
          A useful text for review, continuing education, or be-
          ginning study of maternal-child nursing. Chapters deal
          with the family, sexuality, nursing the pregnant family
          and the growing child, disorders of the fetus, infant
          and child, etc. Appendixes include drug and
          nutritional information. Has a question-essay answer
          format.

9.23 Jensen, Margaret Duncan; Benson, Ralph C.; Bobak,
      Irene M. Maternity Care, the Nurse and the Family.
      St. Louis: Mosby, 1977.
          764 pp. Cloth. Index. References.
          A comprehensive maternity nursing text covering human
          reproduction, family planning, pregnancy (discusses
          nutrition, fathers' roles, and problems), complications
          of pregnancy, postpartum, the newborn, and legal
          issues in maternity nursing. Appendixes include a
          "bill of rights" for the pregnant patient, information
          on nurse-midwife education, and community resources.

9.24 Kalafatich, Audrey J.; Meeks, Dorothy R.; Jones, Barbara M.

Maternal and Child Health: A Handbook for Nurses, rev. ed.
Totowa, N.J.: Littlefield, Adams, 1977.
> 228 pp. Paper. Index. Bibliography. Glossary.
> Stresses the continuity between obstetric and pediatric
> nursing by covering aspects of both in one book. Chap-
> ters include an introduction to maternal and child health;
> pregnancy from the standpoint of the entire family; nurs-
> ing care before, during, and after labor and delivery;
> the various stages of childhood (the newborn, infant,
> toddler, etc.); and handicapped children. Chapters
> are arranged in outline form for easy consultation.

9.25 Lerch, Constance; Bliss, V. Jane. Maternity Nursing, 3d
ed. St. Louis: Mosby, 1978.
> 432 pp. Cloth. Index. Bibliographies. Glossary.
> A text for classroom and/or clinical teaching, divided
> into 5 units: the Preparatory Phase, the Period of
> Pregnancy, the Period of Parturition, the Postpartum
> Period, and the Neonate. Chapters have nursing im-
> plications sections. Appendixes include statistics
> and review questions.

9.26 Lipkin, Gladys B. Parent-Child Nursing; Psychosocial
Aspects, 2d ed. St. Louis: Mosby, 1978.
> 247 pp. Paper. Index. Suggested readings.
> Previously published as Psychosocial Aspects of
> Maternal-Child Nursing (1974). Eleven chapters cover
> trends in maternity care, family planning, the preg-
> nant couple, high-risk pregnancy and birth, the labor-
> ing couple, attachment and separation, the postpartum
> couple, the child from birth to six years, the child
> from six through twelve years, the adolescent, and the
> terminally ill child. Each chapter closes with a nurs-
> ing assessment and care plan that shows the applica-
> tion of the nursing process to a case situation.

9.27 Lytle, Nancy A., ed. Nursing of Women in the Age of Lib-
eration. Dubuque: Wm. C. Brown, 1977.

251 pp. Paper. Name and subject indexes.
Bibliographies.
Focuses on the care of women from puberty through the
reproductive years. Considers the roles of husband,
father, and sexual partner within the framework of an
historical overview, with extensive documentation.
Timely, authentic information asks provocative questions worthy of systematic investigation. A well written
book about women and womanhood, families and parenting, health and hazards to health.

9.28 Malinowski, Janet S.; Burdin, Carolyn P.; Lederman,
Regina P.; et al. Nursing Care of the Labor Patient.
Philadelphia: Davis, 1978.
183 pp. Paper. Index. Bibliography.
Written for the undergraduate nursing student for use
with a comprehensive text on obstetrical nursing. Addresses those concepts that are relevant to the patient
in labor and which the authors believe are most difficult to grasp. Included are measuring contractions,
interpreting fetal heart rates, pelvic measurements,
labor stimulants, premature labor, pain relief, and
the Lamaze technique. Each chapter contains objectives, review questions, and post-tests.

9.29 Malo-Juvera, Dolores; Mason, Diana J.; Blake, Lorraine A.;
et al. Obstetrical Nursing, Continuing Education Review;
Essay Questions and Referenced Answers, 2d ed. [Essay
Question and Answer Review Books.] Garden City: Medical
Examination, 1979.
232 pp. Paper. Index. Bibliography.
Uses an essay question-answer format with sections:
The Antepartum Period; The Intrapartum Period; The
Postpartum Period; The Newborn Period; Fertility
Regulation; Topics of General Interest. Each answer
is footnoted to an original source in either a book or
a journal where the student can look for further infor-
mation.

9.30 Mercer, Ramona Thieme. Nursing Care for Parents at Risk.
Thorofare, N.J.: Charles B. Slack, 1977.
> 178 pp. Paper. Index. References.
> Looks at the disappointments of childbirth when a child
> is born prematurely or with an impairment and also
> addresses the adjustment that is necessary for parents.
> Two sections cover Early Parenting (parenting and
> what it entails, responses to threat or loss by the
> parent) and Situations That Place Parents at Risk (de-
> fect of the infant, mother faces a health problem, pre-
> mature infant, young parents, etc.).

9.31 Miller, Carol L.; Pike, Margaret M.; White, Kathleen J.;
et al. Self-Assessment of Current Knowledge in Maternity
Nursing, 1,227 Multiple-Choice Questions and Referenced
Answers. [Self-Assessment Books.] Flushing, N.Y.:
Medical Examination, 1975.
> 272 pp. Paper (spiral bound). References. Glossary.
> A multiple-choice examination review book for students
> of maternity nursing. An answer key is included at the
> end of the book.

9.32 Miller, Mary Ann; Brooten, Dorothy A. The Childbearing
Family: A Nursing Perspective. Boston: Little, Brown,
1977.
> 495 pp. Cloth. Index. Bibliography.
> A comprehensive text dealing with childbearing, sexual-
> ity, reproduction, pregnancy, postpartum, etc. Gives
> attention to the father and the process of parenting.
> Has a two-page appendix listing certificate and mas-
> ter's degree programs in nurse-midwifery in the
> United States.

9.33 Moore, Mary Lou. Realities in Childbearing. Philadelphia:
Saunders, 1978.
> 772 pp. Cloth. Index. References. Glossary.
> A nursing text on childbearing for the student or prac-
> ticing nurse. Covers physiologic, cultural, emotional,
> developmental, and environmental aspects of the

childbearing family. Each chapter includes a summary. Appendixes include ANA's Standards of
Maternal-Child Health Nursing Practice, Arizona
Nurses' Association—Perinatal Nursing Standards,
lists of journals, audiovisual materials, organizations
concerned with childbearing.

9.34 Phillips, Celeste R.; Anzalone, Joseph T. Fathering: Participation in Labor and Delivery. St. Louis: Mosby, 1978.
151 pp. Paper. References. Glossary.
A text written to supplement books used in nursing and
medical courses on maternity care and obstetrics. It
should be useful for family life classes and prepared
childbirth classes. The focus is on the father in a setting that too often has ignored him. Units are The
Prospective Father; The Physician's Viewpoint;
Family-Centered Care; Birth Experiences; Birth in
Retrospect; and Epilogue. Of special interest are the
descriptions of the birthing experience written by
fathers following the event. Includes photographs of
newborns, fathers and the new child, new families, etc.

9.35 Pillitteri, Adele. Nursing Care of the Growing Family: A
Maternal-Newborn Text. Boston: Little, Brown, 1976.
445 pp. Cloth. Index. References.
Goes into nursing care of the pregnant family and the
newborn infant through the first few weeks of life. Includes chapters on the high-risk pregnancy and the high-
risk infant. Companion volume to Nursing Care of the
Growing Family: A Child Health Text (10.34).

9.36 Reeder, Sharon R.; Mastroianni, Luigi, Jr.; Martin,
Leonide L.; et al. Maternity Nursing, 13th ed. Philadelphia: Lippincott, 1976.
706 pp. Cloth. Index. Bibliographies. Suggested
readings.
First published in 1929, the thirteenth edition of this
comprehensive nursing text has been greatly revised
in light of the changes in today's society. Contains
eight units, most of which have study questions with
answers in the appendix. Major headings to be covered

are listed at the beginning of the chapters. Units cover
current issues, human reproduction, pregnancy, labor
and delivery, the puerperium and the newborn, obstetric
operative procedures, disorders of childbearing, and
home nursing, emergency or disaster situations, and
a brief history of maternity nursing. Illustrated with
good examples. Prior edition by Elise Fitzpatrick.

9.37 Shure, Myrna B.; Spivack, George. Problem-Solving Techniques in Childrearing. [Jossey-Bass Social and Behavioral
Sciences Series.] San Francisco: Jossey-Bass, 1978.
261 pp. Cloth. Index. References.
Interpersonal cognitive problem-solving (ICPS) skills
were found by the authors in earlier studies to be related to healthy adaptive behavior in children. This
book describes a research program with mothers of preschool children. It considered what mothers can do to
stimulate the development of ICPS skills in the child and
which skills were important for the mother to have.
Written for parents, teachers of children and others
who work with them.

9.38 Ziegel, Erna E.; Cranley, Mecca S. Obstetric Nursing, 7th
ed. New York: Macmillan, 1978.
911 pp. Cloth. Index. Bibliography.
The most recent edition of a basic, comprehensive text
for beginning nursing students. Part 1: Scientific Foundations for Perinatal Care; Part 2: The Antepartum
Period; Part 3: Intrapartum Care; Part 4: The Postpartum Family; Part 5: The High-Risk Mother and Baby;
and Part 6: History and Trends. The focus in this book
is on the mother and infant. Only about ten pages are
devoted to the family as the system in which pregnancy
occurs. Earlier editions by C. C. Van Blarcom with
the title Obstetrical Nursing.

Medical

9.39 Greenhill, J. P.; Friedman, Emanuel A. Biological Principles and Modern Practice of Obstetrics. 13th ed.
Philadelphia: Saunders, 1974.

837 pp. Cloth. Index. References.
A standard medical text, based somewhat on the Principles and Practice of Obstetrics by Joseph B. DeLee.
Goes into normal and pathologic states of pregnancy,
labor, and the puerperium.

9.40 Pritchard, Jack A.; MacDonald, Paul C. Williams' Obstetrics, 16th ed. New York: Appleton-Century-Crofts, 1980.
1100 pp. Cloth. Index. References. Reading list.
A standard and extensive medical text in its field.
More detailed than Greenhill as to female reproduction.
Originally authored by J. W. Williams; fourteenth
edition by L. M. Hellman et al.

BATTERED WOMEN

9.41 Walker, Lenore E. The Battered Woman. New York:
Harper & Row, 1979.
270 pp. Cloth. Index.
Explores a problem which has only recently come into
the limelight. Three parts address Psychology of the
Battered Woman; Coercive Techniques in Battering Relationships (sexual abuse, discord in the family, social
battering, etc.); and The Way Out (safe houses, legal
alternatives, medical alternatives, psychotherapy,
etc.). The author draws on cases from her psychotherapy classes in giving examples throughout the book.
Brief information on available resources is at the end
of the book.

BREAST CANCER

9.42 Campion, Rosamund. The Invisible Worm. New York:
Macmillan, 1972.
96 pp. Cloth.
The title, from a poem by William Blake, symbolizes
cancer. The author describes her experience with
cancer and the health care system as she fought for the
right to choose what was done to her.

9.43 Cowles, Jane. Informed Consent. New York: Coward,
McCann & Geoghegan, 1976.
> 224 pp. Cloth. Index. Bibliography. Glossary.
> Attempts to give women the facts about breast cancer
> so they can participate in any decisions being made re-
> lating to their condition. Chapters discuss two cases
> in detail and point up the lack of communication that
> often occurs between doctor and patient or patient and
> spouse. Goes into the anatomy and physiology of the
> human breast and the types of breast cancer.

BREAST FEEDING

9.44 Pryor, Karen. Nursing Your Baby, new rev. ed. New York:
Harper & Row, 1973.
> 289 pp. Cloth. Index. Selected references.
> Examines the relationship between the infant who
> nurses and the mother, how breasts function, the com-
> position of milk, maternal-infant bonding, doctors who
> help and those who do not, the La Leche League, and
> attitudes toward breast feeding. Part 2 discusses
> preparation for breast feeding, what to do in the hos-
> pital, continuation into the home, transitions and
> changes during the first year, and nursing the older
> child.

9.45 La Leche League International. The Womanly Art of Breast-
feeding, 2d ed., rev. and enl. Franklin Park, Ill.: La
Leche League International, 1963.
> 166 pp. Paper. Index. Annotated bibliography.
> This is a readable book for mothers-to-be or the new
> mother, by the La Leche League, which has attempted
> to increase the incidence of breast feeding. Chapters
> cover the rationale for breast feeding; planning for a
> baby; nutrition; worries and old wives' tales; how to
> breast feed; the father's role, etc. Includes
> information about the La Leche League.

FEMINISM

9.46 Arms, Suzanne. Immaculate Deception: A New Look at
Women and Childbirth in America. Boston: Houghton
Mifflin, 1975.
> 318 pp. Cloth. Index. Bibliography.
> Attacks conventional methods of childbirth in hospitals
> and the dehumanizing nature of childbirth in America.
> The author recounts her experience and those of others
> and dwells extensively on the potential and actual role
> midwives can and do play in more satisfying birth ex-
> periences. The book is readable and amply laced with
> quotations from both known authorities and unknown
> citizens.

9.47 Hite, Shere. The Hite Report: A Nationwide Study on
Female Sexuality. New York: Macmillan, 1976.
> 438 pp. Cloth. Bibliography.
> Discusses the results of questionnaires distributed to
> women by the author during study for her Ph.D. in his-
> tory at Columbia University. Chapters are titled Mas-
> turbation, Orgasm, Intercourse, Lesbianism, etc. In-
> cludes the questionnaires as well as information on the
> women who answered them.

9.48 Lanson, Lucienne. From Woman to Woman: A Gynecologist
Answers Questions about You and Your Body. New York:
Knopf, 1975.
> 358 pp. Cloth. Index. Glossary.
> This book, by a female gynecologist, consists of ques-
> tions with essay answers. Designed for the laywoman,
> the parts cover the gynecologic exam, female problems,
> female sexuality, menopause, future developments, and
> the like.

HOME CHILDBIRTH

9.49 Sousa, Marion. Childbirth at Home. Englewood Cliffs:
Prentice-Hall, 1976.

208 pp. Cloth. Index. Footnotes. Bibliography.
A favorable book about a controversial topic. The
author goes into home childbirth as compared to birth
in a hospital, preparing for home childbirth, risks of
home childbirth, etc.

MIDDLE YEARS

9.50 McCauley, Carole Spearin. Pregnancy After 35. New York:
Dutton, 1976.
213 pp. Cloth. Index. Bibliographies.
Explores pregnancy that takes place later than the norm
in a positive, realistic, reassuring fashion. Chapters
deal with genetics, diet during pregnancy, drugs during pregnancy, labor, delivery, etc. Appendixes include nutritional information on various foods, commonly used terms in pregnancy, and addresses of
various agencies.

9.51 Parrish, Louis. No Pause at All. New York: Reader's
Digest Press, 1976.
215 pp. Cloth. Index.
By a physician, this book focuses on and deals positive-
ly with the changes occurring in the middle years of a
woman's life. Dr. Parrish draws on case histories.

MIDWIFERY

9.52 Beischer, Norman A.; Mackay, Eric V. Obstetrics and the
Newborn; for Midwives and Medical Students. Philadelphia:
Saunders, 1976.
532 pp. Cloth. Index. Glossary.
A well-illustrated text for midwives and medical students. Looks at normal pregnancy as well as the disorders of pregnancy. The last section focuses on the
newborn. Authors are from Australia.

9.53   Brennan, Barbara; Heilman, Joan Rattner. The Complete
       Book of Midwifery. New York: Dutton, 1977.
              142 pp. Paper. Index. Selected readings.
              Ms. Brennan is the chief nurse-midwife at New York
              City's Roosevelt Hospital and this book recounts many
              of the experiences she and her patients have had with
              midwife-assisted childbirth. The book also has an ex-
              tensive discussion of the midwife's role and what the
              midwife offers the pregnant mother above and apart
              from the obstetrician. Includes a list by state of
              nurse-midwifery services in the United States.

9.54   Hickman, Maureen A. An Introduction to Midwifery.
       Philadelphia: Lippincott, 1978.
              501 pp. Paper. Index. Bibliography.
              A comprehensive text for midwifery students that ex-
              amines normal and abnormal aspects of pregnancy,
              labor, and puerperium. One section focuses on the
              fetus and the neonate. The last section describes
              health and social services in Great Britain.

9.55   Myles, Margaret F. Textbook for Midwives, with Modern
       Concepts of Obstetric and Neonatal Care, 8th ed. Edinburgh:
       Churchill Livingstone, 1975.
              796 pp. Cloth. Index. Glossary.
              A British text whose eight parts go into female anatomy
              and physiology, pregnancy, problems of pregnancy,
              labor, complications of labor, puerperium, the new
              infant, and miscellaneous problems (e.g., operative
              obstetrics, infertility, etc.). Each chapter includes
              essay and/or fill-in-the-blank questions.

NATURAL CHILDBIRTH

9.56   Bing, Elisabeth D., ed. The Adventure of Birth: Experi-
       ences in the Lamaze Method of Prepared Childbirth. New
       York: Simon and Schuster, 1970.
              192 pp. Cloth. Bibliography. Glossary.
              A series of positive letters from mothers and fathers

describing their experiences with Lamaze childbirth.
Mrs. Bing has been an instructor of prepared childbirth for many years.

9.57 Dick-Read, Grantly. Childbirth Without Fear: The Original
Approach to Natural Childbirth, 4th ed. Revised and edited
by Helen Wessel and Harlan F. Ellis. New York: Harper &
Row, 1972.
   420 pp. Cloth. Index. References. Bibliography.
   Glossary.
   Part 1 discusses the principles behind natural childbirth and Part 2 focuses on the practice of natural childbirth, prenatal health, education, breathing and relaxa-
   tion, labor and delivery. Part 3 discusses the pioneer
   in natural childbirth, Dick-Read. The last section is
   on the physiology of childbirth. Appendixes contain
   sources of information and supplies. Includes illustrations. First published in 1942 as Revelation of Childbirth.

9.58 Karmel, Marjorie. Thank You, Dr. Lamaze: A Mother's
Experiences in Painless Childbirth. Philadelphia: Lippincott, 1959.
   188 pp. Cloth. Suggested readings.
   The author recounts her personal experiences with
   Lamaze childbirth in both France and the United States
   in clear, moving fashion. Includes Manual of Information and Practical Exercises for Painless Childbirth by
   Mmes. Rennert and Cohen.

9.59 Lamaze, Fernand. Painless Childbirth, Psychoprophylactic
Method. Translated by L. R. Celestin. Chicago: Henry
Regerny, 1970.
   192 pp. Cloth. Index.
   The classic on natural childbirth by one of its earliest
   advocates. Gives historical information on the "childbirth without pain" movement, discusses the concept
   and the conditions necessary to achieve it. First published in France in 1956; in Great Britain in 1958.

9.60 LeBoyer, Frederick. Birth Without Violence. New York: Knopf, 1975.
> 114 pp. Cloth.
> Advocates a completely new way of birth and delivery which LeBoyer feels is less traumatic for the child particularly. Originally published in French in 1974, this book is written in a poetic, simple, yet scholarly style with illustrations. A film is also available.

9.61 Salk, Lee. Preparing for Parenthood: Understanding Your Feelings about Pregnancy, Childbirth, and Your Baby. New York: David McKay, 1974.
> 206 pp. Cloth. Index.
> A doctor tells parents a little about their feelings toward parenthood, pregnancy, a new baby, discipline, breast feeding, etc.

9.62 Tanzer, Deborah; Block, Jean Libman. Why Natural Childbirth? A Psychologist's Report on the Benefits to Mothers, Fathers, and Babies. Garden City, N.Y.: Doubleday, 1972.
> 289 pp. Cloth. Index. Footnotes. Further Reading.
> Discusses the psychology of natural childbirth in nontechnical language. Topics include: childbirth throughout history; natural childbirth; effect of drugs; pregnancy and labor; the experience of birth; husbands at delivery; and others. Four women speak about natural childbirth. The appendix contains a list of organizations to contact concerning natural childbirth.

NUTRITION

9.63 Moghissi, Kamran S.; Evans, Tommy N., eds. Nutritional Impacts on Women Throughout Life with Emphasis on Reproduction. Hagerstown, Md.: Harper & Row, 1977.
> 254 pp. Cloth. Index. References.
> This book explores "how best to improve the health of women from early childhood through reproductive years and past menopause." (p. xiii) Individual chapters are by clinicians, nutritionists, and other scientists.

9.64 Slattery, Jill S.; Pearson, Gayle Angus; Torre, Carolyn
Talley; eds. Maternal and Child Nutrition: Assessment and
Counseling. New York: Appleton-Century-Crofts, 1979.
   320 pp. Paper. Index. Bibliography. Glossary.
   A look at nutritional issues in pregnancy, in childhood
   from infancy to adolescence, and in situations of nutritional dysfunction. For professionals involved in practice, this book advocates improving health through good
   nutritional practices. Separate chapters focus on pregnancy, the postpartum period, infants, toddlers and
   preschoolers, the middle years of childhood, and adolescence. The last two chapters look at nutritional
   dysfunction and the effects of hospitalization. Appendixes contain helpful tables.

9.65 Worthington, Bonnie S.; Vermeersch, Joyce; Williams, Sue
Rodwell. Nutrition in Pregnancy and Lactation. St. Louis:
Mosby, 1977.
   223 pp. Paper. Index. References.
   Designed for health professionals who care for mothers
   and infants. Chapters discuss Health Problems of
   Mothers and Infants; Nutritional Guidance in Prenatal
   Care; Lactation, Human Milk, and Nutritional Consid-
   erations, Nutrition and Family Planning, etc.

PARENT EDUCATION

9.66 Brewer, Gail Sforza; Brewer, Tom. What Every Pregnant
Woman Should Know: The Truth about Diets and Drugs in
Pregnancy. New York: Random House, 1977.
   243 pp. Cloth. Index. Bibliography.
   Stresses the need for good nutrition during pregnancy
   rather than being concerned with the amount of weight
   gained. The authors feel that in the past obstetricians
   have been overly preoccupied with controlling weight
   gain during pregnancy. Their feeling is that patients
   should be asked what they eat, not how much they eat.
   Chapters discuss low sodium diets, toxemia, nutrition
   education in medical school, and similar topics.

Includes a listing of some menus during pregnancy, recipes, protein content, and information on various pertinent national organizations concerned with proper nutrition during pregnancy.

9.67 The Boston Children's Medical Center. Pregnancy, Birth & the Newborn Baby: A Publication for Parents. New York: Delacorte Press/Seymour Lawrence, 1972.
474 pp. Cloth. Index.
Written for parents or couples who are parents-to-be, this book deals with pregnancy, birth, the newborn baby, and special problems such as infertility, abortion, etc. More detailed than most such books. Contributors include Richard Chasin, Margaret Mead, Niles Anne Newton, Peter Wolff, and others.

9.68 Clark, Ann L. Leadership Technique in Expectant Parent Education, 2d ed. New York: Springer Publishing, 1973.
118 pp. Paper. References.
A "how-to" book for the education of expectant parents. Chapters deal with reproduction, nutrition, the newborn, the family, contraception, and the like. Chapters include lists of audiovisual material.

9.69 Dickinson, Robert Laton; Belskie, Abram. Birth Atlas, 6th ed. New York: Maternity Center Association, 1968.
40 pp. Cloth (spiral bound).
Consists of black and white plates demonstrating fetal position, birth, pregnancy, labor, twinning, etc. Description is included on the verso of the plates. Oversized format allows viewing by a class or group.

9.70 Dilfer, Carol Stahmann. Your Baby, Your Body, Fitness During Pregnancy. New York: Crown, 1977.
149 pp. Cloth. Index. Bibliography. Annotated suggested readings.
A how-to-exercise book during pregnancy with illustrations, descriptions. Has many varieties of exercises.

9.71   Maternity Center Association.   A Baby Is Born, the Picture
       Story of Everyman's Beginning, 11th ed. New York: Grosset
       & Dunlap, 1975.
             63 pp. Cloth.
             "Gives basic facts about how a baby is conceived and
             what happens physiologically to mother and baby as
             pregnancy advances." (p. vii) Describes labor and
             birth. Really a picture book, often with captions.
             Illustrations present "anatomical sculptures originally
             created for the Maternity Center Association by the
             famous doctor-sculptor team of Robert L. Dickinson
             and Abram Belskie." (p. vii)

9.72   Maternity Center Association.   Guide for Expectant Parents.
       New York: Grosset & Dunlap, 1969.
             182 pp. Paper. Index.
             A book with a question-answer format for expectant
             and new parents. Answers are clear and to the point,
             often supplemented with illustrations.

9.73   Nilsson, Lennart; Furuhjelm, Mirjam; Ingelman-Sundberg,
       Axel; et al. A Child Is Born: New Photographs of Life be-
       fore Birth and Up-to-Date Advice for Expectant Parents,
       completely revised edition. New York: Delacorte Press,
       1977.
             160 pp. Cloth. Index.
             A collection of spectacular photos shows development
             of the fetus in a mother's body. The last chapter pic-
             tures labor and delivery. Text is readable and useful.
             Originally published in Swedish.

9.74   Sasmor, Jeannette L. Childbirth Education: A Nursing
       Perspective. New York: Wiley, 1979.
             322 pp. Cloth. Index. Bibliography.
             For nursing students and nurses in practice as they
             consider childbirth education as part of nursing. This
             book provides a base for knowledgeable decision making
             in practice related to childbirth education. Included are
             an historical perspective, strategies involving the

nursing process, support systems, and a look at the future. Dick-Read, Lamaze, and eclectic approaches are also covered. The chapters on the role of the father and the single parent are especially helpful. Appendixes contain bill of rights for the pregnant patient as well as an outline for teaching a prepared childbirth course.

9.75 U.S. Department of Health, Education and Welfare; Office of Child Development; Children's Bureau. Prenatal Care. DHEW publication no. (OCD) 73-17. Children's Bureau Publication no. 4. Washington: Government Printing Office, 1973.
70 pp. Paper.
First published in 1913 and revised in 1962, this useful booklet answers commonly asked questions about pregnancy and the early days after delivery. Not as comprehensive as Guide for Expectant Parents (9.72) which has more questions.

PSYCHOLOGY

9.76 Bardwick, Judith M. Psychology of Women: A Study of Bio-Cultural Conflicts. New York: Harper & Row, 1971.
242 pp. Cloth. Index. References.
An attempt "to understand the psychological dynamics of middle-class American women." (p. 4) Dr. Bardwick rejects the standard theories on female development and postulates her own. Chapters go into Psychoanalytic Theory, Psychology and the Sexual Body, The Ego and Self-Esteem, The Motive to Achieve, etc.

9.77 Chesler, Phyllis. Women and Madness. Garden City: Doubleday, 1972.
359 pp. Cloth. Index. Footnotes.
This work on female psychology deals with mental asylums, clinicians, female homosexuals, Third World women, feminists, and the like. Appendix on the Female Career as a Psychiatric Patient includes statistics. The book is interlaced with case material and an historical perspective.

9.78 Deutsch, Helene. The Psychology of Women: A Psychoana-
      lytic Interpretation. New York: Grune & Stratton, 1944-45.
          2 vols. Cloth. Index. Bibliography.
          A well-known study on feminine psychology even though
          it is old. Dr. Deutsch was trained by Freud and her
          book reflects much of this viewpoint, as well as her
          own experience with patients. Volume I deals with
          puberty, adolescence, menstruation, homosexuality,
          etc. Volume II, entitled Motherhood, covers concep-
          tion, pregnancy, mother-child interaction, and the like.

9.79 Huber, Joan, ed. Changing Women in a Changing Society.
      Chicago: University of Chicago Press, 1973.
          295 pp. Cloth. References.
          A special issue of the American Journal of Sociology,
          this collection of materials evaluates the status of
          women and new developments in organizations and oc-
          cupational, social, and family life. Provides an over-
          view for the general reader as well as a text for
          courses on sex roles and marriage and the family.

9.80 Williams, Juanita H. Psychology of Women: Behavior in a
      Biosocial Context. New York: Norton, 1977.
          444 pp. Cloth. Index. References.
          The outgrowth of a course on the psychology of women
          taught by the author at the University of South Florida.
          Chapters cover myths and stereotypes, psychoanalysis,
          sex differences, sexuality, sex roles, birth control,
          pregnancy, life styles, mental disorders, aging, and
          so on.

PERIODICALS

Nursing

9.81 Birth and the Family Journal. American Society for Psycho-
      prophylaxis in Obstetrics and the International Childbirth
      Education Association, 110 El Camino Real, Berkeley, Ca.
      94705. Quarterly. 1973 to date.

9.82 Briefs. Charles B. Slack, Inc., 6900 Grove Road, Thorofare, N.J. 08086. (For the Maternity Center Association.)
10 times annually. 1973 to date.

9.83 Childbirth Education. American Society for Psychoprophy-
laxis in Obstetrics, Inc., 1523 L Street, N.W., Washington,
D.C. 20005. Quarterly. 1968 to date.

9.84 Childbirth Without Pain Education Association Newsletter.
Childbirth Without Pain Education Association, 20134
Snowden, Detroit, Mich. 48235. Bimonthly. 1960 to date.

9.85 Current Practice in Obstetric and Gynecologic Nursing.
C.V. Mosby Co., 11830 Westline Industrial Drive, St. Louis,
Mo. 63141. Biannually. 1976 to date.

9.86 Expecting. Parents' Magazine Enterprises, Inc., 52 Vanderbilt Avenue, New York, N.Y. 10017. Quarterly. 1967 to
date.

9.87 ICEA NEWS. International Childbirth Education Association,
195 Waterford Drive, Dayton, O. 45459. Quarterly. 1975
to date.

9.88 Issues in Health Care of Women. McGraw-Hill Book Company, 1221 Avenue of the Americas, New York, N.Y. 10020.
Bimonthly. 1978 to date.

9.89 JOGN Nursing (Journal of Obstetric, Gynecologic and Neo-
natal Nursing). Harper & Row, Medical Department, 2350
Virginia Avenue, Hagerstown, Md. 21740. (For the Nurses
Association of the American College of Obstetricians and
Gynecologists.) Bimonthly. 1972 to date.

9.90 Journal of Nurse-Midwifery. American College of Nurse-
Midwives, 1000 Vermont Avenue, N.W., Washington, D.C.
20005. Quarterly. 1970 to date.

9.91 Midwives Chronicle. Nursing Notes, Ltd., 98 Belsize Lane,
London NW3 5BB, England. (For the Royal College of
Midwives.) Monthly. 1887 to date.

9.92 Nursing Mirror (or Nursing Mirror and Midwives Journal).
IPC Business Press Ltd., 33-40 Bowling Green Lane, London
EC1R 0NE, England. Weekly. 1888 to date.

9.93 Women & Health, The Journal of Women's Health Care.
Haworth Press, 149 Fifth Avenue, New York, N.Y. 10010.
Quarterly. 1976 to date.

Medical

9.94 Abortion Bibliography. Whitson Publishing Company, Inc.,
P.O. Box 322, Troy, N.Y. 12181. Has come out annually
since 1970. World coverage of books and articles for the
preceding year. Arranged by subject with author index.
Covers articles in Hospital Literature Index, Index Medicus,
International Nursing Index, and Cumulative Index to Nursing
and Allied Health Literature.

9.95 American Journal of Obstetrics and Gynecology. C. V.
Mosby Co., 11830 Westline Industrial Drive, St. Louis, Mo.
63141. (For the American Gynecological Society.) Semimonthly. 1920 to date.

9.96 Audio-Digest Obstetrics-Gynecology (on audio cassette and
5-inch reel tape). Audio-Digest Foundation, 1577 E. Chevy
Chase Drive, Glendale, Ca. 91206. Semimonthly. 1954 to
date. (Also available in other areas, e.g., pediatrics,
psychiatry, surgery, etc.)

9.97 Clinical Obstetrics and Gynecology: A Quarterly Periodical.
Harper & Row Medical Department, 2350 Virginia Avenue,
Hagerstown, Md. 21740. Quarterly. 1958 to date.

9.98 Obstetrics and Gynecology. Elsevier-North Holland, Inc.,
52 Vanderbilt Ave., New York, N.Y. 10017. (For the
American College of Obstetricians and Gynecologists.)
Monthly. 1952 to date.

9.99 Surgery, Gynecology & Obstetrics (With International Abstracts of Surgery). Franklin H. Martin Memorial Foundation, 55 E. Erie Street, Chicago, Ill. 60611. (For the American College of Surgeons.) Monthly. 1905 to date.

10
Child Health

In this chapter, we list some of the sources that deal with the growth and development and the medical and nursing care of children in normal and diseased states. For our purposes, we define <u>child health</u> as encompassing the neonate through the adolescent, since this is the usual coverage of pediatric texts.

We have grouped items to include those on growth and development in general, those for parents, those on nursing and medical pediatrics in general, and those on pediatric specialties and other topics: cardiology, death, emergencies, endocrinology, handicapped children, hospitalized children, neurology, newborn, the nurse practitioner, nutrition, ophthalmology, orthopedics, pathology, psychology and psychiatry, renal disease, and surgery. Finally, related periodicals are listed at the end of the chapter.

GROWTH AND DEVELOPMENT

General

10.1 Clarke-Stewart, Alison. Child Care in the Family: A Review of Research and Some Propositions for Policy. [Carnegie Council on Children Publications.] New York: Academic Press, 1977.

151 pp. Cloth. Index. Bibliography.
A "critical review of the research on family influence

on children's development." (p. ix) Explores the
strengths and limitations of current knowledge. Two
parts discuss the research that has been done concerning children from infancy to 9 years of age and the
policy implications of such research.

10.2 Di Leo, Joseph H. Child Development: Analysis and Syn-
thesis. New York: Brunner/Mazel, 1977.
177 pp. Cloth. Name and subject indexes. Bibliography.
Written for those working with children. First examines
affective, social, cognitive, behavioral, and physical
development, then the integrated whole. The World of
Childhood as Seen by Adults and as Seen Through the
Eyes of Children are two main sections.

10.3 Flapan, Dorothy; Neubauer, Peter B. The Assessment of
Early Child Development. New York: Jason Aronson, 1975.
151 pp. Cloth. Index.
Includes charts on various stages of child development
giving typical and atypical behavior ranges. Deals with
the following issues, among others: early child development, social and emotional development, ego and
motor development, superego development, and developmental progression.

10.4 Illingworth, R. S. The Development of the Infant and Young
Child, Normal and Abnormal, 6th ed. Edinburgh: Churchill
Livingstone, 1975.
325 pp. Cloth. Index. Bibliography.
Deals in detail with assessment of the newborn and the
infant with outlines of average development and plates
to show normal and abnormal development. Contains
chapters on Diagnosis of Cerebral Palsy; Mental Retardation.

10.5 Kaluger, George; Kaluger, Meriem Fair. Human Development: The Span of Life, 2d ed. St. Louis: Mosby, 1979.
530 pp. Cloth. Author and subject indexes.
References. Glossary.
Presents a basically chronological sequence approach

to development beginning with the psychology of the life
span and developmental determinants, and moving from
the prenatal period to infancy to childhood, adolescence,
and adulthood. Each chapter has study questions.

10.6 Krajicek, Marilyn J.; Tearney, Alice I., eds. Detection of
Developmental Problems in Children: A Reference Guide for
Community Nurses and Other Health Care Professionals.
Baltimore: University Park Press, 1977.
> 204 pp. Paper. Index. References.
> A collection of papers designed to help the health pro-
> fessional assess developmental problems in children.
> Papers deal with home visits, genetic disorders, vision
> screening, speech and language development, behavior
> modification, child abuse, etc. Includes charts on
> embryonic development and fetal development.

10.7 Lowrey, George H. Growth and Development of Children,
7th ed. Chicago: Year Book, 1978.
> 464 pp. Paper. Index. References.
> By a physician, this text includes material on both nor-
> mal and abnormal growth and development of children.
> Chapters cover both physical and psychological growth
> and development. Appendixes cover physical appraisal
> values.

10.8 Mussen, Paul. The Psychological Development of the Child,
3d ed. [Foundations of Modern Psychology Series.]
Englewood Cliffs: Prentice-Hall, 1979.
> 126 pp. Cloth. Index. References.
> A monograph that focuses "on the major theoretical
> and research trends in contemporary developmental
> psychology." (p. xii) Major topics include language
> and cognitive development, personality development,
> and the development of social behavior.

10.9 Roby, Pamela, ed. Child Care, Who Cares? Foreign and
Domestic Infant and Early Childhood Development Policies.
New York: Basic Books, 1973.
> 456 pp. Cloth. Index. Bibliography.

A collection of papers covering: Who Needs Child
Care?; Child Care: A Basic Right; Does the United
States Care?; and A Look Abroad (Sweden, Finland,
Norway, Israel, Japan, Great Britain, and India).
Calls for the U.S. government to provide more child
care services. Appendixes include cost figures, bud-
gets, lists of pertinent journals and organizations. In-
cludes foreword by Shirley Chisholm.

10.10 Spitz, Rene A.; Cobliner, W. Godfrey. The First Year of
Life: A Psychoanalytic Study of Normal and Deviant Development of Object Relations. New York: International Universities Press, 1965.
394 pp. Cloth. Subject and name indexes.
Bibliography.
The author draws on the psychological literature as
well as on his own data through observations to make
statements concerning early child development and the
mother-child relationship. Preface by Anna Freud.

10.11 Stone, L. Joseph; Church, Joseph. Childhood and Adolescence: A Psychology of the Growing Person, 2d ed. New
York: Random House, 1968.
616 pp. Cloth. Index. References. Bibliographies.
An interesting book replete with examples from our
culture, from other cultures, and from case observations. Chapters go into the stages of childhood (birth,
the infant, the toddler, etc.).

10.12 Valadian, Isabelle; Porter, Douglas; et al. Physical Growth
and Development from Conception to Maturity, A Programmed Text. Boston: Little, Brown, 1977.
539 pp. Paper. Index. Bibliography.
Presents the "common core of knowledge that any person providing health services to children, or planning
such services or policies, should have." (p. ix) Makes
extensive use of charts, graphs, tables, diagrams, and
photographs. The first two chapters cover basic principles of growth and development and methods of
assessment. The remaining chapters discuss specific

body systems. Each chapter presents the basic anatomy
and physiology and the developmental changes to be expected and a brief case presentation for practice in interpretation. The index facilitates the use of this programmed text as a reference. Includes tests and the
answers to the tests.

Books for Parents

10.13 Brazelton, T. Berry. Infants and Mothers, Differences in
Development. New York: Delacorte Press/Seymour
Lawrence, 1969.
> 296 pp. Cloth. Index. Bibliography.
> Chapters deal with the first week of life, the newborn's
> equipment, the next three weeks, and then months 2-12
> in separate chapters. Each chapter (except the equip-
> ment chapter) gives background on average, quiet, and
> active babies. Brazelton has written several other in-
> teresting books for parents.

10.14 Ginott, Haim. Between Parent and Child; New Solutions to
Old Problems. New York: Macmillan, 1965.
> 223 pp. Cloth. Index. Bibliography.
> Parental guide for conversing with children designed for
> the mass popular market, and a companion to Between
> Parent and Teenager (10.15). Includes a brief two-page
> appendix on where to go for help (agencies, directories,
> etc.).

10.15 Ginott, Haim. Between Parent and Teenager. New York:
Macmillan, 1969.
> 256 pp. Cloth. Index. Bibliography.
> Companion volume to Between Parent and Child (10.14).
> Emphasis is on dealing with adolescents. Gives situa-
> tional examples as guides for dealing with teenagers,
> just as Between Parent and Child gives similar exam-
> ples relating to younger children.

10.16 Leach, Penelope. Babyhood, Stage by Stage, from Birth to

Age Two: How Your Baby Develops Physically, Emotionally, Mentally. New York: Knopf, 1976.
344 pp. Cloth. Index. Bibliography.
". . . about being a baby and becoming a toddler. It traces the rapid, varied, but always orderly sequence of changes which take any infant from a helpless parcelled newborn to a roving chattering child." (p. xvi) Includes charts summarizing some chapters.

10.17 Lehane, Stephen. Help Your Baby Learn; 100 Piaget-Based Activities for the First Two Years of Life. Englewood Cliffs: Prentice-Hall, 1976.
205 pp. Cloth. Bibliography.
Contains 100 Piaget-based infant stimulation activities for use by parents to help their newborn to 24-month-old child learn and develop.

10.18 Salk, Lee. What Every Child Would Like His Parents to Know to Help Him with the Emotional Problems of His Everyday Life. New York: McKay, 1972.
239 pp. Cloth. Index.
A question and answer book that addresses many of the questions which come to parents in raising their children. For example, includes chapters on the newborn, toilet training, siblings, death.

10.19 Spock, Benjamin. Baby and Child Care: Completely Revised and Updated for Today's Parents. New York: Hawthorn Books, 1976.
666 pp. Cloth. Index.
Revised edition of The Pocket Book of Baby and Child Care. Also published as The Common Sense Book of Baby and Child Care. The controversial book that guided a whole generation of parents. An excellent reference source for any parent. Centers on newborns and infants, but also deals with puberty and the child through 11 years of age. Points discussed are numbered and in bold type. Cross-indexing between numbers is useful.

10.20 Turtle, William John; Turtle, Lydia Pope. Dr. Turtle's

Babies. Philadelphia: Saunders, 1973.
318 pp. Cloth. Index.
Dr. Turtle was a pediatrician and this book is the out-
growth of his talks and discussion groups with parents
of young children. Entertainingly written, this book is
interspersed with anecdotes and factual information
covering the prenatal period, the child during the first
year of life, and particular problems of young and
older children, i.e., bowel movements, masturbation.

PEDIATRICS

General Sources

Nursing

10.21 Alexander, Mary M.; Brown, Marie Scott. Pediatric History Taking and Physical Diagnosis for Nurses, 2d ed.
New York: McGraw-Hill, 1979.
    529 pp. Cloth. Index. Bibliographies. Glossaries.
The second edition has been expanded to include history
taking and screening tests originally included in Ambulatory Pediatrics for Nurses (10.23). The authors
plan to expand the latter "to deal with common illnesses
in children." (pp. vii-viii) Chapters discuss the physical examination; examination of the various areas:
skin, lymphatic system, eyes, ears, heart, genitalia,
skeletal system, etc.; and the neurologic exam. Includes illustrations and appropriate charts. First edition published as Pediatric Physical Diagnosis for Nurses.

10.22 Broadribb, Violet. Foundations of Pediatric Nursing, 2d ed.
Philadelphia: Lippincott, 1973.
    500 pp. Paper. Index. References.
A basic text which covers pediatric nursing from the
prenatal period to adolescence. Units, often with study
questions, deal with nursing care of children, the hospitalized child, psychosocial development of the child,
the infant, etc. Includes an appendix on pediatric drugs.

234   Child Health

10.23 Brown, Marie Scott; Murphy, Mary Alexander. Ambulatory
       Pediatrics for Nurses. New York: McGraw-Hill, 1975.
           468 pp. Cloth. Index. Bibliographies.
           Discusses history taking, hematology, well-child man-
           agement, screening and diagnosis, growth and develop-
           ment, and common problems. Eleven appendixes con-
           tain such data as nutritional guides, books for children,
           pamphlets and audiovisuals for teaching, and informa-
           tion for parents. Written by two pediatric nurse prac-
           titioners and focuses on preventive pediatrics. Second
           edition due 1980.

10.24 Chinn, Peggy L. Child Health Maintenance: Concepts in
       Family-Centered Care, 2d ed. St. Louis: Mosby, 1979.
           934 pp. Cloth. Index. References.
           This comprehensive pediatric nursing text is divided
           into seven units: Child Health Maintenance; Prenatal
           Development and Care; The Newborn; Infancy and Early
           Childhood; Later Childhood; Adolescence; Serious
           Health Problems During Childhood and Adolescence.
           Stresses specific theory behind nursing practice. Has
           study questions after each chapter.

10.25 Chinn, Peggy L.; Leitch, Cynthia J. Child Health Main-
       tenance: A Guide to Clinical Assessment. St. Louis:
       Mosby, 1974.
           122 pp. Paper. References. Additional resources.
           Primarily for the nursing student and practicing nurse,
           this guide is designed as a learning aid for students
           studying health assessment of the child and as a refer-
           ence source on the care of children. Includes a guide
           for physical assessment; material on immunizations,
           laboratory procedures, etc.; growth and development
           information; home care and hospitalization information;
           information on sexual function; guides for nutritional
           assessment; annotated listing of community and na-
           tional resources. Second edition (1979) not available
           for annotation.

10.26 Chow, Marilyn P.; Durand, Barbara A.; Feldman, Marie N.;
       et al. Handbook of Pediatric Primary Care. New York:
       Wiley, 1979.
       1084 pp. Cloth. Index. References.
       This handbook by four pediatric nurse practitioners is
       designed to bridge the gap between basic nursing texts
       and medical texts which deal with pediatrics. "This
       handbook is designed specifically for use in the clinical
       setting by practicing nurse practitioners who deliver
       comprehensive pediatric primary care from a health-
       oriented, family-centered approach." (pp. vii-viii)
       Divided into two parts: the healthy child (immuniza-
       tion, nutrition, accident prevention, etc.) and the ill
       child (medications, skin, heart, neuromuscular system,
       allergies, etc.). For each category, material is pre-
       sented concisely with ample headings, charts, etc.
       Chapters include lists of other resources (including
       organizations, related books, etc.).

10.27 DeAngelis, Catherine. Pediatric Primary Care, 2d ed.
       Boston: Little, Brown, 1979.
       676 pp. Cloth. Index. References.
       Written by a pediatrician who is also a nurse. This
       book contains specific, pertinent knowledge selected
       from the broad field of pediatrics and is intended for
       non-physician primary health care providers as well as
       primary care physicians. Major section headings are
       Part 1, Data Base (problem-oriented record, physical
       examination, etc.); Part 2, Health Management (nutri-
       tion, immunizations, etc.); Part 3, Common Signs,
       Symptoms and Diseases; and Part 4, Problems of Be-
       havior. Useful for training and as a reference in the
       clinical setting. Title of the first edition was Basic
       Pediatrics for the Primary Health Care Provider.

10.28 Hammar, S. L.; Eddy, Jo Ann. Nursing Care of the Ado-
       lescent. New York: Springer Publishing, 1966.
       232 pp. Paper. Index. Suggested readings.
       A brief book for the nurse involved in care of the ado-
       lescent, problems and their management.

10.29 Hymovich, Debra P. Nursing of Children: A Family-
Centered Guide for Study, 2d ed. Philadelphia: Saunders,
1974.
432 pp. Paper. References.
Uses a workbook or "study guide" approach, i.e., poses
specific questions with space for the student to fill in the
answers. Sheets can also be torn off for separate use.
Presents practical cases relating to the development
of well and ill children.

10.30 Kalafatich, Audrey J., ed. Approaches to the Care of Adolescents. New York: Appleton-Century-Crofts, 1975.
241 pp. Cloth. Index. References. Bibliography.
The focus is on 1) understanding adolescents as they
move toward adulthood, and 2) the therapeutic use of
self with adolescents as they become part of the health
care system. Written for the undergraduate nursing
student, it should also be a helpful reference for a
wider audience. Major topics include the adolescent
stage in life; how teenagers use the health care system;
and specific problem areas such as obesity, venereal
disease, drug abuse, pregnancy, hospitalization, suicide and death. An excellent resource for those who
work with adolescents whose independence, peer group
recognition, and respect for their own identity are
threatened by illness, disability, or other health-
related problems.

10.31 Latham, Helen C.; Heckel, Robert V.; Herbert, Larry J.;
et al. Pediatric Nursing, 3d ed. St. Louis: Mosby, 1977.
605 pp. Cloth. Index. References. Bibliographies.
Divided into two sections: the first one deals with
growth, development, and promotion of the health of
children; the second with the nursing care of the handicapped and ill child. Appendixes include child development tables, and the like.

10.32 Leifer, Gloria. Principles and Techniques in Pediatric
Nursing, 3d ed. Philadelphia: Saunders, 1977.
321 pp. Cloth. Index. References.

This is a selective text rather than a comprehensive
one. It focuses on the growth and development of children in health and illness in terms of the practical aspects of nursing principles needed in order to function
in the clinical setting. This edition expands its treatment of nursing procedures in intensive care units, in-
halation therapy, differences between children and
adults, administration of medicines, and nutrition; and
adds units on cardiopulmonary resuscitation and chest
physiotherapy. Also discusses poison control, oral hygiene, and the adolescent and the needs of parents. Of
particular interest is the new chapter on the pediatric
outpatient and the clinic nurse. Major headings in each
chapter include Principles, Nursing Responsibilities,
Techniques.

10.33   Marlow, Dorothy R. Textbook of Pediatric Nursing, 5th ed.
        Philadelphia: Saunders, 1977.
            949 pp. Cloth. Index. References.
            A basic pediatric nursing text. Arranged broadly by the
            age of the child, e.g., newborn, infant, etc. Includes
            chapters on using the nursing process in caring for chil-
            dren. Teaching aids, including audiovisual media, and
            other information are listed after each chapter.

10.34   Pillitteri, Adele. Nursing Care of the Growing Family: A
        Child Health Text. Boston: Little, Brown, 1977.
            834 pp. Cloth. Index. References.
            Part of the 2-volume set, Nursing Care of the Growing
            Family. The first volume, A Maternal-Newborn Text
            (9.35), focuses on the mother and the newborn; this vol-
            ume centers on the infant, the toddler, and the older
            child.

10.35   Roberts, Florence Bright. Review of Pediatric Nursing,
        2d ed. [Mosby's Comprehensive Review Series.] St. Louis:
        Mosby, 1978.
            213 pp. Paper. References.
            "Comprehensive, but efficient, guide for review of the
            essential elements of pediatric nursing . . . emphasis

. . . on understanding basic pathophysiology and identifying critical details of nursing care." (p. iv)   In
the second edition, new material has been added on
assessment, the high-risk infant, nutrition, ticks and
Rocky Mountain spotted fever, and the battered child.
Has a question and essay answer approach. Questions
are posed and answers are written under them. Chapters are entitled Basic Concepts of Pediatric Care;
Promotion of Health and Prevention of Illness; Special
Needs of the Exceptional Child; Psychological Aspects
of Care; Clinical and Outpatient Care; The Child with
Acute Illness; The Child with Terminal Illness; Common
Dosage Problems, etc. The chapter on dosage first
gives principles and follows with problems and answers
at the end of the chapter.

10.36 Scipien, Gladys M.; Barnard, Martha Underwood; Chard,
Marilyn A.; et al. Comprehensive Pediatric Nursing, 2d ed.
New York: McGraw-Hill, 1979.
1092 pp. Cloth. Index. References. Bibliographies.
A comprehensive approach designed to integrate, discuss, and apply the major content areas essential to
pediatric nursing. These areas include growth; development in children and families; normal and pathophysiology; and the application of the nursing process.
Written for nursing students, practitioners, and educators. A useful reference book, with many charts,
tables, and illustrations.

10.37 Waechter, Eugenia H.; Blake, Florence G.; Lipp, Jane
Phillips, M.D. (medical coordinator). Nursing Care of
Children, 9th ed. Philadelphia: Lippincott, 1976.
834 pp. Cloth. Index. Bibliographies.
Sections include: Introduction to Nursing Care of the
Child; The Newborn; The Infant; The Toddler and the
Preschool Child; Middle Childhood; Puberty and Ado-
lescence. Focuses on normal growth and development,
common and uncommon problems and/or disorders.
Thorough, well-illustrated chapters include situations
for further study. Earlier editions entitled Essentials
of Pediatrics, then Essentials of Pediatric Nursing.

10.38 Whaley, Lucille F.; Wong, Donna L. Nursing Care of Infants and Children. St. Louis: Mosby, 1979.
    1718 pp. Cloth. Index. Bibliography.
    Includes concepts relevant to nursing both well and ill
    children. Units 1 through 9 look at the child and infant
    using a developmental approach to health problems.
    Units 10 through 16 focus on more serious health prob-
    lems that frequently require hospitalization. Has many
    charts, diagrams, photographs, and summaries of con-
    cepts relevant to nursing care.

Medical

10.39 American Academy of Pediatrics, Committee on Standards
of Child Health Care. Standards of Child Health Care, 3d ed.
Evanston: American Academy of Pediatrics, 1977.
    183 pp. Paper. Index. References.
    "This manual is meant to offer guidelines for the deliv-
    ery of quality care rather than to propose rigid cri-
    teria." (Introduction) Chapters cover perinatal care,
    preventive care, care of the child with illness, equip-
    ment and facilities for child health care, use of health
    care personnel who are not physicians, medical records,
    continuing education, the physician and the community,
    and consultations and referrals. Extensive appendixes
    deal with growth charts, emergencies.

10.40 Anyan, Walter R., Jr. Adolescent Medicine in Primary
Care. New York: Wiley, 1978.
    387 pp. Paper. Index. Bibliographies.
    The author, a physician, focuses on the adolescent.
    Parts cover The Organization and Conduct of Adolescent
    Primary Care; Sexual Maturation and Physical Growth:
    A Physiologic Basis for Adolescent Care; and Clinical
    Problems in Adolescence.

10.41 Gellis, Sydney S.; Kagan, Benjamin M. Current Pediatric
Therapy, 8th ed. Philadelphia: Saunders, 1978.
    879 pp. Cloth. Index.

Contains 339 articles prepared by 294 contributors who
are recognized authorities in pediatrics. Chapters
cover Nutrition; Mental and Emotional Disturbances;
Cardiovascular System; Endocrine System; Genitourinary Tract; Muscles; Skin; The Eye; Infectious Diseases; Allergy; Accidents and Emergencies; and the like.

10.42 Green, Morris; Haggerty, Robert J., eds. Ambulatory
Pediatrics II, Personal Health Care of Children in the
Office, 2d ed. Philadelphia: Saunders, 1977.
500 pp. Cloth. Index. References.
Concerned with child health care outside of the hospital.
Three parts include Illnesses and Problems (the longest); Health Promotion (including patient and parent
education); and The Clinician (interviewing, behavior
modification, etc.).

10.43 Hughes, James G. Synopsis of Pediatrics, 5th ed. St.
Louis: Mosby, 1980.
915 pp. Paper. Index. Bibliographies.
A good basic text with both a scientific and clinical
pediatric orientation. Includes chapters on pediatrics
as a discipline, growth and development, specific categories of diseases, child abuse, genetic counseling, etc.
Provides appendixes of blood and cerebrospinal fluid
values and drugs, among others.

10.44 Keay, A. J.; Morgan, D. M.; Stephen, Norah J. Craig's
Care of the Newly Born Infant, 6th ed. New York: Long-
man's, 1978.
508 pp. Paper. Index. Further readings.
Earlier editions by William Stuart McRae Craig. A
British text which gives detailed information relating to
the care of newborns. Chapters discuss the parents,
examining the newborn infant, low birthweight infants,
dyspnea and cyanosis, etc.

10.45 Kempe, C. Henry; Silver, Henry K.; O'Brien, Donough.
Current Pediatric Diagnosis and Treatment, 5th ed.
Los Altos: Lange, 1978.

1102 pp. Paper. Index. References.
Presents basic principles relating to diagnosis and
treatment in pediatrics for medical and nursing students, practitioners in both fields, and other health
professionals. Discusses the physical examination,
growth and development, the newborn, nutrition, adolescence, cardiovascular diseases, orthopedics, poisoning, allergies, etc.

10.46 Rudolph, Abraham M.; Barnett, Henry L.; Einhorn,
Arnold H., eds. Pediatrics, 16th ed. New York:
Appleton-Century-Crofts, 1977.
2198 pp. Cloth. Index. References.
"Concerned with general aspects of normal child growth
and development as well as diseases of infancy and
childhood." (p. xix) Deals with the Health Care System, Assessment and Care of the Child, Development,
Genetics, Allergy, Infections, Metabolism, Skin,
Mouth, Teeth, Gastrointestinal Tract, etc. Very comprehensive. Gives references, explanations of disorders. Fifteenth edition edited by Henry L. Barnett.
Seventeenth edition due 1981.

10.47 Silver, Henry K.; Kempe, C. Henry; Bruyn, Henry B.
Handbook of Pediatrics, 13th ed. Los Altos: Lange, 1980.
735 pp. Paper. Index. Bibliography.
A concise digest of information essential to the diagnosis and management of pediatric disorders. For the
practicing physician and medical student.

10.48 Smith, David W., ed. Introduction to Clinical Pediatrics,
2d ed. Philadelphia: Saunders, 1977.
452 pp. Paper. Index. References.
". . . evolved from a University of Washington, Department of Pediatrics, Student Teaching Synopsis. . ."
(p. ix) Deals with pediatric procedures, drug therapy,
the healthy child, pediatric disorders (i.e., infectious
disease, accident and neglect, endocrine, etc.). Appendixes include growth charts, information on the Denver
Development Screening Test.

10.49 Vaughan, Victor C., III; McKay, R. James, Jr.; Behrman, Richard E. Nelson Textbook of Pediatrics, 11th ed. Philadelphia: Saunders, 1979.
>   2170 pp. Cloth. Index. References.
>   A concise, yet comprehensive, medical text. Helpful for doctors, health professionals, and students who deal with children. Covers every aspect of the field of pediatrics. The senior editor of this and prior editions is Waldo Emerson Nelson.

10.50 Waring, William W.; Jeansonne, Louis O., III. Practical Manual of Pediatrics: A Pocket Reference for Those Who Treat Children. St. Louis: Mosby, 1975.
>   343 pp. Paper. Index.
>   A pocket-sized book with a place for notes at the back and punched holes and perforations for easy removal of pages. An excellent reference source for the pediatric practitioner. Conditions, tests, etc., are printed in bold black type with concise, clear explanations. Uses tables, references in pertinent places.

10.51 Ziai, Mohsen; Janeway, Charles A.; Cooke, Robert E.; eds. Pediatrics, 2d ed. Boston: Little, Brown, 1975.
>   1021 pp. Cloth. Index. References.
>   A basic pediatric text by three physicians. Useful appendixes include differential diagnosis in various situations (i.e., unconsciousness, fever, vomiting, obesity, etc.); information on emergencies, trauma, and poisoning; drug information; laboratory values; data on unusual syndromes.

Specialties and Other Subjects

Cardiology

10.52 Gasul, Benjamin M.; Arcilla, René A.; Lev, Maurice. Heart Disease in Children: Diagnosis and Treatment. Philadelphia: Lippincott, 1966.
>   1363 pp. Cloth. Index. References.

"Primarily a clinical textbook . . . encompassing al-
most all aspects of pediatric cardiology." (Preface)
Gives the prognosis and treatment for many disorders.

Death

10.53   Easson, William M. The Dying Child: The Management of
the Child or Adolescent Who Is Dying. Springfield: Thomas,
1970.
103 pp. Cloth. Index. Bibliography.
A brief book on a difficult subject. Deals with death in
the preschool and school age child and the adolescent.
Includes chapters on the family and the people involved
in treating the dying child.

10.54   Martinson, Ida Marie, ed. Home Care for the Dying Child,
Professional and Family Perspectives. New York: Appleton-
Century-Crofts, 1976.
332 pp. Paper. Index. References.
A very useful book, designed for health professionals
and parents who provide care for terminally ill children
at home. The five sections cover parents' experiences
with dying children at home; nurses' similar experiences; the dying child from the perspective of social
workers and chaplains; technical aspects of medicine
and nursing relating to the dying child; and theoretical
concepts of value to health professionals in this situation.

10.55   Sahler, Olle Jane Z., ed. The Child and Death. St. Louis:
Mosby, 1978.
300 pp. Paper. Index. References.
A collection of papers edited by a physician which covers the child's concept of death, the impact of the fatally ill child on the family, the fatally ill child and the
caregiver, the process after death for the living, ethics
and death education. Contains accounts by parents of
children who are dying or who have died. Includes a
chapter on Books about Death for Children, Young
Adults, and Parents (annotated listing) and lists of

audiovisual materials after some chapters. Based on a symposium held at the University of Rochester Medical Center, September 1977.

Emergencies

10.56 Arena, Jay M.; Bachar, Miriam. Child Safety Is No Accident; A Parents' Handbook of Emergencies. Durham: Duke University Press, 1978.
    292 pp. Cloth. Index.
    Written for parents and others responsible for children as they grow and develop. Includes information on developing a safe life style for children and family, accident prevention, and experience-tested first aid measures. Major headings are Attitudes and Life Styles; Stages of Growth and Development: Hazards and Avoidance; Hazards; Care and Treatment after Injury; Ready Reference Guide. The appendix includes first aid charts.

10.57 Bailey, William Carl, ed. Pediatric Burns. Chicago: Year Book, 1979.
    151 pp. Cloth. Index. References.
    This monograph reports on the Fourth Annual Meeting of the Children's Hospital, Denver, a symposium concerned with the care of burned children. Addresses various issues related to pediatric burn care: metabolic considerations, respiratory concerns, sepsis, topical agents, flammable fabrics, nursing care, psychiatric problems, family considerations, and reconstructive problems. Each chapter has objectives and a self-evaluation quiz.

10.58 Dube, Shiv K.; Pierog, Sophie H., eds. Immediate Care of the Sick and Injured Child. St. Louis: Mosby, 1978.
    309 pp. Paper. Index. References.
    Written for community practitioners to help them improve their care of pediatric emergencies. Part 1 covers the general aspects of emergency services; Part 2

provides an outline for the workup of children with
various symptoms; Part 3 discusses specific emergency
situations (surgical and medical). Five appendixes contain data on procedures, drugs, normal values, and
abbreviations. The outline format in Part 2 includes
the following headings: diagnostic alert, pathophysiology, etiology, workup, and management. A similar
format is used in the specific situations in Part 3.

Endocrinology

10.59 Gardner, Lytt I., ed. Endocrine and Genetic Diseases of
Childhood and Adolescence, 2d ed. Philadelphia: Saunders,
1975.
1404 pp. Cloth. Index. References.
". . . a source of information on the pathophysiology,
diagnosis and therapy of the principal endocrine and
genetic diseases in the pediatric age group." (p. xx)
Chapters deal with growth patterns, pituitary disorders,
sexual disorders, disease states, genetic disorders,
and counseling, etc. Includes appendixes on heights of
boys and girls.

Handicapped Children

10.60 Ayrault, Evelyn West. Growing Up Handicapped: A Guide
for Parents and Professionals to Helping the Exceptional
Child. New York: The Seabury Press, 1977.
216 pp. Cloth. Index. Bibliography.
For parents of handicapped children and the professionals who work with them and their children. Introduces
philosophies basic to raising, training, and handling the
handicapped child through adolescence to adulthood.
Discusses parental responses; family; child's view of
self; discipline; school; play; and other significant topics.
Ten case studies cover children from age 3 months to
16 years and 11 months. Includes a directory of services; local, state, and national offices of a variety of

agencies; and colleges and universities with facilities
for the handicapped.

10.61   Curry, Judith Bickley; Peppe, Kathryn Kluss, eds. Mental
Retardation, Nursing Approaches to Care. St. Louis:
Mosby, 1978.
246 pp. Paper. References.
Presents a series of papers by various authors, including an historical overview of mental retardation nursing; a section on ways for working with mentally re-
tarded persons and their families; and, finally, prevention, identification, and intervention in mental retardation nursing. Each chapter has a brief summary.

10.62   Downey, John A.; Low, Niels L., eds. The Child with
Disabling Illness: Principles of Rehabilitation. Philadelphia: Saunders, 1974.
627 pp. Cloth. Index. References.
A medical text whose major headings include Selected
Chronic Medical Illnesses, Disorders of Neuromuscular
Systems, Disorders of Musculoskeletal Systems and In-
juries, Dentistry, and Psychosocial Aspects. Includes
data for both accurate diagnosis and appropriate care
involving the family to assure a productive life for the
child.

10.63   Siantz, Mary Lou de Leon, ed. The Nurse and the Developmentally Disabled Adolescent. Baltimore: University Park
Press, 1977.
248 pp. Paper. Index. References.
Describes an integrated, comprehensive approach for
nurses and other health care professionals who identify,
plan, and manage problems of the developmentally disabled adolescent. Involves awareness, commitment
toward increasing the quality of life, collaboration, and
interdisciplinary communication as well as knowledge,
skills, and alternative approaches. Contains especially
useful chapters on assessment, teaching plans, legal
aspects, and information from important related discipline areas.

10.64 Steele, Shirley, ed. Nursing Care of the Child with Long-
Term Illness, 2d ed. New York: Appleton-Century-Crofts,
1977.
560 pp. Paper. Index. Bibliographies.
The first part covers the child with a long-term illness
in general and includes a discussion of his perceptions.
The second part goes into the specific illnesses and the
nursing care related to such illnesses. Papers are
clearly written.

Hospitalized Children

10.65 Coffin, Margaret A. Nursing Observations of the Young
Patient. [Foundations of Nursing Series.] Dubuque: Wm. C.
Brown, 1970.
112 pp. Paper. Index. Bibliography.
A brief book designed to help the nurse make meaningful
observations regarding young hospitalized patients.
Chapters include The Young Patient's Family; Nutri-
tional Needs and Responses; Observation of Physical
Responses; Observation of Behavioral Responses; and
Nursing Goals and Problems.

10.66 Hardgrove, Carol B.; Dawson, Rosemary B. Parents and
Children in the Hospital: The Family's Role in Pediatrics.
Boston: Little, Brown, 1972.
276 pp. Cloth. Index. References.
Presents information compiled from questionnaires
which the authors sent to institutions developing programs stressing the psychological and developmental
welfare of children. Discusses actual policies, procedures, and practices of some hospitals. Chapters
cover relations between parents, children, and hospital personnel; living-in by parents and children; hospital planning for parents; facilities; change agents; small
things which hospitals can do to humanize their services
to parents and children; and the future.

10.67 Hofmann, Adele D.; Becker, R. D.; Gabriel, H. Paul. The

Hospitalized Adolescent: A Guide to Managing the Ill and
Injured Youth. New York: The Free Press, 1976.
>249 pp. Cloth. Index. Bibliography.
>A good guide for dealing with the hospitalized adolescent.
>Parts cover Psychodynamic Considerations (illness,
>stress, staff-patient relations, etc.); Basic Manage-
>ment Principles (staff roles, patient care management,
>etc.); and Special Challenges (behavioral problems,
>difficult situations, the adolescent who is dying, etc.).
>Includes case material.

10.68   Klinzing, Dennis R.; Klinzing, Dene G. The Hospitalized
Child: Communication Techniques for Health Personnel.
Englewood Cliffs: Prentice-Hall, 1977.
>168 pp. Paper. Index. Bibliography.
>Written for all those who care for children in hospitals.
>Attempts to "analyze, synthesize, and integrate theory,
>research, and practice from nursing, pediatrics, child
>development, and communication." (p. vii) The goal
>is to help pediatric personnel develop and use appropri-
>ate communicative behaviors and strategies.

10.69   Love, Harold D.; Henderson, Shirley K.; Stewart, Mary K.
Your Child Goes to the Hospital: A Book for Parents.
Springfield: Thomas, 1972.
>103 pp. Paper. Index. References.
>For parents and health professionals working with par-
>ents whose children are in the hospital. Gives an analy-
>sis of the hospitalization procedure (i.e., admission to
>the hospital, etc.) and actual case studies.

10.70   Petrillo, Madeline; Sanger, Sirgay. Emotional Care of Hospitalized Children: An Environmental Approach. Philadelphia: Lippincott, 1972.
>259 pp. Cloth. Index. References. Bibliographies.
>Written by a nursing mental health consultant and a
>liaison child psychiatrist to decrease the gap between
>what is known and what is practiced. It is an "in depth
>guide of just how to deal with common problems" (p. vii)
>of children who are hospitalized. The major sections

cover 1) general knowledge of growth and development; 2) forces of family and culture; 3) human reactions to stress, loss, and separation; and 4) preventive approaches consisting of actual protocols. Uses a systems approach and presents practical, essential knowledge and its direct application to helping the child. For all professionals involved in the management of children. Contains clinical vignettes.

10.71 Plank, Emma N.; Ritchie, Marlene A.. Working with Children in Hospitals: A Guide for the Professional Team, 2d ed., rev. and enl. Cleveland: The Press of Case Western Reserve University, 1971.

> 105 pp. Cloth. Bibliography.
> Examines the psychological effects of hospitalization on the child and suggests practical things which can be done to help the child's growth and development, and relieve anxieties during this time, e.g., drawing, stories, etc. Appendixes include discussions of crafts and experiments; information for parents.

Neurology

10.72 Conway, Barbara Lang. Pediatric Neurologic Nursing. St. Louis: Mosby, 1977.

> 361 pp. Cloth. Index. References.
> By a nurse for the nurse working with pediatric patients. Pulls together into one volume information from many separate sources. Begins with a chapter on Embryonic Development; then covers Physiology; Development of Perception, Integration, and Response; Techniques in Assessment; Static and Developmental Lesions; Genetic and Metabolic Anomalies; Disorders of Neuromuscular Apparatus; Paroxysmal Disorders; Crises in Integrity; Infections and Invasive Disorders; and Adaptive Problems in School and Learning.

10.73 Jabbour, J. T.; Duenas, Danilo A.; Gilmartin, Richard G., Jr.; et al. Pediatric Neurology Handbook, 2d ed. [Medical

Handbooks.] Flushing, N.Y.: Medical Examination, 1976.
521 pp. Paper. Index. Bibliography.
A ready resource that is reasonably comprehensive. Complements existing texts. Includes, among other topics, general aspects of developmental neurology; neurological assessment (infant and child); and major presenting problems: infection, headache, metabolic, systemic, degeneration, and so forth. The appendixes contain charts of normal values and other helpful information.

Newborn

10.74 Aladjem, Silvio; Brown, Audrey K., eds. Perinatal Intensive Care. St. Louis: Mosby, 1977.
447 pp. Cloth. Index. References.
The three major sections contain authoritative essays by various leaders on a wide range of perinatal topics: organization, research, the changing role of the nurse, patient care, and specific problems of this now well-defined medical specialty. Contributors are from obstetrics, pediatrics, anesthesiology, nursing, internal medicine, genetics, radiology, endocrinology, and sociology. For practicing physicians and residents in obstetrics, pediatrics, anesthesiology, and nursing and medical students.

10.75 Klaus, Marshall H.; Fanaroff, Avroy A. Care of the High-Risk Neonate, 2d ed. Philadelphia: Saunders, 1979.
437 pp. Cloth. Index. Bibliography.
A teaching manual using a physiological approach to neonatal care, specifically the care of the fetus and newborn who is sick or at risk. For house officers, nurses, medical students, and pediatricians. Each chapter contains case material and questions to assist application. Not an introductory or a comprehensive text, since it covers major principles only. Considers controversial issues.

10.76   Moore, Mary Lou. The Newborn and the Nurse.
[Saunders Monographs in Clinical Nursing, 3.] Philadelphia:
Saunders, 1972.
290 pp. Cloth. Index. Bibliographies.
Includes chapters on the unborn infant, the newborn,
the healthy and the abnormal newborn, nutrition of newborns, and others.

10.77   Roberts, Florence Bright; Chapman, Judy Cox. Perinatal
Nursing: Care of Newborns and Their Families. New York:
McGraw-Hill, 1977.
282 pp. Paper. Index. References. Bibliographies.
Follows the normal infant from fetus to birth to care
after birth. Chapters also deal with the high-risk infant, the preterm infant, and the infant with other problems (e.g., hyperbilirubinemia and the like). Has a
chapter on the infant's family.

10.78   Schwartz, Jane Linker; Schwartz, Lawrence H., eds.
Vulnerable Infants: A Psychosocial Dilemma. New York:
McGraw-Hill, 1977.
378 pp. Paper. Index. References.
A collection of papers, some reprinted from other
sources, which relate to those interested in "the outcome of pregnancy and/or the subsequent growth and
development of children." (p. xiii) After an introduction, chapters explore Psychosocial Aspects of High-
Risk Pregnancy (e.g., poverty, pregnancy in young
girls); The Crisis of Premature Birth; Effects of Separation on Mother-Infant Bonding; Sequelae (death,
child abuse, low birthweight infants, etc.); Critical
Issues in Comprehensive Care for Mothers and Infants
(the pregnant adolescent, neonatal mortality, newborn
intensive care, euthanasia, etc.).

The Nurse Practitioner

10.79   deCastro, Fernando J.; Rolfe, Ursula T.; Drew, Janice
Kocur; et al. The Pediatric Nurse Practitioner: Guidelines
for Practice, 2d ed. St. Louis: Mosby, 1976.

211 pp. Paper. Index. Bibliographies.
". . . to fill the need for a textbook outlining the training of pediatric nurse practitioners." (p. v) This edition has new chapters on working with parents from the
standpoint of nursing educators, neonatology, hematology, parasitology, and a longer chapter on school health.

Nutrition

10.80 Martin, Ethel Austin; Beal, Virginia A. Roberts' Nutrition
Work with Children, 4th ed. Chicago: University of Chicago
Press, 1978.
312 pp. Cloth. Index. References.
Chapters discuss the definition of nutrition, assessing
nutritional status of children, measurement and standards of growth, developing good nutritional status,
poor nutrition, improving children's nutrition, nutrition programs in schools, nutrition education, etc.
First two editions by Lydia J. Roberts.

10.81 Pipes, Peggy L., ed. Nutrition in Infancy and Childhood.
St. Louis: Mosby, 1977.
205 pp. Paper. Index. References. Additional
readings.
The author, a registered dietitian and master's in public health at the University of Washington, has written
this book for health science students. It contains theoretical nutrition information, including factors in evaluating dietary intakes and planning to resolve nutritional
concerns. Chapters 1 through 4 are a review of nutrition in growth and development and include the recommended nutrient intakes for children. Chapters 5
through 11 discuss the development of feeding behaviors,
factors important in assessing nutritional concerns,
and suggestions for their prevention and resolution.
The contents draw on research and on the clinical
experience of both the author and the contributors.

Ophthalmology

10.82 Jan, James E.; Freeman, Roger D.; Scott, Eileen P.
Visual Impairment in Children and Adolescents. New York:
Grune & Stratton, 1977.
418 pp. Cloth. Index. References.
An extremely useful book dealing with vision problems
in children. Chapters address development of the visually impaired child, care of the visually impaired child,
psychiatric considerations, and the like.

Orthopedics

10.83 Hilt, Nancy E.; Schmitt, E. William. Pediatric Orthopedic
Nursing. St. Louis: Mosby, 1975.
248 pp. Cloth. Index. Bibliography. Glossary.
A thorough book on an evolving nursing specialty. Includes chapters on a history of pediatric orthopedic
nursing, the use of various beds, tools, etc., care of
children with specific handicaps, work with parents.

Pathology

10.84 Kissane, John M. Pathology of Infancy and Childhood, 2d ed.
St. Louis: Mosby, 1975.
1207 pp. Cloth. Index. References.
"Organized along conventional lines of special pathology."
(Preface) Covers diseases related to specific body systems (circulatory, reproductive, etc.), and specific
types of diseases (of the blood, etc.).

Psychology and Psychiatry

10.85 Chapman, A. H. The Games Children Play. New York:
Putnam, 1971.

250 pp. Cloth. Index.
This book outlines various unhealthy games which children can play with their parents. Covers situations where parents are manipulated by their children and then discusses the way to deal with such situations effectively. Topics include sibling rivalry, male and female sexual development, drugs, etc.

10.86 Denzin, Norman K. Childhood Socialization: Studies in the Development of Language, Social Behavior, and Identity. [Jossey-Bass Social and Behavioral Science Series.] San Francisco: Jossey-Bass, 1977.
235 pp. Cloth. Index. Bibliography.
A series of essays with a social-psychological perspective on child development and childhood socialization in particular. The book proposes new directions for theory and research. The author uses a symbolic interactionist approach.

10.87 Fagin, Claire M., ed. Nursing in Child Psychiatry. St. Louis: Mosby, 1972.
183 pp. Paper. Index. Footnotes. Bibliographies.
Deals with child psychiatry for the nurse. Chapters by different authors, written specifically for this book, focus on an introduction to child psychiatry, the disturbed latency-aged child (ages 6-11), racism, the adolescent and independence, the family, etc. Each chapter includes an editor's summary.

10.88 French, Alfred P. Disturbed Children and Their Families: Innovations in Evaluation and Treatment. [Child Psychiatry and Psychology Series.] New York: Human Sciences Press, 1977.
333 pp. Cloth. Index. Bibliography.
The author is a child psychiatrist and the book is "a fresh approach to viewing the evaluation and treatment of children and their families in new and creative contexts." (p. 9) Uses a systems and structural approach to family therapy which integrates developmental and stress variables into systematic evaluation in order

to determine the problem of the child and his family.
Includes a thorough guide to the evaluation of children
and families and two examples illustrating the model.
The book should be useful to both learners and practitioners of child and family therapy.

10.89 Samuels, Shirley C. Enhancing Self-Concept in Early Childhood, Theory and Practice. [Early Education Series.]
New York: Human Sciences Press, 1977.
312 pp. Cloth. Author and subject indexes. Annotated
bibliography.
An extensively referenced study about the concept of
self in the early part of childhood. Part 1: Theoretical
Perspective; Part 2: Review of the Empirical Literature; Part 3: Implications of Research Findings for
Teachers. Includes an annotated bibliography of books
for children about death, sex and reproduction, etc.

10.90 Van Eys, Jan, ed. The Normally Sick Child. Baltimore:
University Park Press, 1979.
188 pp. Cloth. Index. References.
Proceedings of a workshop held in Houston, Texas, in
May, 1978, by the Department of Pediatrics of the University of Texas System Cancer Center, M.D. Anderson
Hospital and Tumor Institute. This is the third workshop in a series, whose other two proceedings have been
published as The Truly Cured Child (10.91) and Research
on Children (see Supplement). This workshop's papers
focus on the care of the child with cancer as a "normally
sick" child, since over 50 percent of the children who
are diagnosed with cancer survive and, therefore, should
ideally not have psychological problems regarding the
nature of their illness. Six sections cover   the child
with cancer, the normal needs of the developing child,
treatment of the child with cancer, children with cancer
and their families, group therapy for children with cancer and/or their families, and summary papers. Contributors include psychiatrists, social workers, physicians, parents, theologians, etc.

10.91 Van Eys, Jan, ed. The Truly Cured Child: The New Challenge in Pediatric Cancer Care: Baltimore: University
Park Press, 1977.
>177 pp. Paper. Index. References.
>This monograph reports on a workshop held in March
>1976 by the Department of Pediatrics, University of
>Texas System Cancer Center, Houston, M.D. Anderson
>Hospital and Tumor Institute for all those involved with
>the children, from laboratory worker to patient. The
>possible development of a therapeutic community and a
>future orientation is stressed. The "truly cured child"
>is defined as one free from disease, on a par with
>peers developmentally, and at ease with having had
>cancer. Brief presentations of topics include conflicts
>between patients and the demands of the institution and
>research and between the personal needs of the staff
>and humane patient care. The last section includes in-
>sights by the participants.

Renal Disease

10.92 James, John A. Renal Disease in Childhood, 3d ed.
St. Louis: Mosby, 1976.
>402 pp. Cloth. Index. Bibliographies.
>A clinical text which covers the whole field of renal
>disease in children and related disorders of the urinary
>tract in a concise and practical manner.

Surgery

10.93 Fochtman, Dianne; Raffensperger, John G., eds. Principles of Nursing Care for the Pediatric Surgery Patient,
2d ed. Boston: Little, Brown, 1976.
>327 pp. Paper. Index. Bibliography.
>Stresses the specific nursing care of the child under-
>going surgery. In addition to discussing general nurs-
>ing care, chapters deal with specific problems, e.g.,
>cardiovascular anomalies, eye surgery, burns,

neurosurgery, trauma, tumors, and the like. Tells a little about the condition and then goes into preoperative and postoperative care. First edition by J. G. Raffensperger and R. B. Primrose entitled Pediatric Surgery for Nurses.

PERIODICALS

Growth and Development

10.94 Adolescence. Libra Publishers, Inc., 391 Willets Road, Roslyn Heights, Long Island, N.Y. 11577. Quarterly. 1966 to date.

10.95 Child Development. University of Chicago Press, 5801 Ellis Avenue, Chicago, Ill. 60637. (For the Society for Research in Child Development, Inc. Quarterly. 1930 to date.

10.96 Child Psychiatry and Human Development; An International Journal. Human Sciences Press, 72 Fifth Avenue, New York, N.Y. 10011. Quarterly. 1970 to date.

10.97 Children Today; An Interdisciplinary Journal for the Professions Serving Children. U.S. Children's Bureau, Administration for Children, Youth, and Families, Department of Health, Education and Welfare, Washington, D.C. 20201. Bimonthly. 1954 to date.

10.98 World's Children; International Journal of Child Care and Development. Save the Children Fund, 157 Clapham Road, London S.W. 9, England. Quarterly. 1920 to date.

Lay

10.99 American Baby: For Expectant and New Parents. American Baby, Inc., 575 Lexington Ave., New York, N.Y. 10022. (For the American Association of Maternal and Child Health.) Monthly. 1938 to date.

10.100 Parents' Magazine: On Rearing Children from Crib to
College. Parents' Magazine Enterprises, Inc., 52
Vanderbilt Avenue, New York, N.Y. 10017. Monthly.
1926 to date.

Nursing

10.101 Baby Care. Parents' Magazine Enterprises, Inc., 52
Vanderbilt Avenue, New York, N.Y. 10017. Quarterly.
1970 to date.

10.102 Current Practice in Pediatric Nursing. C.V. Mosby Co.,
11830 Westline Industrial Drive, St. Louis, Mo. 63141.
Annually. 1976 to date.

10.103 Issues in Comprehensive Pediatric Nursing. McGraw-Hill
Book Co., 1221 Avenue of the Americas, New York, N.Y.
10020. Bimonthly. 1976 to date.

10.104 Maternal-Child Nursing Journal. University of Pittsburgh,
Pediatric and Obstetrical Nursing Departments, 3505 Fifth
Avenue, Pittsburgh, Pa. 15213. Quarterly. 1972 to date.

10.105 MCN: American Journal of Maternal Child Nursing.
American Journal of Nursing Company, 10 Columbus
Circle, New York, N.Y. 10019. Bimonthly. 1976 to date.

10.106 Pediatric Nursing. A. Jannetti and Associates, North
Woodbury Road, Pitman, New Jersey 08071. (For the
National Association of Pediatric Nurse Associates and
Practitioners.) Bimonthly. 1975 to date.

Medical

10.107 American Journal of Diseases of Children. American
Medical Association, 535 N. Dearborn Street, Chicago,
Ill. 60610. Monthly. 1911 to date.

10.108   Journal of Pediatrics; Devoted to the Problems and Dis-
         eases of Infancy and Childhood. C.V. Mosby Company,
         11830 Westline Industrial Drive, St. Louis, Mo. 63141.
         Monthly. 1932 to date.

10.109   Pediatric Clinics of North America. W.B. Saunders Com-
         pany, W. Washington Square, Philadelphia, Pa. 19105.
         Quarterly. 1954 to date.

10.110   Pediatrics. American Academy of Pediatrics, Box 1034,
         Evanston, Ill. 60204. Monthly. 1948 to date.

11
Nursing as a Profession

In this chapter, we have grouped books on the nursing profession in general, books on ethics in the nursing and health professions, books on the expanding role of the nurse, health careers, the history of medicine and nursing, legal aspects of nursing, refresher sources, review books, and women in health. Finally, indexes and periodicals on these areas are listed at the end of the chapter.

NURSING PROFESSION

Worldwide

11.1 Abu-Saad, Huda. Nursing: A World View. St. Louis: Mosby, 1979.
> 227 pp. Cloth. Index. References.
> ". . . intended to orient the reader to past, present, and future nursing practices worldwide." (p. v) Parts cover Origins of the Profession; Europe; The Americas; Near and Middle East; Africa; South Pacific. Includes brief historical and educational information for each geographic region. The appendix is a summary of nursing from ancient to modern times.

11.2 Holland, Walter W.; Ipsen, Johannes; Kostrzewski, Jan, eds. Measurement of Levels of Health. [WHO Regional

Publications European Series, no. 7.] Copenhagen: World
Health Organization, 1979.
> 456 pp. Paper. Index. References.
> The text, written in response to the demand for assess-
> ment methods, focuses on the health problems of
> Europe. As defined for this book, "measurement of
> levels of health is taken to include the incidence and
> prevalence of specific diseases and syndromes, and
> measurements of physical and mental conditions as
> well as the social function of individuals and popula-
> tion and their behaviors or attitudes toward health
> and health-related activities." (p. 9)

11.3 Nursing in the World Editorial Committee. Nursing in the
World: The Needs of Individual Countries and Their Pro-
grammes. Tokyo: International Nursing Foundation of
Japan, 1977.
> 359 pp. Cloth.
> Comprehensive material about nursing on an interna-
> tional basis. Contains entries from countries in Asia,
> the Middle East, Africa, the Americas, Europe, and
> Oceania. Each entry includes social background,
> basic nursing education, midwifery and public health
> education, postgraduate education, and other pertinent
> information. Data were obtained from national or-
> ganizations in each country.

United States

11.4 Ashley, Jo Ann. Hospitals, Paternalism, and the Role of
the Nurse. [Nursing Education Monographs.] New York:
Teachers College Press, 1976.
> 158 pp. Cloth. Index. Footnotes. Bibliography.
> An historical study of the role of nursing in the health
> care environment. The author states that this book
> "which examines discriminatory attitudes toward
> women, can provide both nurses and the public with an
> explanation of why nurses have had so little influence
> on hospital management." (p. x) Chapters include

Hospitals as Schools, Students or Laborers?, Sexism in the Hospital Family, and Nursing and Health Care.

11.5 Auld, Margaret E.; Birum, Linda Hulthen; eds. The Challenge of Nursing: A Book of Readings. St. Louis: Mosby, 1973.

> 247 pp. Paper. References. Bibliographies.
> A collection of papers, mostly reprinted from other sources, by nurses, physicians, educators, students, sociologists, philosophers, researchers, etc., which are designed to give the reader a broad view of the nursing profession. Articles are grouped into five units: introduction, illness, the nursing process, helping the patient, and quality care.

11.6 Benner, Patricia; Benner, Richard V. The New Nurse's Work Entry: A Troubled Sponsorship. New York: Tiresias Press, 1979.

> 160 pp. Cloth. Index. References.
> This monograph reports results of a survey of new nurses, nurse educators, and nursing service personnel on the competencies they expect of new nurses and the discrepancies that exist in the real world. Recommendations speak to activities that can be undertaken by each group to improve the situation.

11.7 Bullough, Bonnie; Bullough, Vern, eds. Expanding Horizons for Nurses. [Issues in Nursing Series, vol. 3.] New York: Springer Publishing, 1977.

> 360 pp. Paper. Index. References. Footnotes.
> Addresses some of the issues of importance to nursing and society today. Included in four parts are articles by various people, usually reprinted from other sources. The expanding nursing profession (e.g., independent practice, nurse midwives); clinical issues in nursing (abortion, mental illness, etc.); legislation and nursing (institutional licensure, labor relations); education for nursing (external degrees, physical diagnosis); and women's liberation.

(sex discrimination, doctor-nurse interactions) are the major themes discussed. Continues <u>New Directions for Nurses</u>.

11.8   Chaska, Norma L., ed. The Nursing Profession: Views Through the Mist. New York: McGraw-Hill, 1978.
  443 pp. Paper. Index. Bibliographies.
  A collection of largely original papers that reflects on the present status of nursing as a profession and provides a base for future planning. Seven parts deal with critical aspects for the nursing profession: professionalism, education, research, theory, practice, interdisciplinary professions, the future in nursing. Part 8 is a summary with questions. Each paper includes editor's questions for discussion. A resource text for both professional nurses and students.

11.9   Davis, Marcella Z.; Kramer, Marlene; Strauss, Anselm L., eds. Nurses in Practice: A Perspective on Work Environments. St. Louis: Mosby, 1975.
  273 pp. Paper. References.
  A collection of clinical experiences by different authors dealing with nurses' work in various environments under various circumstances. This book does not deal with the morality of the care given in any instance, but is seen as a way of examining the delivery of appropriate health care. Two parts explore situations in the hospital (the head nurse, death, pain, the intensive care unit, the pediatric ward, etc.), and situations out of the hospital (clinics, public health nursing, etc.). Each chapter includes discussion questions.

11.10   DeYoung, Lillian. The Foundations of Nursing, As Conceived, Learned, and Practiced in Professional Nursing, 3d ed. St. Louis: Mosby, 1976.
  302 pp. Paper. Index. Suggested readings.
  Deals with many aspects of the profession of nursing, including points of interest to a person just entering nursing (responsibilities, relationships, student

organizations, etc.); developments in nursing (trends
in nursing service and nursing education, future de-
velopments); and, finally, legal aspects, professional
organizations, goals, etc. Appendixes include ANA's
Code for Nurses with Interpretive Statements, ANA's
Educational Preparation for Nurse Practitioners and
Assistants to Nurses, ANA's Standards and Assess-
ment Factors for Organized Nursing Services, and
Abstract for Action: Recommendations from Lysaught's
Report.

11.11 Entry into Nursing Practice. Proceedings of the National
Conference, February 13-14, 1978, Kansas City, Missouri.
Kansas City: American Nurses' Association, 1978.
  163 pp. Paper. Bibliography.
  In 1965 the American Nurses' Association statement,
  Educational Preparation for Nurse Practitioners and
  Assistants to Nurses, recommended two categories
  of nurse manpower in order to improve the quality of
  education for nursing. Since much remains to be done
  in this area, this conference was held in 1978. Proceedings include papers relating to the nursing profession and entry into practice; reports from groups like
  the National League for Nursing and the Southern Regional Education Board; results of small group discussions. Appendixes give a list of participants, resolu-
  tions on entry into nursing practice, etc.

11.12 Hall, Virginia C. Statutory Regulation of the Scope of Nursing Practice—A Critical Survey. Chicago: National Joint
Practice Commission, 1975.
  51 pp. Paper. Footnotes.
  The National Joint Practice Commission was formed
  by the American Medical Association and the American
  Nurses' Association in 1972 to study the roles of the
  medical and nursing professions. This brief document
  includes some background, sections on nurse practice
  acts and medical practice acts, attempts to see the two
  types of acts together, and calls for further study of
  the roles of the two professions vis-à-vis delivery of
  health care.

11.13 Hardy, Margaret E.; Conway, Mary E. Role Theory, Perspectives for Health Professionals. New York: Appleton-
Century-Crofts, 1978.
>354 pp. Cloth. Index. Bibliography.
>Examines roles in nursing and the health profession in
>an attempt to stimulate the reader to a greater knowl-
>edge of the nursing role relative to others. Chapters
>by different authors discuss role theory in general,
>roles in different work situations, the socialization
>process, attitudes toward roles, etc.

11.14 Kelly, Lucie Young. Dimensions of Professional Nursing,
3d ed. New York: Macmillan, 1975.
>573 pp. Cloth. Index. Annotated bibliographies.
>This book gives "an overview of the nonclinical aspects
>of nursing in sufficient detail to be adaptable for use at
>all stages in all types of preservice programs in pro-
>fessional nursing and in continuing education." (p. v)
>Four parts address the history of professional nurs-
>ing; professional nursing as it is now; nursing relative
>to society, religion, and the law; and nursing organi-
>zations and careers. Previous editions by C.W. Kelly.

11.15 Lysaught, Jerome P. Action in Nursing, Progress in Professional Purpose. New York: McGraw-Hill, 1974.
>368 pp. Paper. References. Suggested readings.
>Consists of journal articles, reprinted from other
>sources, and pamphlets outlining many of the state-
>ments and positions taken by the National Commission
>for the Study of Nursing and Nursing Education after
>publication of An Abstract for Action (11.16). Papers
>are organized around seven parts: The Report and Its
>Implementation; Reviews, Critiques, and Commen-
>taries; Research in Nursing Practice; Emerging Pat-
>terns in Nursing Practice; Emerging Patterns in Nurs-
>ing Education; Emerging Patterns in Nursing Careers;
>and Toward the Future in Nursing.

11.16 Lysaught, Jerome P.; National Commission for the Study of
Nursing and Nursing Education. An Abstract for Action.
New York: McGraw-Hill, 1970.

167 pp. Cloth. Footnotes. Glossary.
Reports the results of a study conducted by the National Commission for the Study of Nursing and Nursing Education from 1967 to 1970. The study dealt with
the entire field of nursing, its components, scope,
role in health care delivery, nursing education, and
nursing as a career. Includes recommendations for
the nursing field.

11.17 Lysaught, Jerome P.; National Commission for the Study of
Nursing and Nursing Education. An Abstract for Action:
Appendices. New York: McGraw-Hill, 1971.
509 pp. Cloth.
Appendixes document some of the recommendations in
the original document (11.16).

11.18 Lysaught, Jerome P.; National Commission for the Study of
Nursing and Nursing Education. From Abstract into Action.
New York: McGraw-Hill, 1973.
363 pp. Paper. Footnotes.
Covers implementation of recommendations by the
National Commission for the Study of Nursing and
Nursing Education. Chapters address changes in
nursing organizationally, in the nursing role, in nurs-
ing education, in career development and the like.

11.19 Miller, Michael H.; Flynn, Beverly C.; eds. Current Perspectives in Nursing; Social Issues and Trends. [Current
Practice and Perspectives in Nursing Series.] St. Louis:
Mosby, 1977.
174 pp. Cloth. References.
Focuses on selected social issues in nursing. Includes contributions by experts in "the analysis of the
various forces influencing innovations and change in
nursing." (p. x) Part 1: Ethical Issues; Part 2: Research Issues; Part 3: Issues in Health Care Delivery; Part 4: Issues in Nursing Organization; and
Part 5: Educational Issues.

11.20 Notter, Lucille E.; Spalding, Eugenia Kennedy. Professional
Nursing: Foundations, Perspectives, and Relationships,
9th ed. Philadelphia: Lippincott, 1976.

475 pp. Paper. Index. Bibliographies.
Parts include The Profession of Nursing and Its
Social Setting: Past and Present; Professional, Per-
sonal, and Legal Problems and Relationships; Survey
of Nursing Opportunities; Choosing, Preparing for and
Succeeding in a Field of Nursing; Organizations and
Related Activities (national and international). A basic
text for the nurses' professional development. First
published under the title Professional Adjustments in
Nursing.

11.21   Nursing Development Conference Group. Concept Formali-
zation in Nursing: Process and Product, 2d ed. Edited by
Dorothea E. Orem. Boston: Little, Brown, 1979.
313 pp. Cloth. Index. References.
Presents the further development of the conceptual
structure of nursing in two main sections: an orientation to nursing knowledge and formulations regarding the
structure of nursing knowledge. Uses Orem's general
theory of nursing as a framework and contains useful
summaries of selected nursing theorists from Nightingale to Roy.

11.22   Rowland, Howard S.; Rowland, Beatrice L. The Nurse's
Almanac. Germantown, Md.: Aspen Systems, 1978.
844 pp. Cloth. Index. Footnotes. Glossary.
An extensive reference volume in all areas of the nursing profession. Thirty-eight chapters deal with all
aspects: health care expenditures, jobs and employment for nurses, administration in nursing, professional standards review organization (PSRO), unioni-
zation in nursing, education in nursing, licensing, the
law and nursing, doctors, physician's assistants,
health maintenance organizations (HMO), patients'
rights, the aged patient, males in nursing, and many,
many more.

11.23   Sims, Lillian M.; Lindberg, Janice B. The Nurse Person:
Developing Perspectives for Contemporary Nursing. New
York: Harper & Row, 1978.
243 pp. Cloth. Subject and name indexes. References.

For baccalaureate nursing students as they explore the
role of the professional nurse. Section 1, The Nurse
Person, looks at desirable personal attributes. Section 2, Thinking as a Primary Skill, emphasizes con-
ceptualizing, problem solving, and creative thinking.
Section 3, Communicating as a Human Skill, Section 4,
Facilitating Growth in Self and Others, Section 5,
Reality Issues, and Section 6, Challenges for the Future, all assist students in exploring the world of nursing and their individual places in it.

ETHICS

11.24   Annas, George J.; Glantz, Leonard H.; Katz, Barbara F.
Informed Consent to Human Experimentation: The Subject's
Dilemma. Cambridge: Ballinger, 1977.
    333 pp. Cloth. Index. Bibliography.
    This book "traces and analyzes the legal system's ef-
    forts to articulate the law of informed consent to human
    experimentation for various types of research and with
    various types of subjects." (p. xii) The authors are
    lawyers. Provides a single, comprehensive source
    for both lawyer and layperson. Topics include re-
    search with children; prisoners; fetal research; psycho-
    surgery; and compensation for harm. The appendixes
    contain the Nuremburg Code, the Declaration of
    Helsinki, the American Medical Association's Ethical
    Guidelines for Clinical Investigation, and others.

11.25   Bermosk, Loretta Sue; Corsini, Raymond J., eds. Critical
Incidents in Nursing. Philadelphia: Saunders, 1973.
    369 pp. Cloth. Index.
    Consists of 38 incidents submitted by anonymous nurses
    in which, for one reason or another, the nurses were
    not happy with the outcomes. For each incident, the
    editors give background information and a description
    of the incident, followed by a discussion on the part of
    consultants, including nurses, theologians, social
    workers, educators, physicians, psychiatrists, and
    the like. Each discussion is signed by the specific

consultant writing it. The 38 incidents are grouped
into six sections: The Nurse and the Patient; The
Nurse and Her Peers; The Nurse and the Doctor; The
Nurse and the Family; The Nurse and Supervision;
and The Nurse and the System.

11.26 Davis, Anne J.; Aroskar, Mila A. Ethical Dilemmas and
Nursing Practice. New York: Appleton-Century-Crofts,
1978.
238 pp. Paper. Subject and author indexes.
References.
Aims to increase the awareness of students and graduates alike regarding bioethics in health science and
nursing practice. After a general overview and discussion of traditional approaches, professional ethics,
and institutional constraints, the book focuses on
selected ethical issues.

11.27 Fuchs, Victor R. Who Shall Live? Health, Economics,
and Social Choice. New York: Basic Books, 1974.
168 pp. Cloth. Index. References.
By a medical economist, this intriguing, readable
book explores some of the current issues and problems
in health and medical care. For the lay reader as well
as the health professional. Chapters address Who
Shall Live?; The Physician: The Captain of the Team;
The Hospital: The House of Hope; Drugs: The Key to
Modern Medicine; Paying for Medical Care; and Health
and Social Choice.

11.28 Steele, Shirley M.; Harmon, Vera M. Values Clarification
in Nursing. New York: Appleton-Century-Crofts, 1979.
153 pp. Paper. Index. References. Bibliographies.
Primarily intended for the undergraduate nursing student, this volume deals with the process of values
clarification. Discusses a hypothetical theory of
ethics and poses situations requiring ethical decisions.
Chapters include Medical and Nursing Codes; Morals
and Moral Inquiry; Human Experimentation and
Informed Consent; Euthanasia and Allowing to Die;
Individual Rights; etc.

11.29 Walters, LeRoy, ed. Bibliography of Bioethics. Detroit:
Gale Research, 1975-79.
> 5 vols. Cloth. Title and author indexes.
> A systematic study of value questions which arise in
> the biomedical and behavioral fields. Includes such
> topics as   health care ethics; research ethics; reason-
> able public policies/guidelines for health care deliv-
> ery; and biomedical and behavioral research. At-
> tempts "to identify the central issues of bioethics, to
> develop index language appropriate to the field, and to
> provide comprehensive, cross-disciplinary coverage of
> current English language materials on bioethical topics."
> (p. 3) Lists subject matter consultants, journals cited,
> bioethics thesaurus, subject entries, cross-disciplinary
> fields, print and non-print materials. An ongoing re-
> search project of the Kennedy Institute, Center for
> Bioethics.

11.30 Wojcik, Jan. Muted Consent: A Casebook in Modern Medi-
cal Ethics. [Science and Society: A Purdue University
Series in Science, Technology, and Human Values, vol. 1.]
West Lafayette: Purdue University, Purdue Research
Foundation, 1978.
> 164 pp. Paper. Index. References.
> Explores ethical issues raised by the increasing capa-
> bilities of the medical professions. Covers Experi-
> mentation on Human Subjects; Genetic Counseling and
> Screening; Abortion; Behavior Control; Death and Dy-
> ing; Allocation of Scarce Medical Resources; The
> Eugenic Medicine of the Future Through In Vitro Fer-
> tilization; Genetic Surgery; and Cloning. The begin-
> ning of each chapter examines three fictional cases
> which illustrate ethical dilemmas.

EXPANDING ROLE OF THE NURSE

11.31 Bliss, Ann A.; Cohen, Eva D., eds. The New Health
Professionals: Nurse Practitioners and Physician's Assistants. Germantown: Aspen Systems, 1977.

451 pp. Cloth. Index. References.
The term new health practitioners refers to "midlevel
health practitioners who perform tasks which traditionally have been within the purview of physicians."
(p. 1) The focus is on nurse practitioners and physician's assistants. The five parts: New Health Practitioners; Major Determinants of Practice; NHP Clinical Impact; Evaluative Research on NHP's; Issues and
Conclusions: The Next to Last Word? Appendixes include guidelines for training of physician's assistants
by the American Medical Association, guidelines for
training nurse practitioners from the Nurse Training
Act of 1975, information on legislation for physician's
assistants in 38 states, encounter form for new patient
visit, etc.

11.32 Jacox, Ada K.; Norris, Catherine M., eds. Organizing for
Independent Nursing Practice. New York: Appleton-
Century-Crofts, 1977.
270 pp. Paper. Index. References.
The proceedings of a national invitational conference
held in 1975 at the University of Iowa College of Nursing for independent nurse practitioners. After an overview of the participants and the conference, chapters
address the independent nurse practitioner concept,
forming relationships with other professionals, getting
started, the independent nurse practitioner nationally,
and future directions. Papers include personal experiences of the authors and, often, discussion from
other conference participants. Appendixes give
data from a profile of the participants.

11.33 Kinlein, M. Lucille. Independent Nursing Practice with
Clients. Philadelphia: Lippincott, 1977.
200 pp. Cloth. Index.
Based on the author's own experiences with an independent nursing practice, this book combines theory
and practice. Chapters explore nursing in the past

and the future, initiation of change, setting up independent nursing practice, the philosophy of the nursing
physical exam, general impressions of the author
after having an independent nursing practice, and the
like. The appendix has a discussion of specific client
examples.

11.34 Kohnke, Mary F.   The Case for Consultation in Nursing:
Designs for Professional Practice. New York: Wiley,
1978.
>185 pp. Cloth. Index. Footnotes. Bibliography.
Discusses the professional nurse today, the clinical
nurse specialist, and the clinical nurse consultant.
The author stresses the difference between "nurse
technicians" and professional nurses and urges that
the profession move toward the latter as opposed to
the former. Includes outlines of professional practice
models for several kinds of health care institutions.

11.35 Kohnke, Mary F.; Zimmern, Ann; Greenidge, Jocelyn A.
Independent Nurse Practitioner. Garden Grove, Calif.:
Trainex Press, 1974.
>180 pp. Cloth. Index. Footnotes. Bibliography.
The three authors, all nurses, have operated an independent nursing practice in New York since 1972. In
this book, they address points such as: the general
concept of an independent practice, location of such a
practice, the legal implications of independent nursing
practice, accountability, advocacy, and the future of
independent nursing practice. Appendixes include information on Nurse Practice Acts in the United States,
American Nurses Code of Ethics, and examples of
various forms (e.g., health history, prescriptions,
etc.).

11.36 Maas, Meridean; Jacox, Ada K. Guidelines for Nurse
Autonomy/Patient Welfare. New York: Appleton-Century-
Crofts, 1977.
>352 pp. Paper. Index. References. Bibliography.
Describes a group of nurses who are performing

independent nursing within an existing organization.
Has four parts: Nurses as Aspiring Professionals;
The Pursuit of Autonomy; The Impact of Nurse Autonomy on Others; Significance of the Nurses' Activities
for the Profession. Appendixes include case study
material, peer review documents, etc.

11.37 Rotkovitch, Rachel, ed. Quality Patient Care and the Role
of the Clinical Nursing Specialist. New York: Wiley,
1976.
189 pp. Cloth. Index. Footnotes. Bibliographies.
A series of chapters by various contributors and clinical nurse specialists at Long Island Jewish-Hillside
Medical Center. Addresses the concept of the clinical
nursing specialist in general and then examines specific areas of operation of such a specialist, e.g.,
psychiatry, medical-surgical, pediatrics, obstetrics,
home health, etc. Contributors give historical perspective on their role and the development of their
duties and responsibilities.

11.38 Zahourek, Rothlyn; Leone, Dolores M.; Lang, Frank J.
Creative Health Services: A Model for Group Nursing
Practice. St. Louis: Mosby, 1976.
142 pp. Paper. Annotated bibliography.
Relates the progress of a group of nurses who were
engaged in independent practice. The chapters deal
with setting up the organization, developing it, and
evaluating it. The authors also share recommendations for others who may be interested in similar endeavors. Appendixes include accounting information.

HEALTH CAREERS

11.39 FIND, Financial Information National Directory/'72. Health
Careers. Chicago: American Medical Association, 1972.
232 pp. Paper.
A source for locating funds for careers in health
fields. Separates funds by federal, national, state

(alphabetically by state), and minorities. For each
funding source, gives title, type, qualifications (including specialties, financial need, tests, other criteria), amount of money, length of time, where to
write for further information, etc.

11.40   Frederickson, Keville. Opportunities in Nursing. Louis-
ville: Vocational Guidance Manuals, 1977.
148 pp. Cloth. Index.
Describes nursing, its educational programs, job opportunities, and its professional organizations. Includes names and addresses of nursing associations
and state boards of nursing. Written for high school
students and beginning nursing students.

11.41   Naseem, Attia; Mustafa, Kamil. Medical Careers Planning:
A Comprehensive Guidance Manual on World-Wide Opportunities for Education, Training, Employment, and Financial
Assistance in All Fields of Medicine and Allied Health Professions. Scarsdale: Bureau of Health & Hospital Careers
Counseling, 1975.
872 pp. Cloth. Index. Bibliography.
A comprehensive information source for career planning in medicine and allied health. Divided into two
sections. Career Guidance for the Intending Physician,
Section One, gives the reader factual information concerning licensing of physicians from premedical study
on. Includes information on medical education in the
United States and abroad. Appendixes include hospitals with bed capacity of over 100 beds, a listing of
major allied health and medical careers with addresses
of referral agencies, lists of pharmaceutical companies in North America, and the like. Section Two
deals in general with health organizations and health
careers and then gives basic information on many,
many health careers. Includes duties, education,
necessary to pursue such careers. Appendixes list
organizations for health professions, films dealing
with health careers, etc.

11.42 Nursing Opportunities, 1979: Guide to Professional Hospital
Employment. Oradell, N.J.: RN Magazine, Medical Economics Co., 1979.

      300 pp. Paper. Geographical index.
      "A complete national reference guide to positions now
available for registered nurses in more than 1000
voluntary, proprietary, city, state, and Federal hospitals and the U.S. Armed Forces." (p. 1) Includes
information on how to find a job, licensure, the interview. Hospital listings comprise the large majority of
this compilation. For each hospital, gives information
as to unique features, address, contact person, accreditation, facilities, benefits, and the like. Comes
out every year.

11.43 Nursing 79 Career Directory. Horsham, Pa.: Intermed
Communications, 1979.

      240 pp. Paper. Advertisers' index.
      Published every year, this resource contains adver-
tisements of hospitals arranged by geographic area
(New England, Mid-Atlantic, etc.). For each hospital gives pictures, salary, specialties, continuing
education opportunities, other information. Also includes cultural and recreational information on each
region, information on locating jobs, writing resumes,
interviews, letters of application, licensure, associations, and the like.

11.44 Occupational Outlook Handbook, 1978-79 ed.   U.S. Depart-
ment of Labor, Bureau of Labor Statistics, Bulletin 1955.
Washington, D.C.: Superintendent of Documents, U.S.
Government Printing Office, 1978.

      825 pp. Paper. Dictionary of Occupational Titles
(D.O.T.) Index. Index to occupations and industries.
Bibliography.
      A major source of vocational information for hundreds
of occupations, including nursing and other health professions. Gives some idea of what the job entails, the
training needed, and job availability information.
Gives general job seeking information, local job

information sources. Inexpensive reprints can be purchased concerning the occupations covered from the
Superintendent of Documents using the number designated. Occupations are grouped into 42 sections, one
of which is Health Occupations. A companion to this
Handbook is the Occupational Outlook Quarterly.

HISTORY OF MEDICINE

11.45 Morton, Leslie T. A Medical Bibliography (Garrison &
Morton), An Annotated Check-List of Texts Illustrating the
History of Medicine, 3d ed. Philadelphia: Lippincott, 1970.
  872 pp. Cloth. Index.
  Contains 7,534 entries organized chronologically according to major medical subjects (e.g., biology,
  toxicology, tumors in general, diseases of the genitourinary system). Annotations show the significance of
  the contributions described in the reference cited.
  Useful for researchers, librarians, historians of medicine, students, and others. Second edition entitled
  Garrison and Morton's Medical Bibliography, compiled by Fielding H. Garrison with revisions, addi-
  tions, and annotations by Leslie T. Morton.

11.46 Strauss, Maurice B., ed. Familiar Medical Quotations.
Boston: Little, Brown, 1968.
  968 pp. Cloth. Author and subject indexes.
  Bibliography.
  Includes more than 7,000 quotations, arranged by
  category and listing the source of each where possible.
  Quotes from physicians, patients, scientists, laymen,
  philosophers, clergymen, playwrights, poets, and
  others contribute to the historic picture of medicine.

HISTORY OF NURSING

11.47 Deloughery, Grace L. History and Trends of Professional
Nursing, 8th ed. St. Louis: Mosby, 1977.

277 pp. Paper. Index. References.
This book emphasizes the portions of history with the
greatest impact upon the modern nurse. Discusses
trends that stem from historical material. The recurring theme is the parallel evolution of the role of
women and the modern professional nurse in Western
society. Includes a separate section on Legal Aspects
of the Nursing Profession by Eileen A. O'Neil, J.D.
Has summaries for each chapter. Seventh edition by
Gerald J. Griffin and Joanne K. Griffin.

11.48   Dolan, Josephine A. Nursing in Society: A Historical Perspective, 14th ed. Philadelphia: Saunders, 1978.
402 pp. Cloth. Index. References. Readings.
A systematic yet concise history of nursing for the
student and practitioner. It describes the "evolution,
emergence, and expansion of nursing from a simple
skill to a complex profession." (p. v) Not a chronological account, but rather an interpretation of the responses of nurses to the needs of people in health and
illness against the societal setting and cultural and
scientific background of history. Each chapter has a
helpful summary. Twelfth edition entitled History of
Nursing.

11.49   Fitzpatrick, M. Louise, ed. Historical Studies in Nursing:
Papers Presented at the 15th Annual Stewart Conference on
Research in Nursing, March, 1977. New York: Teachers
College Press, 1978.
130 pp. Cloth. Bibliography.
The importance of historical research in nursing is
reflected in the opening address, comments on the research process, and the reports of several historical
research projects.

11.50   Flanagan, Lyndia, comp. One Strong Voice: The Story of
the American Nurses' Association. Kansas City, Mo.:
American Nurses' Association, 1976.
692 pp. Cloth. Index. Bibliographies.
A history of the American Nurses' Association from

its inception in 1896 to 1976. Includes texts of
speeches at annual meetings by past ANA presidents.
Appendixes cover a chronological listing of ANA activities, and ANA's stand on national health insurance
and other issues, and the like.

11.51   Kalisch, Philip A.; Kalisch, Beatrice J.   The Advance of
American Nursing.   Boston: Little, Brown, 1978.
757 pp.   Cloth.   Index.   References.   Bibliography.
Gives the historical background of the nursing profession with a view to understanding modern nursing.   Begins with Hippocrates and Florence Nightingale and
moves to developments in nursing as late as 1977.
The approach is basically chronologic.

11.52   Safier, Gwendolyn.   Contemporary American Leaders in
Nursing: An Oral History.   New York: McGraw-Hill, 1977.
392 pp.   Cloth.   Bibliography.
Includes interviews with 17 nursing leaders in the
United States during the past several decades.   All
those interviewed were living at the time the book was
published.   The interviews were put on tape and are
transcribed into this volume by the author, a nurse
herself.   The individuals included are Florence G.
Blake, Pearl Parvin Coulter, Ruth Freeman, Lulu K.
Wolf Hassenplug, Virginia Henderson, Eleanor C.
Lambertsen, Lucile Petry Leone, R. Louise McManus,
Mildred L. Montag, Mary Kelly Mullane, Helen Nahm,
Lucille Notter, Estelle Massey Osborne, Martha E.
Rogers, Rozella M. Schlotfeldt, Marion W. Sheahan,
and Dorothy Smith.

11.53   Thompson, Julia.   The ANA in Washington.   Kansas City,
Mo.: The American Nurses' Association, 1972.
147 pp.   Paper.
Discusses ANA's role in federal legislation from approximately 1951 to 1971.   Chapters cover: communication within the nursing profession concerning ANA
activities, specific health legislation, legislation for
nursing education, new directions for the ANA.

LEGAL ASPECTS OF NURSING

11.54 Bernzweig, Eli P. The Nurse's Liability for Malpractice:
A Programmed Course, 2d ed. New York: McGraw-Hill,
1975.
> 290 pp. Paper. Index. Bibliography.
> A programmed approach to law for nurses. Includes
> a discussion of the general principles of the law, the
> rules of liability, the types of negligent conduct, the
> legal aspects of intentional wrongs, proving liability,
> and the principles of malpractice claims prevention.
> Has test questions with answers.

11.55 Bullough, Bonnie, ed. The Law and the Expanding Nursing
Role, 2d ed. New York: Appleton-Century-Crofts, 1980.
> 256 pp. Paper. Index. References. Bibliography.
> A collection of papers focusing on the legal implica-
> tions of the changing role of the nurse in the health
> care setting. The book's three sections cover a his-
> torical perspective on the current legal trends in nurs-
> ing practice, the use of the law for change, and per-
> spectives on the expanding role of nurses and physi-
> cian's assistants. Includes chapters on protocols and
> institutional licensure.

11.56 Cazalas, Mary W., ed. Nursing & the Law, 3d ed.
Germantown, Md.: Aspen Systems, 1978.
> 279 pp. Cloth. Index. Case index. Glossary.
> A book by a nurse-lawyer designed to give a basic in-
> troduction to the legal profession. Three sections
> deal with Nurses and Their Patients (including liabil-
> ity, consent, medical records, drugs and medications,
> intentional wrongs, etc.); Nurses and Their Employers
> (licensing laws, labor, etc.); and The Nurse and So-
> ciety (civil rights, good samaritan laws, abortion,
> etc.). Appendixes include explanation of various
> consent forms, medical malpractice information, sum-
> maries of nurse practice acts, child abuse laws, and
> good samaritan laws by state. Second edition edited
> by Charles J. Streiff.

11.57 Creighton, Helen. Law Every Nurse Should Know, 3d ed.
       Philadelphia: Saunders, 1975.
              327 pp. Cloth. Case and subject indexes. References.
              A "handbook . . . designed to present nurses with the
              basic facts of law in a concise, nontechnical manner."
              (p. v) By a nurse-lawyer, this book gives a thor-
              ough, textbook treatment, liberally laced with exam-
              ples of actual cases. Chapters discuss Law and
              Society; The Practice of Nursing; Contracts for Nurs-
              ing; Breach and Termination of Contract; The Legal
              Status of the Nurse; The Relation of a Nurse's Rights
              and Liabilities to Her Position and Status; Negligence
              and Malpractice; Torts as a Source of Other Civil Ac-
              tions; Crimes: Misdemeanors and Felonies; Wit-
              nesses; Dying Declarations; Wills and Gifts. Most
              chapters have an overview of the laws of all of the
              states in the United States. Also includes a chapter on
              Canadian law relating to nursing. Appendix includes
              excerpts from the author's columns in Supervisor
              Nurse (13.95) and in other journals relating to spe-
              cific problems of law and nursing.

11.58 Hemelt, Mary Dolores; Mackert, Mary Ellen. Dynamics
       of Law in Nursing and Health Care. Reston, Va.: Reston
       Publishing, 1978.
              250 pp. Cloth. Index. Bibliography. Case listing.
              Glossary.
              By a nurse-lawyer and a nurse, this text presents
              principles and theories of law as they relate to medi-
              cine and then discusses these principles and theories
              relative to actual situations. Topics include defini-
              tions; background; doctrine; relevant medical-legal
              issues (abortion, child abuse, confidentiality, medical
              records, etc.). Includes a series of "vignettes" of
              specific situations with answers. The appendixes
              give a brief history of the legal system, the court
              system, and the like. Contains a test on the points
              presented with answers following.

11.59 Murchison, Irene; Nichols, Thomas S.; Hanson, Rachel.

Legal Accountability in the Nursing Process. St. Louis: Mosby, 1978.

> 157 pp. Paper. Index. Bibliography.
> The purpose of this book is "to stimulate a new way of thinking about the law and its relationship to nursing practice." (p. viii) Legal theory is proposed as part of the "interdisciplinary base of nursing science." Sections are Introduction; The Legal Boundaries for Nursing Conduct; The Reasonable, Prudent Nurse; Rights of Patients in Health Care Facilities; and The Nursing Process Legally Revisited. Written for novices and experienced professional nurses. Presents a series of excellent, thought-provoking hypothetical situations. Includes sources of legal authority, standards of care, and ways to analyze litigated cases.

11.60   Rothman, Daniel A.; Rothman, Nancy Lloyd. The Professional Nurse and the Law. Boston: Little, Brown, 1977.

> 185 pp. Cloth. Index. References.
> A text which covers broad areas of the law of concern to the nursing profession. One author is a lawyer and the other is a nurse. Chapters cover rights, laws, government, torts, crime, nurse practice acts, collective bargaining, wills, etc. Appendixes include the ANA guidelines for the individual nurse contract; sample professional liability policy. References include appropriate case citations.

REFRESHER SOURCES

11.61   Cooper, Signe Skott. Contemporary Nursing Practice: A Guide for the Returning Nurse. New York: McGraw-Hill, 1970.

> 348 pp. Cloth. Index. References.
> "This book is designed as a textbook for inactive nurses enrolled in refresher courses." (p. vi) or for those who want to keep abreast of their field of expertise but cannot attend such courses. Four parts include Overview of Nursing Today; Concepts of Nursing

Care (patient education, community health, etc.);
Skills and Equipment; Responsibilities and Opportunities for the Professional Nurse (law and the nurse,
keeping current). Chapters include summaries and
suggested activities.

11.62　U.S. Department of Health, Education, and Welfare, Division of Nursing. A Refresher Course for Registered Nurses,
A Guide for Instructors and Students. DHEW publication
no. (HRA) 74-35. Bethesda, Md., 1974.
　　　318 pp. Paper. References.
　　　Gives guidelines for a refresher course on professional nursing originally developed by the Arizona
State Nurses' Association, specifically for nurses
who have not practiced for many years. Designed to
be used individually or with an instructor, the booklet
is divided into modules (e.g., asepsis, law, etc.)
which take the nurse through various stages in her
educational development and preparation. Includes
an appendix of evaluation forms and instructional
materials.

REVIEW BOOKS

11.63　Brooks, Stewart M., ed. Review of Nursing; Essentials
for the State Boards. Boston: Little, Brown, 1978.
　　　583 pp. Paper. Index. Bibliography. Glossary.
　　　This review book has sections on medical-surgical,
pediatric, maternity, and psychiatric nursing. Each
part is organized into a review section, a section of
questions, and a bibliography. Answers are included.
Appendixes contain information on drugs, nutrition,
communicable diseases, and first aid.

11.64　Gillies, Dee Ann; Alyn, Irene Barrett. Saunders Tests for
Self-Evaluation of Nursing Competence, 3d ed. Philadelphia:
Saunders, 1978.
　　　496 pp. Cloth. Index. Bibliography.
　　　A good source for review prior to licensure examina-

tions. Gives questions and/or situations (and answers) in four broad areas: Maternity and Gynecologic Nursing, Pediatric Nursing, Medical-Surgical Nursing, and Psychiatric-Mental Health Nursing. Includes answer sheets.

11.65 Keane, Claire Brackman; Muhl, Verna Jane. Saunders Review for Practical Nurses, 3d ed. Philadelphia: Saunders, 1977.
490 pp. Paper. Index. Bibliography.
A review text which presents information in concise, outline form and then asks questions with multiple-choice answers on the content previously outlined. Sections cover basic sciences, nutrition, nursing, drugs and their administration, etc. Includes answer sheets for student use and answers to questions.

11.66 Lagerquist, Sally L., ed. Addison-Wesley's Nursing Examination Review. Menlo Park: Addison-Wesley, 1977.
454 pp. Cloth. Index. Bibliographies.
Five units cover Psychiatric Nursing, Medical Nursing, Surgical Nursing, Maternity Nursing, and Pediatric Nursing. Each unit includes multiple-choice questions and a bibliography with answers and rationale. Contains information on orientation to the examinations and trends in nursing. Appendixes include Erickson's Stages of Personality Development, information on diets, intravenous therapy, diagnostic tests, positioning the patient, drugs, etc. Provides blank answer sheets.

11.67 Lewis, LuVerne Wolff. Lippincott's State Board Examination Review for Nurses. Philadelphia: Lippincott, 1978.
745 pp. Paper. References.
After an introduction, presents multiple-choice questions on Medical Nursing; Surgical Nursing; Obstetric Nursing; Nursing of Children; and Psychiatric Nursing. Provides answers with the reasoning behind them after each section. Answer sheets for student use are included. Questions and answer sheets approximate the State Board Test Pool Examinations.

11.68 Mosby's Comprehensive Review of Nursing, 9th ed.
St. Louis: Mosby, 1977.
609 pp. Cloth. Index. Bibliography.
Presents didactic material followed by multiple-choice
questions relating to anatomy and physiology, physical
sciences, nutrition, behavior, pharmacology, history,
nursing fundamentals, psychiatric nursing, medical-
surgical nursing, rehabilitation and nursing, etc.
Each chapter includes a summary. Accompanied by
Test Papers and Answer Book (39 pp.), which includes
blank test forms for the student to use and answers to
questions with information as to the level of difficulty
of the question based on field test data.

11.69 Nursing Examination Review Books Series.
Several of these spiral booklets, which include
multiple-choice questions for review of the entire
field of nursing, are listed in this volume under their
respective topic headings. Available from Medical
Examination Publishing Company, Inc., 969 Stewart
Avenue, Garden City, N.Y. 11530.

11.70 PreTest for Students Preparing for the State Board Examinations for Registered Nurse Licensure, 4th ed.
Wallingford: PreTest Service, 1979.
67 pp. Paper. Bibliography.
Consists of tests divided into five sections (Medical
Nursing, Surgical Nursing, Nursing Care of Children,
Maternal-Newborn Nursing, and Psychiatric Nursing)
similar to the State Board Test Pool Examinations for
registered nurse licensure. Exams in each category
are multiple-choice and last approximately the same
length of time and cover the same type of items covered on the state board exams. No answers are included with the tests. However, answer sheets,
which the student is to mark and mail back to the
PreTest Service, are included. The student will receive notification (within three weeks throughout the
year) of her score according to PreTest.

11.71   Smith, Sandra Fucci, ed. Review of Nursing for State Board
        Examinations, 2d ed. Los Altos: National Nursing Review,
        1979.
                399 pp. Paper. Annotated bibliography.
                A review book for state boards, divided into eight chap-
                ters, each of which covers a content area from the
                board examinations. Included are: Nursing Through
                the Life Cycle, Medical Nursing, Surgery, Emergency
                Interventions and Nursing Procedures, Maternity Nurs-
                ing, Pediatric Nursing, Psychiatric Nursing, and
                Legal Issues in Nursing. Each chapter includes a
                brief introduction, outline of content, and multiple-
                choice review questions with answers following.

WOMEN IN HEALTH

11.72   Bermosk, Loretta S.; Porter, Sarah E.; et al. Women's
        Health and Human Wholeness. New York: Appleton-Century-
        Crofts, 1979.
                266 pp. Paper. Index. References. Bibliography.
                For women, particularly those in the health profes-
                sions. Has three parts: background on women's
                health (holistic approach to health, women in the health
                care system, feminism, nursing, etc.); a model for
                women's health and services; and holistic health. In-
                cludes a brief conclusion at the end of the book.

11.73   Grissum, Marlene; Spengler, Carol. Womanpower and
        Health Care. Boston: Little, Brown, 1976.
                314 pp. Paper. Index. References.
                Addresses many issues confronting nurses as women
                today. Chapters discuss the female role in society;
                the nurse's role in society; saying no; power; changing
                the traditional role of nursing; etc. The authors are
                registered nurses with master's degrees.

11.74   Hughes, Marija Matich. The Sexual Barrier: Legal, Medi-
        cal, Economic, and Social Aspects of Sex Discrimination,

rev. and enl. Washington, D.C.: Hughes Press, 1977.
844 pp. Cloth. Index. Bibliography.
A "compilation of English language sources on issues
of special interest to women." (p. ix) Seventeen
categories (Aging, Child Care, Economic Status,
Health, Minority Women, Religion, Sex Roles, etc.)
are arranged alphabetically and list resources (books,
articles, pamphlets, government documents, etc.)
from 1960 to 1975. Includes over 8,000 entries which
are annotated when necessary.

11.75 Kjervik, Diane K.; Martinson, Ida M., eds. Women in
Stress: A Nursing Perspective. New York: Appleton-
Century-Crofts, 1979.
342 pp. Cloth. Index. Footnotes.
By two nurses, this book addresses stress in women
and in nursing in four major parts. Part 1 concerns
Florence Nightingale and the image of nursing. Part
2 covers the responses to stress of the two sexes,
sexuality, women's mental health, etc. Part 3 discusses crises in women (e.g., rape, child abuse,
battered women). Part 4 deals with loss (e.g.,
divorce, hysterectomy, widowhood, etc.).

INDEXES

11.76 Henderson, Virginia. Nursing Studies Index: An Annotated
Guide to Reported Studies, Research Methods, and Historical and Biographical Materials in Periodicals, Books, and
Pamphlets Published in English. Philadelphia: Lippincott,
1963-1972.
Gives retrospective access to literature pertinent to
nursing history which is not indexed elsewhere. Includes abstracts relative to the studies, and often
gives study methods, background of the author and
the study. Four volumes cover the periods 1900 to
1929, 1930 to 1949, 1950 to 1956, and 1957 to 1959.
Arranged by subject with author access.

PERIODICALS

11.77   American Nurse. American Nurses' Association, 2420
Pershing Rd., Kansas City, Mo. 64108. Monthly. 1975
to date.

11.78   Current Perspectives in Nursing. C.V. Mosby Co., 11830
Westline Industrial Drive, St. Louis, Mo. 63141. Biannually.
1977 to date.

11.79   Image. Sigma Theta Tau, National Honor Society of Nursing,
1100 W. Michigan St., Indianapolis, Ind. 46202. Three
times a year. 1967 to date.

11.80   Imprint. National Student Nurses' Association, 10 Columbus
Circle, New York, N.Y. 10019. Quarterly. 1968 to date.

11.81   International Nursing Review. International Council of
Nurses, Box 42, 1211 Geneva 20, Switzerland. Six times
annually. 1926 to date.

11.82   League Exchange. National League for Nursing, 10
Columbus Circle, New York, N.Y. 10019. Irregularly,
latest 1975. 1952 to date.

11.83   Medicolegal News. American Society of Law and Medicine,
Inc., 454 Brookline Ave., Boston, Mass. 02215. Quarterly.
1973 to date.

11.84   New York State Nurses Association Journal. New York
State Nurses' Association, 2113 Western, Guilderland, N.Y.
12084. Quarterly. 1929 to date.

11.85   NLN News. National League for Nursing, 10 Columbus
Circle, New York, N.Y. 10019. Monthly. 1952 to date.

11.86   Nurse Practitioner: A Journal of Primary Nursing Care.
Health Sciences Media and Research Services, Inc., 4311
37th N.E., Seattle, Wash. 98105. Bimonthly. 1975 to date.

11.87 Nursing Dimensions. Nursing Resources, Inc., 12 Lakeside Park, 607 North Avenue, Wakefield, Mass. 01880. Quarterly. 1973 to date.

11.88 Regan Report on Hospital Law. Medica Press, Inc., 1231 Industrial Bank Bldg., Providence, R.I. 02903. Monthly. 1960 to date.

11.89 Regan Report on Medical Law. Medica Press, Inc., 1231 Industrial Bank Bldg., Providence, R.I. 02903. Monthly. 1968 to date.

11.90 Regan Report on Nursing Law. Medica Press, Inc., 1231 Industrial Bank Bldg., Providence, R.I. 02903. Monthly. 1960 to date.

11.91 Reports. American Nurses' Association, House of Delegates. American Nurses' Association, 2420 Pershing Rd., Kansas City, Mo. 64108. Biannually. 1954 to date.

11.92 Summary Proceedings. American Nurses' Association, House of Delegates, 2420 Pershing Rd., Kansas City, Mo. 64108. Biannually. 1898 to date.

12
Education and Nursing

In recent years, the field of nursing has attempted to improve the quality of the teaching and learning process for its students. In this chapter, we have grouped reference books on nursing education, other books on nursing education, and books on education in general. There follow books arranged by subject categories: educational administration, audiovisual materials, behavioral objectives, clinical teaching, evaluation, graduate education, medical education, open curriculums, research in nursing education, students, and testing. Finally, pertinent indexes and periodicals are listed. The National League for Nursing publishes hundreds of its own publications each year. It has been impossible for us to include all of their publications. We recommend that you write for their most recent catalog of available publications, many of which deal with important aspects of nursing education: 10 Columbus Circle, New York, N.Y. 10019.

NURSING EDUCATION

Reference Sources

12.1 A Directory of Expanded Role Programs for Registered Nurses. Health Manpower References; DHEW publication no. HRA 79-10. Washington, D.C.: U.S. Government Printing Office, 1979.

30 pp. Paper. Index.
Lists programs awarding a certificate, bachelor's degree, or master's degree. Arranged according to state, with addresses.

12.2 Directory of Schools of Nursing, With Pre-Basic, Basic and Post-Basic Nursing and Midwifery Training Schemes and Educational Career Opportunities, 3d ed. London: Her Majesty's Stationery Office, 1977.
374 pp. Paper. Index.
A directory of educational programs in nursing in the United Kingdom. This edition issued by the Department of Health and Social Security. Earlier editions by King Edward's Hospital Fund for London.

12.3 National League for Nursing, Division of Baccalaureate and Higher Degree Programs. Baccalaureate Education in Nursing; Key to a Professional Career in Nursing 1979-80: Information about NLN-Accredited Baccalaureate Programs in Nursing. NLN publication no. 15-1311. New York: NLN, 1979.
28 pp. Paper.
An annual publication which gives information concerning addresses, requirements, number of students, administrative officials of baccalaureate programs accredited by the National League for Nursing.

12.4 National League for Nursing, Division of Research. State Approved Schools of Nursing—Registered Nurses; Meeting Minimum Requirements Set by Law and Board Rules in the Various Jurisdictions, 37th ed. NLN publication no. 19-1780. New York: NLN, 1979.
73 pp. Paper.
An annual publication which gives information (addresses, administrative officials, enrollment, financial support, number of graduates, etc.) about registered nurse programs accredited in the various states.

12.5 World Directory of Post-Basic and Post-Graduate Schools of Nursing. Geneva: World Health Organization, 1965.
223 pp. Cloth.

Old, but the only book to cover schools of nursing all over the world. Useful as a starting point, but all data listed must be verified by writing the appropriate school.

Non-reference Sources

12.6 Bevis, Em Olivia. Curriculum Building in Nursing: A Process, 2d ed. St. Louis: Mosby, 1978.
> 242 pp. Paper. Index. Bibliographies.
> A book intended "to provide a source for those engaged in the process of nursing curriculum formation, revision, or study." (p. vii) Includes examples of questionnaires and extensive tables, models, and the like dealing with nursing education, teaching strategies, students, evaluating change, etc.

12.7 Clark, Carolyn Chambers. Classroom Skills for Nurse Educators. [Springer Series on the Teaching of Nursing, vol. 4.] New York: Springer Publishing, 1978.
> 310 pp. Paper. Index. References.
> Written for instructors in nursing, this book's goal is "to provide nurse educators with legitimate classroom experiences that involve nursing students in active independent learning methods and have the potential to promote independent graduates and practitioners." (p. vii) The objective is to provide an efficient but humanistic way to apply theory. Topics include effective learning system design, role playing, simulations and gaming, peer learning, values clarification, and individualized learning.

12.8 Conley, Virginia C. Curriculum and Instruction in Nursing. Boston: Little, Brown, 1973.
> 673 pp. Cloth. Index. References. Supplementary readings.
> A thorough text, whose 5 parts are entitled Dynamics of Curriculum Development; Sources of Curriculum Decisions; Process of Curriculum Development; The

Instructional Process; Strategies and Processes for
Curriculum Change. Each chapter has a summary.

12.9   De Tornyay, Rheba. Strategies for Teaching Nursing.
[Wiley Paperback Nursing Series.] New York: Wiley, 1971.
145 pp. Paper. Index. References.
By a registered nurse and doctor of education, this
brief book gives information on various teaching
strategies. Part 1 deals with general aspects of
teaching (e.g., using examples and models, asking
questions), and Part 2 covers various methods of
teaching (e.g., seminar teaching, individualized instruction). Each chapter has a short summary.

12.10   Guinée, Kathleen K. Teaching and Learning in Nursing: A
Behavioral Objectives Approach. New York: Macmillan,
1978.
196 pp. Paper. Index. References.
Chapters discuss roles of the learner and teacher;
deriving and analyzing competencies; evaluation;
writing behavioral objectives; the learning process
and the learner; learning resources and grading. Each
chapter includes behavioral objectives; a summary.

12.11   National League for Nursing. Coping with Change Through
Assessment and Evaluation. NLN publication no. 23-1618.
New York: NLN, 1976.
104 pp. Paper. Bibliographies.
Includes the following papers by various authors:
Theory and Process of Change; Changing the Method-
ology of Learning; Change and the Developmental
Student; Nurses in Today's Changing Society; etc.
Focus is on associate degree nursing in many cases.

12.12   National League for Nursing. Instructional Innovations:
Ideals, Issues, Impediments. NLN publication no. 16-
1687. New York: NLN, 1977.
165 pp. Paper. Footnotes.
These papers from an NLN Council of Diploma Programs conference are grouped by 5 categories: The

"Ideal" Teacher in the Teaching/Learning Situation;
Enhancing and Limiting Factors in the Role of the Instructor; Realities and Ground Rules for Initiating Instructional Innovations; Innovative Uses of Supportive
Services; Innovative Instructional Patterns. The appendix includes a type of self-improvement form for
teachers.

12.13 National League for Nursing. Scholarships, Fellowships,
Educational Grants and Loans for Registered Nurses.   NLN
publication no. 41-408.   New York: NLN, 1979.
11 pp. Paper. Bibliography.
Lists sources of funding for registered nurses pursu-
ing baccalaureate, master's, or doctoral degrees.

12.14 Shaffer, Stuart M.; Indorato, Karen L.; Deneselya, Janet A.
Teaching in Schools of Nursing. St. Louis: Mosby, 1972.
110 pp. Paper. Index. Bibliography.
The authors feel that nursing school often does not allow for thorough background in educational problems
and teaching. Thus, the "purpose of this book is to
teach nurses how to teach." (p. vii) Discusses
the history of nursing education, the design
and evaluation of teaching, aids to teaching (e.g.,
programmed instruction, media, etc.), and the like.
Appendixes include evaluative questions.

12.15 Smeltzer, C. H. Psychological Evaluations in Nursing Education. New York: Macmillan, 1965.
249 pp. Cloth. Index. Bibliography.
This book, by a professor of psychology, discusses
human needs; aptitude and nursing; selection of nursing students; the teaching/learning process; student
evaluation, including testing and grading; counseling
of student nurses; "morale" in nursing, and the like.
An appendix includes questions and problems for each
chapter.

EDUCATION IN GENERAL

12.16 American Universities and Colleges, 11th ed. Edited by
       W. Todd Furniss, et al. Washington, D.C.: American
       Council on Education, 1973.
       1879 pp. Cloth. Institutional index.
       Gives brief essays on over 1440 American colleges
       and universities. Includes information on enrollment,
       address, background, accreditation, history, govern-
       ing board, calendar, admission information, publica-
       tions, finances, administrative officials, and the like.

12.17 Galli, Nicholas. Foundations and Principles of Health Edu-
       cation. New York: Wiley, 1978.
       389 pp. Cloth. Index. References.
       A book for the health education profession which, ac-
       cording to the author, draws on knowledge from many
       disciplines and has no unique body of knowledge of its
       own. Principles are drawn from law, science, educa-
       tion, psychology, sociology, and anthropology. Sec-
       tion 1 examines the history, philosophy, and objectives
       of health education; Section 2 discusses the foundations
       of health education; Section 3 looks at the competencies
       of the health educator. The only mention of nursing is
       that health educators must know how each of the health
       professions contributes to health care.

12.18 Mood, Alexander M. The Future of Higher Education; Some
       Speculations and Suggestions; A Report for the Carnegie
       Commission on Higher Education. New York: McGraw-
       Hill, 1973.
       166 pp. Cloth. Index. Bibliography.
       Chapters cover the climate of higher education,
       problems in higher education, new technology in
       higher education, students and new directions in
       higher education.

12.19 Segall, Ascher J.; Vanderschmidt, Hannelore; Burglass,
       Ruanne; et al. Systematic Course Design for the Health
       Fields. New York: Wiley, 1975.

406 pp. Paper. Index. References.
Based on a course on curriculum design in the Harvard
School of Public Health. Units deal with design, implementation, and methods used in course design. Includes examples, illustrations.

12.20 Smith, G. Kerry, ed. New Teaching, New Learning.
[Jossey-Bass Series in Higher Education.] San Francisco:
Jossey-Bass, 1971.
261 pp. Cloth. Index. Bibliography.
Chapters, by different authors, cover teaching; the
teaching environment; admissions policies; policy-
making on the campus; the professor; and future directions for higher education. A publication of the American Association for Higher Education from the 26th
National Conference on Higher Education held in
Chicago, 1971.

EDUCATIONAL ADMINISTRATION

Nursing

12.21 National League for Nursing, Department of Baccalaureate
and Higher Degree Programs. Quality Assurance: Models
for Nursing Education. Papers Presented at the Fourteenth
Conference of the Council of Baccalaureate and Higher Degree Programs, Washington, D.C., November, 1975. NLN
publication no. 15-1611. New York: NLN, 1976.
65 pp. Paper. Bibliographies.
Papers by such people as Mabel Wandelt, Maria
Phaneuf, and Nancy A. Lytle discuss "high-risk students" at various levels of the nursing education process, involvement by faculty in quality assurance,
assessing nursing care, and the like. Includes a list
of readings on the nursing audit, quality assurance.

12.22 U.S. Department of Health, Education and Welfare, Division
of Nursing. The Decanal Role in Baccalaureate and Higher
Degree Colleges of Nursing. Health Manpower Refer-

ences; DHEW pub. no. (HRA) 75-11.   Bethesda:
DHEW, 1975.
59 pp. Paper. References.
Includes four seminal papers from the proceedings of
a conference sponsored by the Division of Nursing and
held in Virginia in 1974 designed to explore the dean's
role in baccalaureate and graduate nursing education.
Dr. Irene S. Palmer: The Decanal Role in Academic
and Institutional Leadership; Dr. Virginia R. Jarratt:
The Decanal Role in the Enhancement of Educational
Institutions; Dr. A. D. Albright: Educational Administration—A Look to the Future; and Dr. Rozella M.
Schlotfeldt: Opportunity in the Decanal Role.

Other

12.23   Commission on Academic Tenure in Higher Education.
Faculty Tenure; a Report and Recommendations. [The
Jossey-Bass Series in Higher Education.] San Francisco:
Jossey-Bass, 1973.
276 pp. Cloth. Index. Selected bibliography.
Glossary.
A sourcebook on tenure that gives historical data and
explores the legal implications as well. Includes
recommendations based on this commission's study.

12.24   Patterson, Franklin. Colleges in Consort, Institutional Cooperation Through Consortia. [The Jossey-Bass Series in
Higher Education.] San Francisco: Jossey-Bass, 1974.
182 pp. Cloth. Index. Bibliography.
". . . one interested observer's look at the status,
problems, and prospects of cooperative groups of institutions in higher education." (p. xi) Chapters are
entitled History and Overview; Getting and Spending;
The Economics of Consortia; Governance and Decision-
Making; Reality and Possibility, etc. Includes data on
various consortia.

AUDIOVISUAL MATERIALS

Medical and Nursing

12.25 Ash, Joan; Stevenson, Michael. Health: A Multimedia
Source Guide. New York: Bowker, 1976.
> 185 pp. Cloth. Source index. Index to free or inex-
> pensive material. Subject index. Bibliography.
> For librarians, health professionals, and laypeople,
> this annotated guide directs seekers to organizations
> which deal with health-related matters—publishers,
> audiovisual dealers and distributors, libraries, socie-
> ties, government agencies, pharmaceutical companies,
> book dealers, and research institutes.

12.26 Eidelberg, Lawrence, ed. The Health Sciences Video
Directory, 1977. New York: Shelter Books, 1977.
> 270 pp. Paper.
> An annotated listing of over 4400 videotaped programs
> from some 120 producers and/or distributors. Each
> title is indexed according to MeSH (Medical Subject
> Headings) in the first section. The second section is
> an alphabetical listing by title of each program. Titles
> are in bold black type with producer/distributor infor-
> mation; order number if any; date of production; tar-
> get audience; series if applicable; program content
> person; length of program; the format of video on
> which the program is available; color or black and
> white information; sale, rental, preview, lease price
> or distribution information; other material available
> with the unit; and brief summary. Includes both com-
> mercial and university distributors. Has abbrevia-
> tions for producers/distributors with keys by abbre-
> viated and full name, including address, phone num-
> ber, and contact person where applicable. To be up-
> dated annually with supplements. Later edition en-
> titled The Videolog: Programs for the Health Sciences
> (Esselte Video, 1979) not available for annotation.

12.27 Lange, Crystal M. Autotutorial Techniques in Nursing Education. Englewood Cliffs: Prentice-Hall, 1972.
> 105 pp. Cloth. Footnotes.
> The author, a nurse-educator, outlines her multisen-
> sory, autotutorial approach to nursing education.
> Covers Autotutorial Approaches; Environmental De-
> sign; The Faculty Team: Design for Student Learning;
> Student Performance; Design and Equipping of Auto-
> tutorial Laboratories; and the like. Appendixes am-
> plify the text.

12.28 National Information Center for Educational Media. Index
to Health and Safety Education, 3d ed. Los Angeles:
NICEM, 1977.
> 1141 pp. Paper.
> Has over 33,000 entries of media (16 mm films, film-
> strips, slide sets, transparencies, 8 mm cartridges,
> videotapes, audio tapes, records) in health and re-
> lated areas. Material ranges in level from preschool
> to professional. Includes subject listing, alphabetic
> listing, and listing of producers and distributors.

12.29 The National Survey of Audiovisual Materials for Nursing,
1968-1969. Conducted by ANA-NLN Film Service. New
York: National League for Nursing, American Journal of
Nursing Co., 1970.
> 243 pp. Paper. Index.
> Gives results of a survey of schools of nursing, some
> hospitals, schools of public health, and the like, which
> tried to determine what audiovisual software materials
> were available for nursing personnel. Items are listed
> by format (includes almost every conceivable format
> then in use) with subject indexes. Appendixes include
> forms, criteria, used in the survey. Now quite out of
> date, but included, since it is the only survey of this
> kind.

12.30 Roth, Dorothea H.; Price, Donel W. Instructional Television: A Method for Teaching Nursing. St. Louis: Mosby,
1971.

186 pp. Paper. Index. Bibliography. References.
Deals with the use of television as a teaching tool in
nursing. Chapters go into Instructional Script Writing; Television Production; Clinical Television Instruction; Educational Accountability; and the like. For
someone highly interested in using television as an instructional medium. Includes samples of scripts and
authorization forms. Provides a summary after each
chapter.

12.31 U.S. National Medical Audiovisual Center. National Medical
Audiovisual Center Catalog; Audiovisuals for the Health
Scientist. DHEW publication no. (NIH) 77-506. Atlanta:
NMAC, 1977.
　　　352 pp. Paper. Index.
Catalog of audiovisual software available on free loan
from the National Medical Audiovisual Center. Arranged by broad subject categories (key in front of the
book) with title index included. Supplements appear
several times a year.

Other

12.32 Audiovisual Market Place: A Multimedia Guide. New York:
Bowker, 1980.
　　　432 pp. Paper. Index. Bibliography.
Comes out annually. Lists audiovisual software and
hardware producers, distributors, companies, reference sources, periodicals, associations, and the like.
A good sourcebook of information in the audiovisual
areas.

12.33 Educational Film Locator of the Consortium of University
Film Centers and R. R. Bowker Company. New York:
Bowker, 1978.
　　　2178 pp. Cloth.
A union list of some 37,000 film titles held by mem-
ber libraries of the Consortium of University Film
Centers (approximately 50 libraries from all over the
United States). Includes all types of educational films

on medical and non-medical subjects (e.g., agriculture, biological sciences, education, medical sciences, social sciences, geographic areas, etc.). Bibliographical elements are standardized with authority files, International Standard Book Numbers, etc. The materials listed are available from the Consortium members, and extensive information as to availability of the items (including fees, restrictions, loss information, return, etc.) is given. Includes Series Listing, Foreign Film Title Index, producer/distributor addresses, and the like.

12.34   Kemp, Jerrold E.; Carraher, Ron; Szumski, Richard F.; et al. Planning and Producing Audiovisual Materials, 3d ed. New York: Crowell, 1975.

320 pp. Cloth. Index. Bibliography. Glossary.
A comprehensive text, first published in 1963. Four parts deal with: Background in Audiovisual Communications; Planning Your Audiovisual Materials; Fundamental Skills (e.g., recording, taking pictures, etc.); and Producing Your Audiovisual Materials. Chapters are practically oriented and end with review questions and answers. Appendixes include lists of various sources and services relating to audiovisual materials. Fourth edition due 1980.

12.35   National Audio-Visual Association. The Audio-Visual Equipment Directory, 1978–79, 23d ed. Fairfax: NAVA, 1978.

482 pp. Paper. Index.
Published every two years. Gives specifications on all varieties of audiovisual hardware. Arranged by category of equipment, e.g., slide projectors, 16 mm projectors, etc.

12.36   Strohlein, Alfred. The Management of 35mm Medical Slides. New York: United Business Publications, 1975.

128 pp. Paper. Index. Bibliography.
A thorough, practical book covering acquisition, indexing, cataloging, circulation, legal aspects of

maintaining slide collections, etc. Has lists of
sources for slides, equipment, manufacturers. For
someone who wishes to organize a slide collection
systematically.

12.37 U.S. National Audiovisual Center. A Reference List of
Audiovisual Materials Produced by the United States Government, 1978. Washington, D.C.: National Audiovisual
Center, 1978.
354 pp. Paper.
Contains information on over 6,000 audiovisual items
(primarily 16 mm films) produced by some 175 federal
agencies on a variety of subjects, including the health
sciences, education, safety, and science. Loan, rental,
or sales information is given on each program. Consists of a listing by broad subject, then by title.

12.38 Zuckerman, David W.; Horn, Robert E. The Guide to Simu-
lations/Games for Education and Training. Lexington,
Mass.: Information Resources, 1973.
501 pp. Paper. Index.
An unusual book which lists games and simulated exercises with a description and note as to availability
and address. Arranged in alphabetical order by the
name of the game with subject index.

BEHAVIORAL OBJECTIVES

12.39 Mager, Robert F. Preparing Instructional Objectives,
2d ed. Belmont: Fearon, 1975.
136 pp. Paper.
First published in 1962, this book was one of the first
to go into detail about writing behavioral objectives.

12.40 Reilly, Dorothy E. Behavioral Objectives in Nursing:
Evaluation of Learner Attainment. New York: Appleton-
Century-Crofts, 1975.
178 pp. Paper. Index. References. Recommended
readings.

Stresses the use of behavioral objectives as a means of evaluating learning, thus facilitating the teaching-learning process. Chapters give a practical approach while at the same time laying a theoretical background. Covers accountability in instruction, developing behavioral objectives, the taxonomy in developing such objectives, and evaluating the attainment of the various objectives.

12.41 Vargas, Julie S. Writing Worthwhile Behavioral Objectives. New York: Harper & Row, 1972.

175 pp. Paper. Index. Bibliography.
A self-instructional text on the writing of behavioral objectives in the cognitive domain. The format includes pretests, exercises, and post-tests. Chapter headings include How Objectives Help the Teacher, Identifying Behavioral Objectives, Making Objectives Behavioral, and Writing Worthwhile Objectives. Uses examples from elementary school.

CLINICAL TEACHING

12.42 Infante, Mary Sue. The Clinical Laboratory in Nursing Education. New York: Wiley, 1975.

102 pp. Cloth. Index. Bibliography.
This book, by an R.N.-Ed.D., discusses the use of the "clinical laboratory" in nursing education and tries to "cast a new perspective on this sphere of preparation for practice." (p. vi) Two parts explore the laboratory in the educational process and research relating to this concept.

12.43 Lenburg, Carrie B. The Clinical Performance Examination: Development and Implementation. New York: Appleton-Century-Crofts, 1979.

334 pp. Cloth. Index. Bibliography.
Using the Clinical Performance in Nursing Examination developed for the New York External Degree Nursing Program, the author describes the process

of development and implementation of such examinations. Discusses the basic concepts, content determination, scheduling, uses, validity, and reliability of the examination. Provides useful information for nursing education and nursing service personnel as they plan the assessment of competencies of students or graduates.

12.44 Schweer, Jean E.; Gebbie, Kristine M. Creative Teaching in Clinical Nursing, 3d ed. St. Louis: Mosby, 1976.
216 pp. Paper. Index. References. Suggested readings.
"The primary aim of this book is to assist the nursing teacher in exploring the concept of creativity as it applies to the function of clinical teaching." (p. v) Four units explore Foundations of Teaching in Clinical Nursing, Climate for Creative Teaching in Clinical Nursing, Aspects of Design for Teaching Programs in Clinical Nursing, and Professional Responsibilities for Fostering Creative Teaching in Clinical Nursing.

12.45 Smith, Dorothy W.; et al. Perspectives on Clinical Teaching, 2d ed. [Springer Series on the Teaching of Nursing, vol. 2.] New York: Springer Publishing, 1977.
266 pp. Paper. Author and subject indexes. References. Suggested readings.
Designed primarily for clinical teachers in undergraduate nursing programs. Chapters cover: values and clinical teaching, trends, student-faculty relations, prejudices in clinical teaching (e.g., racism, sexism, ageism), integrated curricula, audiovisuals in clinical teaching, small group conferences, professionalism in nursing, etc.

12.46 Wiedenbach, Ernestine. Meeting the Realities in Clinical Teaching. New York: Springer Publishing, 1969.
166 pp. Paper. Index. References.
A companion to the author's Clinical Nursing: A Helping Art (1964). Deals with the whys of clinical teaching, the logistics of teaching, and how to do clinical teaching. Brief but outcome-oriented.

EVALUATION

12.47 Bloom, Benjamin S.; Hastings, J. Thomas; Madaus,
George F. Handbook on Formative and Summative Evaluation of Student Learning. New York: McGraw-Hill, 1971.
    923 pp. Cloth. Name and subject indexes.
    References.
    A textbook on the evaluation of student learning. Part
    1 gives background on evaluation and methods of evalu-
    ation; part 2 discusses evaluation in various teaching
    environments. The focus is on preschool and second-
    ary education.

12.48 Cook, Thomas D.; Del Rosario, Marilyn L.; Hennigan,
Karen M.; et al; eds. Evaluation Studies Review Annual,
Vol. 3. Beverly Hills: Sage Publications, 1978.
    783 pp. Cloth. References.
    The third volume in a series of reports of evaluation
    studies among evaluators in diverse fields. The
    series has been published yearly since 1976. The
    studies in this volume are arranged under 8 parts:
    The Policy and Political Context of Evaluation;
    Methodology; Health; Income Maintenance; Criminal
    Justice; Education; Mental Health; and Evaluation in
    the Public Interest.

12.49 Green, Joan L.; Stone, James C. Curriculum Evaluation:
Theory and Practice, With a Case Study From Nursing Edu-
cation. [Springer Series on the Teaching of Nursing.] New
York: Springer Publishing, 1977.
    271 pp. Cloth. Index. Bibliography.
    A comprehensive formulation of evaluation theories;
    major models of assessment process; requirements
    for appropriate methods, technology, and instruments;
    and analysis and interpretation of the data obtained.

12.50 Morgan, Margaret K.; Irby, David M. Evaluating Clinical
Competence in the Health Professions. St. Louis: Mosby,
1978.
    316 pp. Cloth. Index. Bibliographies.
    Written for health educators in order to improve

skills and procedures in evaluating student performance. Four sections discuss the systematic
collection of data and the judgment of the worth of particular samples of student knowledge, skills, and attitudes. Section 1 contains general directions for beginning the evaluation process; Section 2 takes an in-depth
look at techniques of assessment; Section 3 considers
implementation; and Section 4 describes modes of
clinical evaluation from nine professions.

12.51 Reilly, Dorothy E., ed. Teaching and Evaluating the Affective Domain in Nursing Programs. Thorofare, N.J.:
Slack, 1978.
        75 pp. Paper. References.
        This book addresses an extremely important area for
        nursing education. The monograph includes papers
        presented at a workshop for faculty on critical issues
        of ethical, moral, and value development. These are
        areas that can be taught and evaluated. Includes moral
        and value exercises as well as a taxonomy of behaviors
        with evaluation strategies.

12.52 Schneider, Harriet L. Evaluation of Nursing Competency.
Boston: Little, Brown, 1979.
        162 pp. Paper. Index. References.
        After a brief review of the relevant literature, the
        author discusses several methods of assessing the
        knowledge base of nurses. These methods include
        tests based on films, direct observation of perfor-
        mance, videotape recordings, written simulations,
        and clinical lab simulations.

12.53 Steele, Shirley, et al. Educational Evaluation in Nursing.
Thorofare, N.J.: Slack, 1978.
        160 pp. Paper. References. Bibliography. Glossary.
        Uses the content, input, process, product (CIPP)
        model of evaluation and documents the process in
        a systematic evaluation of a graduate program in
        child health nursing. Discusses context and in-
        put evaluation, process evaluation (courses, teaching

put evaluation, process evaluation (courses, teaching strategies), and product evaluation. Chapters examine specifics such as looking at student progress and test construction. The book closes with a summary, conclusions, and recommendations. The appendixes contain examples of context, process, and product evaluation instruments.

GRADUATE EDUCATION

12.54   National League for Nursing. Developing a Master's Program in Nursing. NLN publication no. 15-1747. New York: NLN, 1978.

        37 pp. Paper. Bibliography.
        Contains papers presented at a conference held in Minneapolis in 1978. Topics include feasibility; philosophy, objectives, and conceptual frameworks; role development and cognates; and clinical specialization.

12.55   National League for Nursing. Doctoral Programs in Nursing, 1979-80. NLN publication no. 15-1448. New York: NLN, 1978.

        8 pp. Paper.
        Lists doctoral programs in nursing by state. Information given includes the institution, administrator, areas of study, and degrees offered.

12.56   National League for Nursing. Department of Baccalaureate and Higher Degree Programs. Master's Education in Nursing; Route to Opportunities in Contemporary Nursing 1979-80; Information about NLN-Accredited Master's Programs in Nursing. NLN publication no. 15-1312. New York: NLN, 1979.

        26 pp. Paper.
        Comes out annually. Gives information on NLN accredited schools of nursing which offer master's degrees: address, curriculum information, enrollments, fees, administrative officials.

12.57 Peterson's Annual Guides to Graduate Study, 1979. Book 3:
       Graduate Programs in the Biological, Agricultural, and
       Health Sciences in the U.S. and Canada. Princeton:
       Peterson's Guides, 1979.
              1466 pp. Paper. Index.
              A comprehensive reference guide to graduate pro-
              grams in the United States and Canada. Includes pro-
              files of the institutions, distribution of programs, and
              abstracts or descriptions of particular programs.

12.58 U.S. Department of Health, Education and Welfare, Division
       of Nursing. The Doctorally Prepared Nurse, Report of Two
       Conferences on the Demand for and Education of Nurses with
       Doctoral Degrees.   Health Manpower References; DHEW
       pub. no. (HRA) 76-18.   Bethesda: DHEW, 1976.
              104 pp. Paper.
              The proceedings of two Division of Nursing conferences
              focusing on doctoral training for nurses. Part 1 dis-
              cusses trends, issues, and projected developments;
              Part 2 covers manpower.

MEDICAL EDUCATION

12.59 American Medical Association. Medical Education in the
       United States. Chicago: AMA, 1900-1980.
              Bibliographies.
              A yearly issue of the Journal of the American Medical
              Association. For the year covered, gives extensive
              statistical data relative to medical education, medical
              schools, students, continuing medical education, allied
              health education, programs sponsored by various gov-
              ernment agencies, etc.

12.60 Association of American Medical Colleges. AAMC Direc-
       tory of American Medical Education, 1979-80. Washington,
       D.C.: AAMC, 1979.
              387 pp. Paper. Name index.
              Contains alphabetical and geographical listings of
              medical schools with addresses and names of admin-

istrative official for the medical schools and universities. Also describes the Association of American Medical Colleges' (AAMC) organization, activities, and membership.

OPEN CURRICULUMS

12.61   Cross, K. Patricia. Beyond the Open Door: New Students to Higher Education. [Jossey-Bass Series in Higher Education.] San Francisco: Jossey-Bass, 1971.
200 pp. Cloth. Index. References.
". . . seeks to shed some light on the critical task of developing an education that will serve the needs of new students to higher education." (p. xi) Defines the category "new students" and delves into their needs, education, career motivation, etc., before making recommendations. Appendixes list characteristics of these students, etc. A study sponsored by the Educational Testing Service; the Center for Research and Development in Higher Education, University of California, Berkeley; and the College Entrance Examination Board.

12.62   Hastings, Glen E.; Murray, Louisa, eds. The Primary Nurse Practitioner: A Multiple Track Curriculum. Miami: Banyan Books, 1976.
225 pp. Cloth. References. Bibliography.
"This monograph describes a program, jointly administered by the Department of Medicine of the School of Medicine and by the School of Nursing of the University of Miami, to prepare registered nurses to provide primary health care in a variety of community settings." (p. vii) Goes into the curriculum, justification for the curriculum, evaluation, etc. Appendixes include examples of course outlines, forms, etc.

12.63   Lenburg, Carrie B., ed. Open Learning and Career Mobility in Nursing. St. Louis: Mosby, 1975.
397 pp. Paper. Index. References.

". . . presents new curriculum designs and new learning methods put together in different ways to provide a
diversity of educational opportunities not experienced
before in this country." (p. xi) Six parts are entitled
Nontraditional Study Comes of Age; Issues and Problems Related to Career Mobility in Nursing; Type I.
The Licensure Based Model; Type II. The Advanced
Placement Model; Type III. The Multiple Exit-Reentry
Models; Type IV. The Assessment Model.

12.64 National League for Nursing, Division of Research. Directory of Career Mobility Programs in Nursing Education.
NLN publication no. 19-1605. New York: NLN, 1976.
263 pp. Paper. School index.
A listing of nursing schools in the United States which
offer open curriculums for students interested in fur-
thering their nursing education. Based on survey data
compiled by the NLN, it gives background on schools,
types of programs, and types and numbers of students.
Arranged alphabetically by state.

12.65 Notter, Lucille; Robey, Marguerite C.; Weinstein, Mark H.;
et al. Guidelines for Implementation of Open Curriculum
Practices in Nursing Education. NLN publication no. 19-
1701. New York: National League for Nursing, 1978.
24 pp. Paper. Bibliography.
Gives guidelines for open curriculum programs based
on the first phase of a study by the NLN.

12.66 Searight, Mary W., ed. The Second Step: Baccalaurate
Education for Registered Nurses. Philadelphia: Davis, 1976.
252 pp. Cloth. Index. References. Bibliographies.
Explores the concept of the open curriculum in nursing
education. Chapters include Pressures for Opening
the Curriculum; Strategies for Organizing Learning;
Preceptorship Study: Contracting for Learning; Faculty
Group and Interpersonal Processes; Curriculum Evaluation Research, etc. Most of the contributors are
from California State College, Sonoma, California,
and the book draws on their experience with an upper

division baccalaureate program for associate degree
or diploma nurses.

12.67 Story, Donna Ketchum. Career Mobility: Implementing the
Ladder Concept in Associate Degree and Practical Nursing
Curricula. St. Louis: Mosby, 1974.
206 pp. Paper. Index. References.
First discusses the career ladder concept, then goes
on to outline such a program in Foundations of Nursing; Science; Nutrition; Behavioral Science; Maternal
and Child Health Nursing; Medical-Surgical Nursing.
Includes course outline, behavioral objectives, learning experiences (including texts, films, etc.) for each
category.

12.68 Treece, Eleanor Walters. Internship in Nursing Education:
Technoterm. New York: Springer Publishing, 1974.
122 pp. Paper.
"Technoterm is a block of practical or work experience
offered to senior student nurses with the objective of
preparing them for the responsibilities and activities
they will encounter in their first positions as professional nurses." (p. 1) This book reports the results of
this type of program in various settings since approximately 1969. Technoterm was implemented with practical and diploma programs, but the author also
stresses its usefulness in other settings.

RESEARCH IN NURSING EDUCATION

12.69 Ward, Mary Jane; Fetler, Mark E. Instruments for Use in
Nursing Education Research. Boulder: Western Interstate
Commission for Higher Education, 1979.
846 pp. Paper. Author and subject indexes.
References. Annotated bibliographies.
A compilation of information on published and unpub-
lished test instruments used in research in nursing
education in a wide variety of areas. In many cases,
includes the instrument itself, information regarding

scoring, reliability, validity, and the like. Subjects covered include: administrative style, death and dying, nursing students, job satisfaction, nursing profession, leadership, values, attitudes toward the elderly, self-concept, and many more. Includes information on the use of certain well-known tests in nursing, such as the Edwards Personal Preference Schedule, the Minnesota Multiphasic Personality Inventory, and the Torrance Tests of Creative Thinking, to mention only a few. Appendixes contain sample letters and materials used in compiling the instruments, lists of persons using the instruments, etc.

STUDENTS

12.70 Aiken, Eula; Stathas, John J. The Different Student. Philadelphia: Davis, 1978.
>157 pp. Paper. Bibliography.
>Designed to facilitate the "different" student's acceptance into and performance in the new teaching/learning environment. "Different" students are defined by the authors (one an RN, the other a counselor at a school of nursing) to include those who "reflect ethnic, cultural, and sexual differences or life styles." (p. 2) Presents 38 brief vignettes with space provided for reader response. The authors themselves have written their own "responses, issues, and proposed actions." Can be used in teaching, at workshops, etc. Includes vernacular and drawings to add to the attitudes conveyed.

12.71 Litwack, Lawrence; Sakata, Robert; Wykle, May. Counseling, Evaluation, and Student Development in Nursing Education. Philadelphia: Saunders, 1972.
>243 pp. Cloth. Index. Bibliographies.
>Three parts, Counseling, Evaluation, and Student Development, discuss such topics as group approaches in guidance and counseling; testing; clinical evaluation; and attrition in nursing schools. The appendix includes a statement on the rights and freedom of students.

12.72 Smeltzer, C. H. The Interview in Student Nurse Selection.
New York: Putnam, 1968.
>185 pp. Cloth. Index. Bibliography.
>Chapters deal with justification of the interview pro-
>cess, persons doing the interviewing, types of inter-
>viewing, conducting the interview, evaluating the in-
>terview, etc. Appendix includes a readiness test for
>interviewing.

TESTS

12.73 Buros, Oscar K., ed. The Eighth Mental Measurements
Yearbook. Highland Park, N.J.: Gryphon Press, 1978.
>2 vols. Cloth. Index. Bibliographies.
>Designed to assist test users in education, psychology,
>and industry to locate information on standardized
>tests of every description. Contains bibliographies
>for each test. First published in 1938, it is supple-
>mented by its seven predecessors.

12.74 Sax, Gilbert. Principles of Educational Measurement and
Evaluation. Belmont: Wadsworth, 1974.
>642 pp. Cloth. Index. Bibliography. Suggested
>readings.
>A practical book with chapters on construction of
>tests, problems with various types of tests, analyzing
>test results, etc. Includes appendixes on computation
>of various types of scores.

INDEXES

12.75 Current Index to Journals in Education. Macmillan Information, 866 Third Avenue, New York, N.Y. 10022. Monthly
with semiannual cumulations. 1969 to date.

12.76 *Education Index; An Author-Subject Index to Educational
Publications in the English Language. H. W. Wilson Co.,

---

*See Chapter 16 for detailed explanation of this index.

950 University Ave., Bronx, N.Y. 10452. Monthly with
annual cumulations. 1929 to date.

12.77 Hospital/Health Care Training Media Profiles. Olympic
Media Information, 71 West 23rd Street, New York, N.Y.
10010. Bimonthly. 1974 to date.

12.78 Index to Audiovisual Serials in the Health Sciences. Medical
Library Association, 919 North Michigan Avenue, Suite 3208,
Chicago, Ill. 60611. Quarterly with annual cumulation.
1977 to date.

12.79 *National Library of Medicine Audiovisuals Catalog. National
Library of Medicine, 8600 Rockville Pike, Bethesda, Md.
20209. Quarterly with annual cumulation. 1977 to date.

PERIODICALS

Nursing Education

12.80 Current Perspectives in Nursing Education. C. V. Mosby
Co., 11830 Westline Industrial Drive, St. Louis, Mo. 63141.
Biannually. 1976 to date.

12.81 Journal of Audiovisual Media in Medicine. Update Publishing International, Inc., 2337 LeMoine Ave., Fort Lee, N.J.
07024. Quarterly. 1951 to date.

12.82 Journal of Continuing Education in Nursing. Charles B.
Slack, Inc., 6900 Grove Road, Thorofare, N.J. 08086.
Bimonthly. 1970 to date.

12.83 Journal of Nursing Education. Charles B. Slack, Inc., 6900
Grove Road, Thorofare, N.J. 08086. Nine times per year.
1962 to date.

---

*Order from Superintendent of Documents, Washington,
D.C. 20402.

12.84   Nurse Educator. Concept Development Company, 12 Lakeside Park, 607 North Avenue, Wakefield, Mass. 01880. Bimonthly. 1976 to date.

12.85   Nursing Outlook. American Journal of Nursing Company, 10 Columbus Circle, New York, N.Y. 10019. (For the American Nurses' Association and the National League for Nursing.) Monthly. 1953 to date.

Other

12.86   Academe; Bulletin of the AAUP. American Association of University Professors, One Dupont Circle, Washington, D.C. 20036. Quarterly. 1915 to date.

12.87   Change Magazine. Change Magazine, NBW Tower, New Rochelle, New York 10801. Monthly. 1969 to date.

12.88   Chronicle of Higher Education. Editorial Projects for Education, 1333 New Hampshire Ave., N.W., Washington, D.C. 20036. Weekly (biweekly during summer months). 1966 to date.

12.89   Graduate Woman. American Association of University Women, 2401 Virginia Avenue N.W., Washington, D.C. 20037. Six times per year. 1882 to date.

12.90   Journal of Higher Education. Ohio State University Press, 2070 Neil Avenue, Columbus, Ohio 43210. (For the American Association for Higher Education.) Bimonthly. 1930 to date.

12.91   Journal of Medical Education. Association of American Medical Colleges, One Dupont Circle N.W., Washington, D.C. 20036. Monthly. 1926 to date.

13

Administration and Nursing

The direction and management of personnel to provide high quality nursing care to patients/clients in diverse settings has always been an important aspect of nursing. This chapter lists books using general and nursing approaches to administration; change; health care delivery; personnel; quality assurance, including peer review programs; and staff development. Relevant periodicals are listed at the end of the chapter.

ADMINISTRATION

Nursing

13.1 Alexander, Edythe L. Nursing Administration in the Hospital Health Care System, 2d ed. St. Louis: Mosby, 1978.
289 pp. Cloth. Index. Bibliography.
Written for nurses preparing for roles in nursing service administration. Attempts to increase the awareness of factors that affect problems in organization and management. The information is presented operationally by relating concepts and methodologies to nursing management. Chapters include an historical perspective on concepts of administration as well as current administrative theories and principles.

13.2 Arndt, Clara; Huckabay, Loucine M. Daderian. Nursing
      Administration: Theory for Practice with a Systems Ap-
      proach. St. Louis: Mosby, 1975.
              292 pp. Cloth. Index. Bibliography.
              Includes the major components of administration, using
              a systems approach. For both the novice and experi-
              enced administrator. Combines major schools of thought
              and research findings to provide a conceptual framework
              for administrative action. Second edition due 1980.

13.3 Bailey, June T.; Claus, Karen E. Decision Making in
      Nursing: Tools for Change. St. Louis: Mosby, 1975.
              167 pp. Paper. Index. References.
              For nurses who must solve patient care and manage-
              ment problems and bring about change. Presents a
              systems approach to problem solving. Uses a series
              of case studies to explicate relevant problems. Part
              1 presents a decision-making framework and Part 2
              illustrates the use of the Claus–Bailey model in nurs-
              ing care problems.

13.4 Barrett, Jean; Gessner, Barbara A.; Phelps, Charlene.
      The Head Nurse; Her Leadership Role, 3d ed. New York:
      Appleton-Century-Crofts, 1975.
              450 pp. Cloth. Subject and author indexes. Annotated
              references.
              For the head nurse or clinical specialist with admin-
              istrative responsibilities or the nursing student in her
              senior year in college. Contents include The Patient
              and the Nurse; The Nursing Process; Organization and
              Administration of the Hospital for Delivery of Patient
              Care; and The Head Nurse's Responsibility for Staff
              Development. Also contains exercises and questions
              for discussion.

13.5 Beyers, Marjorie; Phillips, Carole. Nursing Management
      for Patient Care, 2d ed. Boston: Little, Brown, 1979.
              292 pp. Cloth. Index. Bibliography.
              A text for nursing students and graduates to facilitate
              their roles as managers. Discusses theories of

management and develops a framework for their application. Includes case studies to provide opportunities for application of content.

13.6 Broadwell, Martin M. The Practice of Supervising: Making Experience Pay. Reading, Mass.: Addison-Wesley, 1977.
169 pp. Paper. Index.
Focuses on the importance of experienced supervisors and the need to help them keep up-to-date with newer practices.

13.7 Clark, Carolyn Chambers; Shea, Carole A. Management in Nursing: A Vital Link in the Health Care System. New York: McGraw-Hill, 1979.
308 pp. Cloth. Index. References.
Uses a systems framework to present the knowledge and skills needed for effective management in the complex, changing health care system. Written for senior baccalaureate nursing students or graduate students. Useful in continuing education also. Part 1 is entitled Management: Theory and Process; Part 2, Nursing Alternatives Within the System. Of special interest is the presentation of the nurse-manager in different organizational settings.

13.8 Diekelmann, Nancy L.; Broadwell, Martin M. The New Hospital Supervisor. Reading, Mass.: Addison-Wesley, 1977.
155 pp. Paper. Index.
A guide for the new supervisor that contains little theory but provides practical applications of many theories. Major headings: Attitudes and Feelings, Supervisory Skills, Supervisory Activities.

13.9 DiVincenti, Marie. Administering Nursing Service, 2d ed. Boston: Little, Brown, 1977.
467 pp. Cloth. Index. References.
A useful reference for the nurse director with or without formal preparation or experience. Provides a comprehensive look at the patient and his needs, the nurse director's role and management functions,

management tools, and nursing's involvement in the physical and human environment in which care is delivered. Contains 25 appendixes covering patients' rights, guides for implementing change, etc.

13.10   Donovan, Helen M. Nursing Service Administration: Managing the Enterprise. St. Louis: Mosby, 1975.
   271 pp. Paper. Index. References.
   Written for nurses at all levels who are responsible for the work of others. This monograph provides the fundamental structure for understanding administrative concepts and theories.

13.11   Douglass, Laura M. Review of Leadership in Nursing, 2d ed. [Mosby's Comprehensive Review Series.] St. Louis: Mosby, 1977.
   173 pp. Paper. Index. References.
   A short monograph which provides a careful analysis of the nurse leader now and in the future. Consists of discussion questions with answers. First edition entitled Review of Team Nursing.

13.12   Douglass, Laura Mae; Bevis, Em Olivia. Nursing Management and Leadership in Action, 3d ed. St. Louis: Mosby, 1979.
   289 pp. Paper. Index. Bibliography.
   Discusses the functions that assist in the delivery of nursing care. Leadership activities under whatever mode of patient assignment require skills found in this book. Includes a theoretical framework, teaching-learning principles, communication skills, as well as delegation, evaluation, change, and other leadership behaviors. Previous edition entitled Nursing Leadership in Action.

13.13   Ganong, Joan M.; Ganong, Warren L. Nursing Management: Concepts, Functions, Techniques and Skills. Germantown, Md.: Aspen Systems, 1976.

343 pp. Cloth. Index. Notes. Suggested readings.
Glossary.
A book covering effective management of patient/client
care and services for nurse managers and nursing
students. The authors assert that all nurses use the
process of management in their work and thus could
profit from this book. Uses Maslow's hierarchy of
human needs as a base for the philosophy of management developed. Part 1: Workworld of the Nurse
Manager; Part 2: Patient Care Management; Part 3:
Operational Management; and Part 4: Human Resources
Management.

13.14   Kron, Thora. The Management of Patient Care: Putting
Leadership Skills to Work, 4th ed. Philadelphia: Saunders,
1976.
247 pp. Paper. Index. Bibliography.
For beginning practitioners of nursing, focuses on the
responsibilities of nurses for the management of patient
care and on ways to exercise leadership in this regard.
Part 1: Leadership—The Greatest Challenge in Nursing
Today; Part 2: Managing Yourself and Others; Part 3:
Putting Your Leadership Skills to Work; Part 4: Patient Care Management and Team Nursing. Earlier
editions entitled Nursing Team Leadership.

13.15   Levine, Harry D.; Phillip, P. Joseph. Factors Affecting
Staffing Levels and Patterns of Nursing Personnel. DHEW
pub. no. (HRA) 75-6. Bethesda: U.S. Department of Health,
Education and Welfare, Division of Nursing, 1975.
110 pp. Paper. Bibliography.
Builds on "the 1970 American Hospital Association -
Division of Nursing joint survey of nursing personnel
employed in hospitals; the Association's 1970 annual
survey of hospitals, Health Resources Statistics, 1971;
and Census of Population: 1970." (p. iii) A study of
nurse staffing patterns and needs.

13.16   McQuillan, Florence L. Fundamentals of Nursing Home Administration, 2d ed. Philadelphia: Saunders, 1974.

403 pp. Cloth. Index. References.
Discusses the theory and planning of the nursing home
facility; the administrator's functions; rehabilitation
and patient care planning in the nursing home setting;
services available in the nursing home (laundry, dietary, etc.); and evaluation of the nursing home. Appendixes include information on fatty acid, cholesterol,
sodium and potassium content of foods, Medicare certification guidelines.

13.17 McQuillan, Florence L. The Realities of Nursing Management: How to Cope. Bowie, Md.: Brady, 1978.
372 pp. Cloth. Index. References.
Examines management roles in nursing both for simi-
larities as well as differences. Major headings are
leadership and self-direction, the nurse-manager, the
director of nurses, supervisory levels, etc. Case
studies illustrate management concepts.

13.18 Moloney, Margaret M. Leadership in Nursing: Theory,
Strategies, Action. St. Louis: Mosby, 1979.
221 pp. Paper. Index. References.
Looks at nursing leadership from its behavioral aspects and as an interactional process. For graduate
and undergraduate nursing students as well as nurses
in practice. Major segments are Introduction to
Nursing Leadership; Theory: Leadership Theories,
Selected Theorists, and Process in Leadership; Strategies: Nursing Leadership Process and Behavior; Action: Leadership Behavior in Selected Disciplines and
Nursing; and Preparation for Nursing Leadership and
Predictions for Its Future.

13.19 Stevens, Barbara J. First-Line Patient Care Management.
Wakefield, Mass.: Contemporary Publishing, 1976.
182 pp. Paper. Index. Bibliography.
For head nurses and teachers of nursing leadership,
this book focuses on the supervision of the actual delivery of patient care. This level is different from the
middle (supervisor) or top (nurse executive) manage-

ment. Headings: First-Line Managers, Managerial
Methods, Patient Management, and Staff Management.

13.20 Stevens, Barbara J. The Nurse as Executive. Wakefield,
Mass.: Contemporary Publishing, 1975.
260 pp. Paper. Index. Bibliography.
A text for administrators in nursing education or nursing service who are relatively new in their fields. The
major section headings are General Management
Skills, Management Applications in Nursing, and Theoretical and Educational Aspects. Uses examples from
nursing.

13.21 Stevens, Warren F. Management and Leadership in Nursing.
New York: McGraw-Hill, 1978.
270 pp. Cloth. Index. Bibliography.
Uses a theoretical approach to discuss organization
and management as related to the roles and functions
of professional nursing. Applies systems theory in
examining topics in major units: planning, organizing,
directing, and controlling. Includes an approach to
assessment of the formal and informal structure of an
organization and factors influencing each function.

13.22 Stone, Sandra; Berger, Marie S.; Elhart, Dorothy; et al.;
eds. Management for Nurses: A Multidisciplinary Approach.
St. Louis: Mosby, 1976.
280 pp. Paper. Index. Bibliography.
A collection of readings for nursing students in leadership courses, graduate students, and nurses in practice who need to know and use management concepts.
Unit 1: Structural Factors and Their Influence on Effi-
cient Organizational Functioning; Unit 2: Personnel
Factors; Unit 3: Economic or Extrinsic Factors.
Articles are reprinted from a variety of sources, both
nursing and non-nursing. Topics include Power and
Accountability; Leadership; and Budget Planning,
among others. Second edition due 1980.

13.23 Yura, Helen; Ozimek, Dorothy; Walsh, Mary B. Nursing
       Leadership: Theory and Process. New York: Appleton-
       Century-Crofts, 1976.
              237 pp. Paper. Index. Bibliography.
              Explores the state of nursing leadership and nursing
              leadership process. The six chapters include an in-
              troduction which contains some historical data; con-
              cepts and theories related to nursing leadership; nurs-
              ing leadership process with its related theory; educa-
              tional preparation for nursing leadership; application
              of the leadership process; and steps in the development
              of nursing leadership. The major focus is on the need
              to identify, develop, and nurture nurse leaders and to
              use the leadership process effectively.

General

13.24 Brown, Bernard L. Risk Management for Hospitals: A Prac-
       tical Approach. Germantown, Md.: Aspen Systems, 1979.
              186 pp. Cloth. Index. Bibliography. Glossary.
              Covers a timely area in a practical fashion. By the ad-
              ministrator of Kennestone Hospital, Marietta, Georgia.
              Chapters cover risk management in hospitals; design,
              organization, implementation, philosophy of a risk
              management program; and self-insurance. The last
              chapter includes a summary. Each chapter has a con-
              clusion and a checklist of questions. Includes samples
              of forms throughout and a glossary at the end of the
              book. Appendixes contain case studies information,
              trustee agreement, etc.

13.25 Harris, O. Jeff, Jr. Managing People at Work: Concepts
       and Cases in Interpersonal Behavior. New York: Wiley,
       1976.
              581 pp. Cloth. Index. Bibliography.
              A look at important, relevant concepts about managing
              people that directly links management theory with ap-
              plication. First presents the concepts, illustrates
              them, and then provides opportunities to use the con-

cepts in the cases included. A thorough, interesting approach to this topic.

13.26 Hodge, Melville H. Medical Information Systems: A Resource for Hospitals. Germantown: Aspen Systems, 1977.
201 pp. Cloth. Index. Bibliography.
Aims to "assist men and women who run our hospitals in understanding the rationale behind medical information systems and major management issues in selection, implementation, and benefit realization." (p. x)

13.27 Likert, Rensis. The Human Organization. New York: McGraw-Hill, 1967.
258 pp. Cloth. Index. Bibliography.
Looks at quantitative research and its application to the improvement of human resource management and proposes a "science-based system of management." (p. 2) Examines organizational characteristics and variables and ways to study them.

13.28 McCool, Barbara; Brown, Montague. The Management Response: Conceptual, Technical and Human Skills of Health Administration. Philadelphia: Saunders, 1977.
248 pp. Cloth. Index. References. Selected readings.
A series of learning modules that provide objectives, examples, exercises, and questions. The three main sections concentrate on conceptual, technical, and human skills. The book is written for middle management, i.e., department heads, supervisors, head nurses, team leaders, etc. Includes a discussion of planning, strategy, decision-making, training, communication, and motivation, among other skills. Utilizes a very interesting model to organize the book. Contains reprints of selected readings for each section.

13.29 McMillan, Norman H. Planning for Survival: A Handbook for Hospital Trustees. Chicago: American Hospital Association, 1978.
114 pp. Paper.
An exceedingly readable book by an advocate of busi-

ness techniques for long-term planning by the hospital.
Includes segments on Getting Organized, Getting the
Facts Together, Sizing Up the Facts, Putting the Plan
on Paper, and Putting the Plan to Work.

13.30 Mathieu, Robert P. Hospital and Nursing Home Management: An Instructional and Administrative Manual.
Philadelphia: Saunders, 1971.
> 280 pp. Cloth. Index.
> For the administrator, details the requirements for
> an extended care facility, including all the various
> policies such as personnel, nursing service, dietary,
> business, pharmaceutical, housekeeping, etc., as well
> as rules for accreditation. Within each category dis-
> cusses job descriptions, forms, training requirements,
> as appropriate.

13.31 Mehr, Robert I.; Hedges, Bob A. Risk Management: Concepts and Applications. [Irwin Series in Insurance and Economic Security.] Homewood, Ill.: Irwin, 1974.
> 726 pp. Cloth. Index. Footnotes.
> Loss prevention and control are essential elements of
> all organizations. This book explores the manage-
> ment and achievement of organizational objectives and
> their relationship to risks that may occur.

13.32 Metzger, Norman. The Health Care Supervisor's Handbook.
Germantown: Aspen Systems, 1978.
> 137 pp. Cloth. Author and subject indexes. Footnotes.
> Approaches management skills on the supervisory level
> from a "how-to" perspective. Topics include manag-
> ing, interviewing, turnover, evaluation, communica-
> tion, disciplining, unions, and self-assessment. Ap-
> pendixes contain supervisory evaluations checklists.

13.33 Plovnick, Mark S.; Fry, Ronald E.; Rubin, Irwin M.
Managing Health Care Delivery: A Training Program for
Primary Care Physicians. Cambridge: Ballinger, 1978.
> 130 pp. Paper. References.
> A training manual which contains sessions for varying

size groups of residents, faculty, and co-workers.
Topics are: Factors Influencing the Coordination of
Care; Managing Goal Conflicts; Managing Role Conflicts; Allocating the Decision–Making Authority; Organization Structure and Design; and Managing the
Change Process. Provides guidelines and instructions
for the session leader. The focus is on the day-to-day
management of health workers, not on budgeting. Includes objectives, a session outline, reading lists for
use before and after class, and a discussion guide.

13.34 Rakich, Jonathan S.; Longest, Beaufort B., Jr.; O'Donovan,
       Thomas R. Managing Health Care Organizations. [Saunders
       Series in Health Care Organization and Administration.]
       Philadelphia: Saunders, 1977.
         350 pp. Cloth. Index. Footnotes.
         For persons who are, or are aspiring to be, managers
       in health care organizations. The authors describe
       their approach as a "broad process approach." (p. vi)
       Includes a frame of reference for coping with external
       forces and organizations and a set of skills for manag-
       ing internal complexities. Part 1, Setting and Frame-
       work; Part 2, Output-Input Determination; Part 3, Or-
       ganizational Design and Structure; Part 4, Organiza-
       tional Dynamics; and Part 5, Organizational Control
       and Change. Each chapter has a summary and dis-
       cussion questions.

13.35 Rubin, Irwin M.; Fry, Ronald E.; Plovnick, Mark S. Man-
       aging Human Resources in Health Care Organizations: An
       Applied Approach. Reston: Reston Publishing, 1978.
         317 pp. Cloth. Bibliographies.
         For students and practitioners in health care delivery
       management. Each chapter provides essential con-
       cepts, guidelines, and directions for experiential
       learning on each topic. Useful in both academic and
       continuing education settings. Topics include Organi-
       zational Planning and Goal Setting; Performance Ap-
       praisal; Clarifying and Negotiating Role Responsibili-
       ties; Managerial Decision-Making; Value and Value
       Conflicts; and others.

13.36 Schmied, Elsie, ed. Maintaining Cost Effectiveness. [The
       Management Anthology Series; Theme 3, Product and Service
       Cost Effectiveness.] Wakefield, Mass.: Nursing Resources,
       1979.
            259 pp. Paper. Index. References.
            An anthology of previously published articles for the
            nurse administrator focusing on product and service
            cost effectiveness. Major sections are: Planning for
            Cost Effectiveness; Forecasting; Preparation of the
            Budget; Feedback and Control; and Developing an Ac-
            curate Nursing Service Budget: A Case Study.

13.37 Selbst, Paul L.; Launer, Deborah J.; et al. Modern Health
       Care Forms; Hospital and Nursing Home Administration.
       Boston: Warren, Gorham & Lamont, 1976.
            1 vol. (various pagings). Cloth. Index.
            Gives examples of actual forms used in health care in-
            stitutions. Forms are organized in six sections: or-
            ganization and management, financial management,
            personnel and labor relations, medical and profes-
            sional affairs, physical facilities, and support ser-
            vices. Sources of forms are given and supplemented
            yearly with looseleaf page inserts.

13.38 Steffl, Bernita M.; Eide, Imogene. Discharge Planning
       Handbook. Thorofare, N.J.: Charles B. Slack, 1978.
            81 pp. Paper. Index. Bibliography.
            A manual for health professionals focusing on dis-
            charge planning that provides continuity of care, sup-
            ports quality assurance, and is cost effective. Chap-
            ters include the definition of and a rationale for dis-
            charge planning. Also covers alternatives for care,
            implementation of discharge planning, roles and re-
            sponsibilities, managerial strategies, and evaluation
            of discharge plans. Includes a guide for discharge
            planning in an emergency room.

13.39 Southwick, Arthur F. The Law of Hospital and Health Care
       Administration. Ann Arbor: University of Michigan, School
       of Public Health, Health Administration Press, 1978.
            500 pp. Cloth. Index. References. List of cases.

Written for health administration students as a classroom text on the legal aspects of health care to help
them recognize legal problems and to know when and
how to obtain legal counsel. Part 1: Introduction to
Law and the Legal System; Part 2: The Hospital as a
Corporation; Part 3: The Physician-Patient Relationship—Professional Liability; Part 4: The Hospital-
Patient Relationship; and Part 5: The Hospital-
Physician Relationship. The text is limited to "private" law and does not cover "public" law; that is, the
law of governmental regulation of the health care system. Includes the private law of contract, tort, and
property, and constitutional law as relevant. Contributions on the Anglo-American legal system and professional liability by George J. Siedel, III.

13.40 Warner, D. Michael; Holloway, Don C. Decision Making
and Control for Health Administration: The Management of
Quantitative Analysis. Ann Arbor: Health Administration
Press, 1978.
427 pp. Cloth. Index. Bibliography.
Presents a conceptual decision-making framework at
a mathematical level for the health administrator
using applications from the health field. Major sections are Introduction, Analysis for Decision Making,
Forecasting and Measurement, Cybernetic Control.
A complex, difficult book.

13.41 Warren, David G. Problems in Hospital Law, 3d ed.
Germantown, Md.: Aspen Systems, 1978.
339 pp. Cloth. Index. References. List of cases.
Provides a basic orientation to the field of hospital
law to assist health care personnel in understanding
the legal aspects of the hospital's operation. Topics
include rights, responsibilities, and liabilities of hospital staff; concerns related to hospital activities (admission, discharge, treatment, etc.); and financial
management including tax exemption. The first chapter is especially helpful to those not familiar with law
in general. Second edition compiled by the Health and
Law Center of Aspen Systems Corporation.

CHANGE

13.42   Brooten, Dorothy A.; Hayman, Laura Lucia; Naylor,
Mary Duffin. Leadership for Change: A Guide for the
Frustrated Nurse. Philadelphia: Lippincott, 1978.
> 172 pp. Paper. Index. Bibliography.
> For graduates and students in schools of nursing. Pro-
> vides a helpful examination of theory and practical skill
> in planning and directing change as an integral part of
> leadership in nursing. It could also serve as a text
> for management or other staff development efforts.
> The book opens with an historical review of change in
> nursing followed by a discussion of the need for further
> change and of a theoretical framework for planning and
> implementing it.

13.43   Claus, Karen E.; Bailey, June T. Power and Influence in
Health Care: A New Approach to Leadership. St. Louis:
Mosby, 1977.
> 191 pp. Paper. Index. References. Suggested
> readings.
> The authors have developed a model of Power/Author-
> ity/Influence that they believe nurses can use to in-
> crease their power and become more effective leaders.
> A text for leadership courses in schools of nursing or
> for continuing education programs. Part 1: A Frame-
> work for Power and Influence; Part 2: Developing
> Power and Influence. Examines power, authority,
> and influence in an operational context. Also dis-
> cusses personal, interpersonal, organization, and
> social power.

13.44   Deloughery, Grace L.; Gebbie, Kristine M. Political Dynamics: Impact on Nurses and Nursing. St. Louis: Mosby,
1975.
> 236 pp. Cloth. Index. References.
> Recognizing that involvement in political activity is
> essential, the authors have written this call to action
> for nurses. Units are the American Political System,
> Power, The Nurse's Dilemma, and Preparation for

Action. Theoretical presentations provide a framework for understanding specific problems and possible actions. Covers a wide range of theories, concepts, examples, and comments. Mentions sources of data.

13.45 Jewell, Donald O., ed. Women and Management: An Expanding Role. Atlanta: Georgia State University, School of Business Administration, Publishing Services Division, 1977.
413 pp. Cloth. Footnotes. Sources for further reading.
A collection of articles (original and reprinted) that cover relevant ideas, research, and experience and reflect the multifaceted difficulties of advancing a woman in management. Headings include Perspectives on Women in a Changing Society, Women and Management, and Gearing Up—A Positive Response.

13.46 Lippitt, Gordon L. Visualizing Change: Model Building and the Change Process. LaJolla: University Associates, 1973.
370 pp. Paper. Index. Bibliography.
Suggests ways to anticipate and cope creatively with change. Proposes the use of models to conceptualize problem situations, focusing on planned change for individual, group, and community.

13.47 Watzlawick, Paul; Weakland, John H.; Fisch, Richard. Change: Principles of Problem Formation and Problem Resolution. New York: Norton, 1974.
172 pp. Cloth. Index. References.
Discusses change as a phenomenon, its nature and types. Parts cover Persistence and Change, Problem Formation, and Problem Resolution. Based on the authors' work at the Brief Therapy Center of the Mental Research Institute in Palo Alto, California.

HEALTH CARE DELIVERY

13.48 Elinson, Jack; Mooney, Anne; Siegmann, Athilia E.; eds. Health Goals and Health Indicators: Policy, Planning, and Evaluation. [AAAS Selected Symposia.] Boulder: Westview

Press, American Association for the Advancement of
Science, 1977.
> 137 pp. Cloth. Index. Bibliography.
> Combines the expertise of the medical and social
> sciences in establishing criteria for determination of
> health goals, conducting analyses of health policies,
> studying indicators of health status, and exploring the
> consequences of health practices and policies.

13.49   Feldstein, Martin S.; Lindsay, Cotton M.; et al.; eds.
New Directions in Public Health Care: An Evaluation of Pro-
posals for National Health Insurance, 2d ed. San Francisco:
Institute for Contemporary Studies, 1976.
> 277 pp. Paper. Bibliography.
> A series of essays by various economists which dis-
> cuss national health insurance. Chapters deal with
> Government and Health, The Market for Medical Care,
> Public Sector Medicine: History and Analysis, etc.

13.50   Health: United States, 1978. Washington, D.C.: U.S. Department of Health, Education and Welfare, 1978.
> 488 pp. Paper. Bibliography.
> The third annual report from the Secretary of Health,
> Education and Welfare to the President and Congress
> on the status of the nation's health. Part A contains
> analytic review chapters on cost containment, disease
> prevention, children and youth, mental disorders,
> long-term care, and quality of medical care. Part B
> is a series of 188 statistical tables with interpretations
> organized by Health Status and Determinants, Utiliza-
> tion of Health Resources, Health Care Resources, and
> Health Care Costs and Financing. A guide to the tables
> is included.

13.51   Joint Commission on Accreditation of Hospitals. Accreditation Manual for Hospitals. Chicago: JCAH, 1978.
> 193 pp. Paper. Index. Footnotes. Glossary.
> The Joint Commission on Accreditation of Hospitals is
> committed to the "development of national standards of
> structure, function, staffing, and procedure for

hospitals." (Foreword) This manual provides guidelines for hospitals working for accreditation by the
JCAH. After an introduction and information regarding the rights and responsibilities of patients, and administrative procedures, the materials on standards
follow. Aspects covered include anesthesia, building and grounds, dietetics, emergency, safety and sani-
tation, management and control, home care, infection
control, medical records, medical staff, nuclear medicine, nursing, outpatient services, pathology, pharmaceutical systems, libraries, professional services,
radiology, rehabilitation, respiratory care, social services, special care facilities, and the like. Appendixes
give accreditation and appeal procedures, audit information. Includes emergency services standards
at the back of book. The Manual is published August
1 of each year effective for all visits by January 1 of
the succeeding year.

13.52   Jonas, Steven, et al. Health Care Delivery in the United
        States. New York: Springer Publishing, 1977.
        492 pp. Cloth. Index. Bibliography.
        A text for an introductory course in health care deliv-
        ery that provides basic knowledge required by present
        and future decision-makers in the health care system.
        Describes the various elements of the system. In-
        cludes the economic and political ramifications. Ap-
        pendixes contain sources of data and additional topics
        such as occupational safety and health, and school
        health care.

13.53   National Health Directory, 3d ed. Bethesda: Science and
        Health Publications, 1979.
        636 pp. Cloth. Name and agency indexes.
        Contains key information sources (name, title, ad-
        dress, and phone number) regarding health programs
        and legislation. Major units are: Congressional Name
        Index; Key Congressional Health Subcommittees; Con-
        gressional Delegations; Congressional Committees;
        Federal Health Agencies; Federal Regional Health

Officials; State Health Officials; City and County
Health Officials.

13.54 Roemer, Ruth; Kramer, Charles; Frink, Jeanne E. Planning Urban Health Services: From Jungle to System. New
York: Springer Publishing, 1975.
> 351 pp. Cloth. Index. Bibliography.
> Gives an overview of the American health system by
> discussing the historical development and the prob-
> lems of fragmentation of services. Includes brief re-
> views of health systems in other countries as well.
> The authors present a proposal for a realistic system
> of health maintenance organizations in a regional
> framework.

13.55 Somers, Anne R.; Somers, Herman M. Health and Health
Care: Policies in Perspective. Germantown, Md.: Aspen
Systems, 1977.
> 528 pp. Cloth. Index. Footnotes.
> Looks at old and persistent problems of today and yes-
> terday. Some selections were written for the book;
> other pieces of historical value are reprinted. Topics
> examined are medicine, health care professionals,
> access to care, inflation, public policy. The authors
> propose a framework for health and health care policies.

13.56 Thompson, John D. Applied Health Services Research.
Lexington, Mass.: Lexington Books, 1977.
> 199 pp. Cloth. Index. Bibliography.
> "Health services research is an organized and rigor-
> ous inquiry primarily concerned with the effectiveness
> of the delivery of medical care to groups of people."
> (p. 1) It is an area of multidisciplinary research.
> Topics include Research on Nurse Staffing, Economics
> of Hospital Care, The Quality of Nursing Care, and
> others.

13.57 Torrens, Paul R. The American Health Care System:
Issues and Problems. St. Louis: Mosby, 1978.
> 120 pp. Paper. References.

The author, a physician with a master's in public
health, discusses history, background information,
and organizational data on the American health care
delivery system; issues in the American health care
system (measurement, purpose, the role of government, technology, control, the role of change); and an
"ideal" model for a future system of health care in
America. The discussion of the ideal health care
model is theoretical rather than practical.

PERSONNEL

13.58 American Nurses' Association. Facts About Nursing,
       1976-77; A Statistical Summary. Kansas City, Mo.: ANA,
       1977.
              330 pp. Paper. Index.
              A periodic publication (irregular, usually every two
              years) that provides all sorts of statistical informa-
              tion relating to nursing. Includes information on areas
              such as nursing resources, education, economics, and
              vital statistics. Began publication in 1935.

13.59 Applied Management Sciences, Inc. Review of Health Man-
       power Population Requirements Standards. DHEW publica-
       tion no. (HRA) 77-22; Health Manpower References. Rock-
       ville, Md.: U.S. Department of Health, Education and Wel-
       fare, Bureau of Health Manpower, 1977.
              70 pp. Paper. References.
              A report that provides health systems agencies with
              technical assistance for planning by presenting an
              analysis of existing studies of health manpower/
              population requirement standards found in the litera-
              ture. Includes suggested ways in which requirement
              ratios may be used.

13.60 Foerst, Helen V.; Gareau, Florence E.; Levine, Eugene.
       Planning for Nursing Needs and Resources. DHEW publica-
       tion no. (NIH) 72-87. Bethesda: U.S. Department of
       Health, Education and Welfare, Division of Nursing, 1972.

204 pp. Paper. Index. Annotated bibliographies.
An attempt to give guidelines to those involved in improving health care, services, and education. Discusses the nature, design, and organization of planning, and assessing needs and requirements. Appendixes include information on historical and state surveys or studies, other materials useful for planning, and location of statistical data.

13.61 Kramer, Marlene. Reality Shock: Why Nurses Leave Nursing. St. Louis: Mosby, 1974.

249 pp. Paper. Index. References.
A highly publicized, readable report of an eight-year study of new graduates in nursing. Discusses the Anticipatory Socialization program and the experiment in the study developed as a solution to the problems faced by the new graduates when the reality of their positions finds them unprepared. Describes an emerging theory of postgraduate professional socialization. The target audience is faculty and students (graduate and undergraduate) as well as nurses in the work setting.

13.62 Millman, Michael L., ed. Nursing Personnel and the Changing Health Care System. Cambridge: Ballinger, 1978.

287 pp. Cloth. Index. Footnotes.
Papers presented at a conference in Glen Cove, N.Y., in 1977, sponsored by the Conservation of Human Resources Project, Columbia University. The papers cover health manpower; nursing manpower, supply and distribution; nursing staffing, etc. The book is intended more as a point of departure on this subject rather than as a definitive answer to the points discussed.

13.63 U.S. Department of Health, Education and Welfare, Division of Nursing. Second Report to the Congress, March 15, 1979 (revised), Nurse Training Act of 1975. Report of the Secre-

tary of Health, Education and Welfare on the Supply and
Distribution of and Requirements for Nurses as Required by
Section 951, Nurse Training Act of 1975, Title IX, Public
Law 94-63.   DHEW publication no. (HRA) 79-45; Health Man-
power References.   Hyattsville, Md.: DHEW, 1979.

> 160 pp. Paper. Bibliography.
> Introduction gives the plan for this data collection re-
> quired by law. Seven chapters include national re-
> quirements for nursing personnel, projected supply
> and requirements, conclusions, and summary. Ap-
> pendixes include statistical tables.

13.64   U.S. Department of Health, Education and Welfare, Division
of Nursing. Survey of Foreign Nurse Graduates.   DHEW
publication no. (HRA) 76-13; Health Manpower References.
Bethesda: DHEW, 1976.

> 112 pp. Paper.
> Results of a survey of foreign nurse graduates done by
> the American Nurses' Association. Describes the
> methodology of the survey, various laws and regula-
> tions pertaining to foreign nurses, and delineates the
> survey findings. Appendixes give forms used and in-
> formation necessary for data collection.

13.65   Yett, Donald E. An Economic Analysis of the Nurse Short-
age. Lexington, Mass.: Lexington Books, 1975.

> 324 pp. Cloth. Index. Bibliography.
> Report of ten years of research by an economist on the
> market for nurses. Chapters discuss: Contemporary
> Views on the Employment Outlook for Nurses; Demand
> and Supply: The Economics of Skills Manpower Short-
> ages; Trends in the Employment of Nurses; Trends in
> the Remuneration of Nurses; Application of Alternative
> Labor Market Models to the Data on Nursing: Results
> and Policy Implications. The author emphasizes the
> need to consider the future demand for nurses in plan-
> ning nurse training.

QUALITY ASSURANCE

13.66 Cantor, Marjorie Moore, et al. Achieving Nursing Care
Standards: Internal and External. Wakefield, Mass.:
Nursing Resources, 1978.
> 180 pp. Cloth. Index. References.
> For nurses with administrative responsibilities in
> nursing care delivery systems who must set standards
> for themselves and also must meet those set by other
> governmental, accrediting, and professional agencies.
> Sections cover Programming for Establishing and
> Maintaining High Standards of Nursing Care; Standards
> of Patient Welfare; Standards of Process; and Stan-
> dards of Structure. Especially useful since it looks at
> resources and constraints in setting and meeting stan-
> dards.

13.67 Carter, Joan Haselman; Hilliard, Mildred; Castles, Mary
Reardon; et al. Standards of Nursing Care: A Guide for
Evaluation, 2d ed., enl. New York: Springer Publishing,
1976.
> 292 pp. Cloth. Index. Bibliographies.
> ". . . a guide for persons who seek to provide quality
> nursing care and who desire specific tools designed to
> help meet the goal." (p. x) Consists of written stan-
> dards for providing nursing care in general, and in re-
> lation to specific cases, such as cardiac difficulties,
> obstetrics. Chapters discuss evaluation and adminis-
> tration relating to these types of standards. Appen-
> dixes include procedures, forms relating to activities
> reports, and the like. This book is an outgrowth of a
> program by the St. Louis University Hospital, Nurs-
> ing Service Department.

13.68 Davidson, Sharon Van Sell; Burleson, Bette C.; Crawford,
Jean E. S.; et al. Nursing Care Evaluation: Concurrent
and Retrospective Review Criteria. St. Louis: Mosby, 1977.
> 420 pp. Cloth. Index. Bibliography.
> Presents guidelines for involvement in professional
> standards review organization (PSRO) activities.
> First, presents an introduction and overview of quality

assurance, then, model nursing criteria arranged in alphabetical order, and lastly, a section on complications. Written primarily for nurses and nurse administrators.

13.69 Doughty, Dorothy Beckley; Mash, Norma Justus. Nursing Audit. Philadelphia: Davis, 1977.
    225 pp. Paper. Index. References.
    A practical, readable book about audit programs in nursing. Discusses audit programs, implementation of such programs, construction of criteria. Includes samples.

13.70 Jacobs, Charles M.; Christoffel, Tom H.; Dixon, Nancy. Measuring the Quality of Patient Care: The Rationale for Outcome Audit. Cambridge: Ballinger, 1976.
    183 pp. Cloth. Index. Footnotes. Bibliography.
    Discusses medical audits as required by the Joint Commission on the Accreditation of Hospitals. Includes forms and audit examples.

13.71 Jelinek, Richard C.; Dennis, Lyman C., III. A Review and Evaluation of Nursing Productivity. DHEW publication no. (HRA) 77-15; Health Manpower References. Bethesda: U.S. Department of Health, Education and Welfare, Division of Nursing, 1977.
    380 pp. Paper. Index. Bibliography.
    A thorough review of studies of nursing productivity, the "state-of-the-art summation of ways in which nursing productivity has been defined, researched, and enhanced through innovations in the organization and delivery of nursing care." (p. iii) Useful for administrators, educators, and researchers. Uses a systems model to organize a review of the studies. Includes recommendations. Study conducted by Medicus Systems Corporation.

13.72 Kraegel, Janet M.; Mousseau, Virginia S.; Goldsmith, Charles; et al. Patient Care Systems. Philadelphia: Lippincott, 1974.

219 pp. Cloth. Index. References. Bibliography.
Proposes that "the use of the science of design in patient care will put an end to the haphazard, confused,
chaotic and often purposeless approaches that have
emerged in hospitals." (p. v) Presents a rational approach to the design of complex health care systems.
The book grew out of a research project undertaken by
the authors using a systems methodology. Besides reporting their methods, experience, and results, they
present implications for change in future health care
delivery.

13.73 Mason, Elizabeth J. How to Write Meaningful Nursing
Standards. New York: Wiley, 1978.
355 pp. Paper (spiral bound).
A workbook written for nurses responsible for developing standards for quality assurance programs. Uses a
step-by-step approach. Chapters cover Setting the
Stage; Writing Process Standards; Writing Outcome
Standards; Writing Content Standards; Validating Standards; Organizing the Task.

13.74 Mayers, Marlene G.; Norby, Ronald B.; Watson, Annita B.
Quality Assurance for Patient Care: Nursing Perspectives.
New York: Appleton-Century-Crofts, 1977.
300 pp. Paper. Index. Bibliography.
The aim of this book is "to assist nursing service personnel to apply effectively the principles of evaluation
to the patient care setting." (p. ix) For students and
graduates. Topics include The Evaluation Process,
Quality Assurance Mechanisms, Documentation of
Patient Care, and Implementation of a Quality Assurance Program.

13.75 Nicholls, Marion E.; Wessells, Virginia G., eds. Nursing
Standards & Nursing Process. Wakefield, Mass.: Contemporary Publishing, 1977.
164 pp. Paper. Index. Bibliography.
For students and beginning practitioners as they look
at the standard-setting function of the nursing manage-

ment role. The units are Terminology and Standard
Setting; Factors Affecting Nursing Standards; Nursing
Process, Nursing Standards, and Quality Control; and
Case Studies. The case studies represent actual situations in which standards were set, the means of
achieving them were identified, and the outcome evalu-
ated.

13.76 Phaneuf, Maria C. The Nursing Audit: Self-Regulation in
Nursing Practice, 2d ed. New York: Appleton-Century-
Crofts, 1976.
>204 pp. Paper. Index. References.
Chapters discuss quality performance and appraisal of
nursing care, the audit, the instrument itself, planning
for the audit, the audit committee, experiences of
auditing in university hospitals and visiting nurse
agencies, the Slater Nursing Competencies Rating
Scale, etc. Appendixes include random number tables,
audit forms, explanations of the audit. Subtitle of the
first edition was Profile for Excellence.

. 13.77 Rezler, Agnes G.; Stevens, Barbara J., eds. The Nurse
Evaluator in Education and Service. New York: McGraw-
Hill, 1978.
>333 pp. Cloth. Author and subject indexes.
Bibliography.
Includes materials essential for prospective nursing
instructors, clinical specialists, and nursing admin-
istrators. Covers basic ideas about evaluation in
nursing in a clear, concise way, using relevant exam-
ples. Part 1: Basic Concepts of Evaluation; Part 2:
Evaluation in Nursing Education; Part 3: Evaluation in
Nursing Service; and Part 4: Reporting and Analyzing
Evaluation Data.

13.78 Schwirian, Patricia M. Prediction of Successful Nursing
Performance, Part I and Part II. DHEW publication no.
(HRA) 77-27; Health Manpower References. Hyattsville,
Md.: U.S. Department of Health, Education and Welfare,

Public Health Service, Health Resources Administration,
Bureau of Health Manpower, Division of Nursing, 1978.
226 pp. Paper. Author index. Annotated bibliography.
Results of a study done by The Ohio State University
Research Foundation. Part I is a comprehensive literature review from 1965-1975 of "literature relevant
to academic and clinical selection and prediction criteria in nursing that could serve as a reference for
researchers and educators, and suggest areas for
future research." (p. iii) Part II consists of
results from a questionnaire sent to 151 nursing
schools which requested information on their prediction and measurement of nursing performance as well
as names of specific "effective performers." Plans
are to undertake a third part to report on actual job
performance by those named as well as of a random
sample from among those not nominated. Parts III
and IV (one volume, 1979) not available for annotation.

13.79 Wandelt, Mabel A.; Stewart, Doris Slater. Slater Nursing
Competencies Rating Scale. New York: Appleton-Century-
Crofts, 1975.
101 pp. Paper. References. Bibliography.
The Slater Nursing Competencies Rating Scale consists of 84 items which are designed to rate actions by
nurses as they care for patients. This book contains
information on the scale and its use in general, how to
measure an individual by using the scale, tests of reliability and validity relating to the scale, and evaluation and the experience of others regarding the scale.

STAFF DEVELOPMENT

13.80 Cooper, Signe Skott; Hornback, May Shiga. Continuing
Nursing Education. New York: McGraw-Hill, 1973.
261 pp. Cloth. Index. Footnotes. References.
"This book is designed primarily for nurse faculty
members responsible for continuing education in institutions of higher learning." (p. vii) A readable

book on a topic of growing importance to all nurses.
Covers definition and justification of continuing education, history of continuing education, the design and
implementation, teaching methodology, and evaluation
of continuing education. Other chapters deal with refresher courses, inservice education, and self-directed
learning.

13.81 Eng, Evelyn. Staff Development in a Hospital Nursing Service. NLN publication no. 20-1447; League Exchange, no.
95. New York: National League for Nursing, 1972.
77 pp. Paper.
Contains practical information relating to nursing service personnel development and administration. Includes statements and/or guidelines on the philosophy
and purpose of hospital nursing service, orientation of
new employees, employee evaluation, guidelines for
staff reporting, meetings attended, ward conferences,
retention and recruitment of personnel, and public relations. The last chapter gives job descriptions for
various nursing service personnel.

13.82 Lasdon, Gail S., ed. Improving Ambulatory Health-Care
Delivery: Multidisciplinary Applications. Lexington, Mass.:
Heath, 1977.
209 pp. Cloth. References.
A report of a conference on improving ambulatory
health care delivery. Looks at current problems,
and at feasible and practical solutions for decision making in the short run. Topics include manpower and technology, quality assessment, cost analysis, regional planning, patient-oriented care, and the
perspective of the administrator.

13.83 MacVicar, Jean; Boroch, Rose. Approaches to Staff Development for Departments of Nursing: An Annotated Bibliography. NLN publication no. 20-1658. New York: National
League for Nursing, 1977.
38 pp. Paper.
This brief collection of annotated references is com-

prised of citations to general articles on continuing
education, methods, expanded roles for nurses, refresher programs, nurse internships, and the continuing education unit. A brief listing of films and
audio cassette tapes is also included.

13.84 Popiel, Elda S., ed. Nursing and the Process of Continuing
Education, 2d ed. St. Louis: Mosby, 1977.
249 pp. Paper. Selected bibliography.
Five parts are entitled What Is Continuing Education?;
Implementation of Continuing Education; Who Is Involved?; Evaluation of Continuing Education Programs;
and Examples of Continuing Education Programs.
Parts include papers by various nurse, adult, or other
educators.

13.85 Price, Elmina Mary. Learning Needs of Registered Nurses.
[Nursing Education Monographs.] New York: Teachers College Press, Department of Nursing Education, Teachers
College, Columbia University, 1967.
111 pp. Paper. Bibliography.
Gives the results of a study the author did of hospital
personnel (nurses, aides, orderlies) which attempted
to ascertain their weaknesses in terms of training and
their needs in terms of inservice programs. Goes
into the methodology, participants, conclusions of the
study. Appendixes include instruments used and the
coded results.

13.86 Swansburg, Russell C. Inservice Education. New York:
Putnam, 1968.
340 pp. Paper. Index. Bibliography.
A programmed text designed to delineate some of the
basics related to inservice people. Chapters are entitled What Is Inservice Education and Who Should Receive It?; Why Do We Need Inservice Education?; How
Do We Get Inservice Education off the Ground?; What
Shall the Program Be?; What Responsibility Do People
Have for Continuing Their Own Education? Appendixes
include information on teaching techniques, etc.

13.87 Tobin, Helen M.; Wise, Pat S. Yoder; Hull, Peggy K. The
Process of Staff Development: Components for Change.
2d ed. St. Louis: Mosby, 1979.
> 248 pp. Cloth. Index. Bibliography.
> Written for staff development educators primarily,
> this book looks at the development, process, and con-
> cepts of staff development education. Reflects the
> changes related to agency responsibility and practi-
> tioner responsibility for continuing education. Topics
> include philosophy and goals, organization and admin-
> istration, concepts related to learning, and evaluation.
> Appendixes contain useful samples ranging from a
> year's staff development schedule, to an orientation
> program, to offerings developed for varying levels of
> nursing personnel.

PERIODICALS

13.88 Health Care Dimensions. F. A. Davis Co., 1915 Arch
Street, Philadelphia, Pa. 19103. Semiannually. 1974 to
date.

13.89 Health Care Education. Rienhardt-Keymer Publishing Co.,
Inc., 60 East 42nd Street, New York, N.Y. 10017. Quarterly. 1972 to date.

13.90 Health Care Management Review. Aspen Systems Corporation, 20010 Century Boulevard, Germantown, Md. 20767.
Quarterly. 1976 to date.

13.91 Hospitals. American Hospital Association, 840 North Lake
Shore Drive, Chicago, Ill. 60611. Biweekly. 1936 to date.

13.92 Journal of Nursing Administration. Journal of Nursing Administration, Inc., 12 Lakeside Park, 607 North Avenue,
Wakefield, Mass. 01880. Monthly. 1971 to date.

13.93   Nursing Administration Quarterly. Aspen Systems Corpora-
        tion, 20010 Century Boulevard, Germantown, Md. 20767.
        Quarterly. 1976 to date.

13.94   Nursing Leadership. Charles B. Slack, Inc., 6900 Grove
        Road, Thorofare, N.J. 08086. Quarterly. 1978 to date.

13.95   Supervisor Nurse. S-N Publications, Inc., 18 S. Michigan
        Avenue, Chicago, Ill. 60603. Monthly. 1970 to date.

13.96   Vital Statistics of the United States. U.S. National Center
        for Health Statistics, U.S. Public Health Service, Health
        Resources Administration, 5600 Fishers Lane, Rockville,
        Md. 20857. Annually. 1937 to date.

14
Research and Nursing

Research in nursing practice areas is growing. The use of
research from relevant fields of knowledge continues to be
important. As nursing develops its own body of knowledge
and theory to explain and predict nursing phenomena, nursing researchers will continue to use knowledge and theory
from the natural sciences, social sciences, and humanities.
This chapter is divided into the following sections: the research process, government documents, grants, research
conference reports, statistical sources, and writing for publication. Periodicals in these areas are listed at the end of
the chapter.

RESEARCH PROCESS

Abdellah, Faye G.; Levine, Eugene. Better Patient Care
Through Nursing Research, 2d ed. New York: Macmillan,
1979.
> 753 pp. Cloth. Author and subject indexes.
> References. Glossary.
> A practical, but theoretically based book on research
> that focuses on the problems and approaches that are
> unique to nursing, using nursing and health care situa-
> tions as examples. Part 1 introduces research in
> nursing; Part 2 describes research methodology; Part
> 3 discusses numerous studies; and Part 4 looks at the
> current status of nursing research. The book is com-
> prehensive, unique, up-to-date, and attempts to

answer troublesome questions of the beginning researcher.

14.2 American Journal of Nursing Co. Approaches to Nursing
Research and Theory Development in Nursing. New York:
AJN Co., 1969.
>   92 pp. Paper. References.
>   Articles reprinted from the journal, Nursing Research
>   (14.51). Examines thinking on important questions: How
>   will nursing define research? How can theories in
>   nursing be developed? What is the role of the nurse
>   researcher? Useful for researchers and consumers
>   of research.

14.3 Brink, Pamela J.; Wood, Marilynn J. Basic Steps in Planning Nursing Research: From Question to Proposal. North
Scituate, Mass.: Duxbury Press, 1978.
>   214 pp. Paper. Index. Bibliography.
>   A text for the beginning researcher that provides an
>   introduction to the research process by examining in
>   detail the research plan. Useful for either graduate
>   or undergraduate courses introducing students to re-
>   search.

14.4 Diers, Donna. Research in Nursing Practice. Philadelphia:
Lippincott, 1979.
>   290 pp. Cloth. Index. Bibliography.
>   This text, written for nursing students (graduate and
>   undergraduate) and faculty, is based on the premise
>   "that all nurses can, and should, do research." (p. 2)
>   After discussing research problems and the research
>   process, the author describes various study designs:
>   factor-searching studies, association-testing studies,
>   and others. The final four chapters look at measure-
>   ment, data collection, the rights of subjects, and the
>   evaluation and writing of research.

14.5 Downs, Florence S.; Fleming, Juanita W. Issues in Nursing Research. New York: Appleton-Century-Crofts, 1979.
>   191 pp. Paper. Index. References.

The issues selected lie close to the heart of the research process and knowledge of them by consumers
of nursing research, researchers, educators, administrators, and graduate students should help "create
an atmosphere more conducive to and supportive of
research in nursing." (p. ix) Topics range from the
research process to the future of nursing research.
Contributors include Susan Gortner, Virginia Cleland,
Joanne Stevenson, Carolyn A. Williams, and Jean
Hayter.

14.6   Downs, Florence S.; Newman, Margaret A.; comps.   A
Source Book of Nursing Research, 2d ed.   Philadelphia:
Davis, 1977.
> 200 pp.   Paper.   Bibliography.
> After opening with the Elements of a Research Critique,
> the book is divided into two parts.   Part 1: Evaluation
> of Nursing Intervention includes research reports and
> focuses on nursing approaches.   Part 2: Exploration
> of Indices of Health includes reports that look at rela-
> tionships between client characteristics and behaviors.
> The appendix contains an appraisal of An Abstract for
> Action (11.16).   The reports reflect a variety of focuses,
> designs, and methodologies useful to students and other
> beginning researchers.

14.7   Drew, Clifford J.   Introduction to Designing Research and
Evaluation.   St. Louis: Mosby, 1976.
> 223 pp.   Cloth.   Index.   Bibliographies.   Glossary.
> A general introduction to research with an emphasis
> on design of an investigation.   Contains practice prob-
> lems to provide opportunities to simulate research
> situations.

14.8   Fox, David J.   Fundamentals of Research in Nursing, 3d ed.
New York: Appleton-Century-Crofts, 1976.
> 313 pp.   Cloth.   Index.   Bibliography.
> A basic text intended to familiarize the nurse, what-
> ever her role, with concepts which will enable her to
> read, do, and evaluate research.   Includes chapters

on research design, research process, problem-
solving, descriptive statistics, correlational procedures, inferential statistical concepts and procedures,
sampling, data-gathering, research instruments, and
analysis of qualitative data. Includes a reading list
designed to give more extensive background in terms
of already published studies.

14.9   Gallant, Donald M.; Force, Robert; eds. Legal and Ethical
Issues in Human Research and Treatment: Psychopharma-
cologic Considerations. New York: SP Medical & Scientific, 1978.
    186 pp. Cloth. Index. References.
    Presents practical guidelines for maintaining the pri-
    mary ethical values of the physician scientist. These
    values include obligation to patient, duty to humanity,
    and adherence to truth. (p. xix) Discusses the inter-
    play among science, philosophy, and law. The four
    major topics are science and the law, science and
    ethics, impact of litigation on psychopharmacology,
    and legislative and administrative constraints on
    psychopharmacology. Based on a symposium spon-
    sored by the American College of Neuropsychopharma-
    cology held in New Orleans, December 1979.

14.10   Krueger, Janelle C.; Nelson, Allen H.; Wolanin, Mary
Opal. Nursing Research: Development, Collaboration, Utilization. Germantown: Aspen Systems, 1978.
    424 pp. Cloth. Index. References.
    A report of a project, conducted over six years, on
    the feasibility of increasing nursing research activities
    on a regional basis. Of special interest are the dis-
    cussions of collaborative research, the approaches to
    research on quality of nursing care, and the problems
    of utilization of research findings. For those persons
    who use and/or conduct research.

14.11   Notter, Lucille E. Essentials of Nursing Research. New
York: Springer Publishing, 1974.
    147 pp. Cloth. References. Glossary.

Gives a brief historical perspective on research in
nursing and then goes on to discuss the meaning and
purpose of research, selecting a problem, the literature search, the hypothesis, the research method, data
collection and analysis, drawing conclusions, communicating the findings, and evaluating the research process.

14.12 Pavlovich, Natalie. Nursing Research: A Learning Guide.
St. Louis: Mosby, 1978.
265 pp. Paper. Selected readings.
For undergraduate nursing students as they learn the
basic concepts of nursing research. Provides problems and exercises to give the readers practice in
using their knowledge and skills in nursing research.
Each chapter includes the following sections: objectives, selected readings, definitions of terms, discussion questions, application, implications for nursing,
and review. Topics included are problems, literature
review; hypothesis; research methods; data collection;
data analysis; findings, conclusions, recommendations,
and implications; and research report.

14.13 Phillips, Bernard S. Social Research: Strategy and Tactics, 3d ed. New York: Macmillan, 1976.
365 pp. Cloth. Index. References. Annotated
bibliography.
The author views theory as the most important research tool, and research methods as the strategies
and tactics of scientists. For the student and beginning researcher as they look at the research process,
data collection, measurement and scaling, analysis of
data, and application of logic and mathematics. Includes exercises.

14.14 Polit, Denise F.; Hungler, Bernadette P. Nursing Research:
Principles and Methods. Philadelphia: Lippincott, 1978.
663 pp. Cloth. Index. References.
A basic text on methods and techniques of research,
for undergraduate and graduate students in introductory courses and as a reference for the nursing

community. A book for both the consumer and pro-
ducer of nursing research. The relevancy of the book
is increased by the liberal use of nursing research as
examples. Major headings include The Scientific Research Process; Preliminary Research Steps; Types
of Nursing Research Approaches and Research Design
Considerations; Data Collection Methods; Measurement
and Sampling; The Analysis of Research Data; Communication in the Research Process.

14.15   Riehl, Joan P.; Roy, Callista. Conceptual Models for Nursing Practice, 2d ed. New York: Appleton-Century-Crofts,
1980.
432 pp. Paper. Index. References.
A text which looks at models and their conceptual
frameworks and the implementation of theory into
practice. Includes The Nature of Nursing Models,
Conceptual Frameworks, Developmental Models for
Nursing Practice, Systems Models for Nursing Practice, Interaction Models for Nursing Practice, and
the Coalition of Nursing Models. Especially useful for
graduate and undergraduate nursing students.

14.16   Selltiz, Claire; Wrightsman, Lawrence S.; Cook, Stuart.
Research Methods in Social Relations, 3d ed. New York:
Holt, Rinehart and Winston, Society for the Psychological
Study of Social Issues (SPSSI), 1976.
624 pp. Cloth. Index. Bibliography.
A tried and true text for the social sciences that presents a thorough discussion of research methods including ethical concerns. Useful for nurse researchers as they examine social relationships involving
clients.

14.17   Stevens, Barbara J. Nursing Theory: Analysis, Application, Evaluation. Boston: Little, Brown, 1979.
280 pp. Cloth. Subject and author indexes.
Bibliography.
A look at the nursing theories proposed by several
nursing authors in order to make explicit the under-

lying structures and meanings. The goal is to develop
the ability to understand theories and their implications as the body of nursing theory develops. For
nursing students and practitioners who wish to learn
how to analyze theoretical works.

14.18 Susser, Mervyn. Causal Thinking in the Health Sciences:
Concepts and Strategies of Epidemiology. New York:
Oxford University Press, 1973.
181 pp. Cloth. Index. References.
An attempt "to develop causal models in a manner that
will foster understanding of the relationships between
states of health and environment." (p. viii) Written
for students in epidemiology as well as in other applied social science endeavors. After an historical
overview of cause in the health sciences, the author
discusses strategies for establishing cause by using
causal models. The focus is on research design and
analysis.

14.19 Treece, Eleanor Walters; Treece, James William, Jr.
Elements of Research in Nursing, 2d ed. St. Louis:
Mosby, 1977.
349 pp. Paper. Index. Bibliography.
A readable, concise, and practical text for a course
in research methodology. The book should help persons reach the point where they can conduct a study,
as well as read and critique research reports. Sections of the book focus on: research process, theory
and method, preparation for and collection of data,
analysis of data, and presentation of findings.

14.20 U.S. Department of Health, Education and Welfare, Division
of Nursing. Instruments for Measuring Nursing Practice
and other Health Care Variables. Edited by Mary Jane Ward
and Carol Ann Lindeman. DHEW pub. no. (HRA) 78-53,54;
Health Manpower References. Hyattsville, Md.: DHEW,1979.
828 pp. (2 vols.). Paper. Index. References.
A much-needed and useful compilation and critique of
both psychosocial and physiological instruments used

in nursing research. Includes the following data for each instrument: Author(s), variable(s) description, development, use in research, comments, references, source of information, instrument copyright.

14.21   Verhonick, Phyllis J., ed. Nursing Research I. Boston: Little, Brown, 1975.
      240 pp. Cloth. Index. Bibliography.
      The first volume in a series on nursing research. Section 1 addresses the conceptual framework of nursing research, and Section 2 discusses the behavioral science application in nursing research. Contributors include, among others, Jeanne Quint Benoliel, Imogene M. King, Rozella M. Schlotfeldt, and James K. Skipper.

14.22   Verhonick, Phyllis J., ed. Nursing Research II. Boston: Little, Brown, 1977.
      266 pp. Cloth. Index. References.
      The second volume (see 14.21) of a series that focuses on clinically oriented research in nursing. Its target is the beginning researcher who has a master's or doctoral degree. Section 1: Nursing Research in a Clinical Setting; Section 2: Models for Data Analysis. Contributing authors include Faye Abdellah, Virginia Cleland, Donna Diers, and Daniel Howland.

14.23   Verhonick, Phyllis J.; Seaman, Catherine C. Research Methods for Undergraduate Students in Nursing. New York: Appleton-Century-Crofts, 1978.
      154 pp. Paper. Index. Bibliography.
      An introduction to the rudiments of the research process written for undergraduates and practitioners of nursing. Discusses the main steps in the process of research. Recommended for a one-semester course in which the student completes a circumscribed study in some aspect of nursing.

14.24   Wandelt, Mabel A. Guide for the Beginning Researcher. New York: Appleton-Century-Crofts, 1970.
      322 pp. Paper. Index. References. Glossary.

An introduction to research problem-solving. Outlines and elucidates the "13 steps" of the research process, including defining the problem; stating the purpose of the study; making assumptions; collecting, organizing, and analyzing data; and reporting outcome. Marginal highlighting makes points easily distinguishable.

14.25 Werley, Harriet H.; Zuzich, Ann; Zajkowski, Myron; et al.; eds. Health Research: The Systems Approach. New York: Springer Publishing, 1976.
       330 pp. Cloth. Index. References.
       Includes papers presented at a March 1971 conference of health professionals and systems specialists commemorating the twenty-fifth anniversary of the Wayne State University College of Nursing, sponsored by their Center for Health Research. Begins with a discussion of general systems theory, then health professionals as subsystems, and administrative subsystems. Further papers concentrate on designing research using systems theory, using a systems approach to client and practitioner interaction, and the application of systems concepts to health care delivery.

14.26 Wooldridge, P. J.; Leonard, R. C.; Skipper, J. K. Methods of Clinical Experimentation to Improve Patient Care. St. Louis: Mosby, 1978.
       244 pp. Paper. Index. References. Glossary.
       "This book was written to help promote the use of clinical experiments for testing patient care procedures and developing general principles of more effective practice." (p. ix) It is a companion to the forthcoming volume, Behavioral Science and Nursing Theory, by the same authors. This text expands the Clinical Experimental Method (CLEM), as it is dubbed by the authors, and has three parts: Basic Concepts and Principles; Design and Data Analysis; Philosophy, Methodology, and Application. Includes an outline of strategies and techniques for CLEM, and discussion of actual experimental design studies.

GOVERNMENT DOCUMENTS

14.27 Jackson, Ellen. Subject Guide to Major United States Government Publications. Chicago: American Library Association, 1968.

> 175 pp. Cloth. Bibliography.
> An annotated listing by subject of major government documents. Subjects covered include: Education, Food, Health, Medicine, Research, Statistics, Vital Statistics, etc. Under each subject, lists title of publication, issuing agency, and Superintendent of Documents number. Includes an annotated bibliography of governmental guides, catalogs, and indexes by W. A. Katz.

14.28 Morehead, Joe. Introduction to United States Public Documents, 2d ed. [Library Science Text Series.] Littleton, Colo.: Libraries Unlimited, 1978.

> 377 pp. Cloth. Subject index. Selected title/series index. References.
> "The purpose of this work is to set forth an introductory account of public documents, their locus, diffusion, habitation, and use." (p. 5) Sections cover the Government Printing Office, Superintendent of Documents, Depository Library System, Non-Depository Publications, Selected General Guides to Federal Publications, Legislative Branch Materials, Publications of the Presidency, Department and Agency Publications, Publications of the Judiciary, Documents of Independent and Regulatory Agencies, and Reports of Advisory Committees and Commissions. A readable, organized book on a difficult subject. Appendixes include information for documents librarians, abbreviations.

14.29 U.S. Office of the Federal Register, National Archives and Records Service. United States Government Manual, 1979–80. Washington, D.C.: Government Printing Office, 1979.

> 914 pp. Paper. Name, subject, agency indexes.

This is the "official handbook of the Federal Government." (p. iii) Gives information on programs of governmental agencies, some quasi-official agencies, and some international organizations.

14.30 Wynkoop, Sally. Subject Guide to Government Reference Books. Littleton, Colo.: Libraries Unlimited, 1972.
276 pp. Cloth. Index. Bibliography.
An annotated guide to major reference books published by both federal agencies and the Government Printing Office. Consists of four parts covering works of general interest, works on the social sciences, works on science and technology, and works on the humanities. The science and technology section includes the medical sciences, arranged by broad categories. Listings include title, issuing agency, number of pages, price, Library of Congress catalog card number, Superintendent of Documents number, and annotation. Entries are numbered.

GRANTS

14.31 Annual Register of Grant Support, 1979-80, 13th ed. Chicago: Marquis Academic Media, 1979.
743 pp. Cloth. Indexes by subject, program and organization, personnel, geographic region.
Details the grant support programs of government agencies, public and private foundations, corporations, community trusts, unions, educational and professional associations, and special-interest organizations. Useful for academic scholars and researchers as well as for persons in business, civic improvement, and social welfare. Each program description includes type, purpose, duration of grant, funding available, eligibility requirements, deadlines, and other pertinent information.

14.32 Lewis, Marianna O., ed. The Foundation Directory, 7th ed. New York: The Foundation Center, 1979.

594 pp. Cloth. Indexes of foundations (alphabetically and by state and city); donors, trustees, and administrators; and fields of interest.

A standard reference for information about non-governmental sources of grant-making foundations. Included are some 3,138 private, company-sponsored, and community foundations which have a certain level of assets and annual contributions. Useful for fund seekers of all kinds.

14.33 Noe, Lee, ed. The Foundation Grants Index, 1977. New York: The Foundation Center, 1978.

443 pp. Cloth. Indexes by recipients, key words and phrases, subject categories.

In the first section, grants are described and listed by states of the recipients. Section 2 lists both domestic and foreign recipients of grants. Section 3 lists key words or phrases, and Section 4 is a subject index. Last is a list of foundations with addresses. Can be used in conjunction with the Foundation Directory (14.32) by persons seeking funding for various projects.

RESEARCH CONFERENCE REPORTS

14.34 Batey, Marjorie V., ed. Conference on Communicating Nursing Research. Boulder: Western Interstate Commission on Higher Education (WICHE), 1968-78.

11 vols. Paper. References.

Reports from a conference on nursing research held each year since 1968. The research report is followed in each case by a critique.

14.35 Nelson, M. Janice, ed. Clinical Perspectives in Nursing Research: Relevance, Suffering, Recovery. New York: Teachers College Press, 1978.

94 pp. Paper. References.

This monograph contains the three papers (with critiques) presented at the fourteenth annual Stewart Conference on Research in Nursing. Topics include The

Relevance and Use of the Clinical Laboratory, Nurses'
Inferences of Suffering, and Patients' Definitions of
Recovery from Acute Illness.

14.36 Semradek, Joyce A.; Williams, Carolyn A.; eds. Resolving
Dilemmas in Practice Research: Decisions for Practice.
Chapel Hill: University of North Carolina, School of Nurs-
ing, 1976.
    110 pp. Paper. References.
    Reports on a symposium held at the School of Nursing,
    March 1974, which "was designed to provide a forum
    for interdisciplinary discussion of issues of practice
    research." (p. iii) Invited papers include Dickoff and
    James, "From Dilemmas to Presets Through Design";
    Spitzer, "Canadian Studies of Primary Care Delivery
    by Nurse Practitioners"; Jacox, "Development of a
    Rationale for Practice: A Study of Pain Experience";
    Lindeman, "Case Studies of Practitioner Research."
    Includes summaries of panel discussions in response
    to the papers.

STATISTICAL SOURCES

14.37 American Hospital Association. Hospital Statistics, 1979:
Data from the American Hospital Association 1978 Annual
Survey. Chicago: AHA, 1978.
    216 pp. Paper. Index to statistical tables.
    "Presents detailed statistical data, in tabular form,
    on registered hospitals in the United States and its
    associated areas." (p. iv) An annual publication that
    began in 1972.

14.38 Statistical Services of the United States Government, rev. ed.
Washington, D.C.: U.S. Government Printing Office, 1975.
    234 pp. Paper. Bibliography.
    Part 1 describes the organization of statistical ser-
    vices in the federal government. Part 2 describes
    the principal economic and social statistics series
    collected by government agencies. Part 3 describes

agency statistical responsibilities and their principal
statistical publications.

14.39 U.S. Department of Commerce, Bureau of the Census.
Statistical Abstract of the United States, 1979, 100th ed.
Washington, D.C.: Government Printing Office, 1979.
   1057 pp. Cloth. Index. Bibliography.
   The "standard summary of statistics on the social,
   political, and economic organization of the United
   States." (p. ix) Of special interest to nursing are
   sections on population, vital statistics, health and
   nutrition, education, and social insurance and welfare
   services. Appendixes include Guide to Sources of Statistics and Guide to State Statistical Abstracts. Comes
   out annually.

14.40 Wasserman, Paul; Bernero, Jacqueline, eds. Statistical
Sources: A Subject Guide to Data on Industrial, Business,
Social, Educational, Financial, and Other Topics for the
United States and Internationally, 5th ed. Detroit: Gale
Research Co., 1977.
   976 pp. Cloth. Index.
   Sources of information about the United States and foreign countries are indexed under specific subjects.
   International statistical sources are included. Entries
   are arranged alphabetically by subject. Both publications and source agencies are included. Also contains
   a selected bibliography of key statistical sources. Subjects are not exclusively medical.

WRITING FOR PUBLICATION

14.41 King, Lester S. Why Not Say It Clearly: A Guide to Scientific Writing. Boston: Little, Brown, 1978.
   186 pp. Paper. Index. References.
   Written by a retired editor with 16 years experience
   for all who wish to improve their expository writing
   skills. Contents use examples from medical and
   English literature. Contains useful sections on begin-

ning to write and on editing and revising. Closes with
an outline for a course in medical writing.

14.42 O'Connor, Andrea B. Writing for Nursing Publications.
Thorofare, N.J.: Charles B. Slack, Inc., 1976.
>99 pp. Paper.
>Designed to help nurses share their knowledge, obser-
>vations, and expertise through the medium of writing.
>Provides information for selected journals of relevance
>to nursing for those wishing to have articles published,
>including procedures, types of articles, the scope of
>the journal, and so on. Appendix has a limited list
>of journals. Many of the specialty journals are not
>included.

14.43 University of Chicago Press. A Manual of Style: For
Authors, Editors, and Copywriters, 12th ed., rev. Chicago:
University of Chicago Press, 1969.
>546 pp. Cloth. Index. Bibliography.
>A reference book in three parts: Bookmaking, Style,
>and Production and Printing. Includes information on
>the preparation of a manuscript, proofs, copyright,
>punctuation, bibliographies, typography, etc. Some-
>times referred to as the Chicago Manual of Style.

14.44 U.S. Government Printing Office. Style Manual, Issued by
the Public Printer under Authority of Section 1105 of an Act
of Congress Approved October 22, 1968, rev. ed. Washington, D.C.: Government Printing Office, 1973.
>548 pp. Cloth. Index.
>The official style manual which is used in government
>printing. Previous editions entitled Manual of Style.

INDEXES

14.45 *American Statistics Index: A Comprehensive Guide and Index to the Statistical Publications of the U.S. Government.

---

*See Chapter 16 for a detailed explanation of this index.

Congressional Information Service, 7101 Wisconsin Ave.,
Washington, D.C. 20014. Monthly with quarterly and annual
cumulations. 1973 to date.

14.46 Excerpta Medica Abstracting Journals. Excerpta Medica,
Inc., P.O. Box 3085, Princeton, N.J. 08540.*

14.47 *Monthly Catalog of United States Government Publications.
Superintendent of Documents, Government Printing Office,
Washington, D.C. 20402. Monthly with annual cumulations.
1895 to date.

14.47 Public Affairs Information Service Bulletin. PAIS, 11 West
40th Street, New York, N.Y. 10018. Weekly. Cumulated
5 times per year and annually. 1915 to date.

PERIODICALS

14.49 ANS; Advances in Nursing Science. Aspen Systems Corporation, 20010 Century Boulevard, Germantown, Md. 20767.
Quarterly. 1978 to date.

14.50 International Journal of Nursing Studies. Pergamon Press,
Inc., Journal Department, Maxwell House, Fairview Park,
Elmsford, N.Y. 10523. Quarterly. 1964 to date.

14.51 Nursing Research. American Journal of Nursing Co. (for
the American Nurses' Association and National League for
Nursing), 10 Columbus Circle, New York, N.Y. 10019.
Bimonthly. 1952 to date.

14.52 Nursing Research Report. American Nurses Foundation,
Inc., 2420 Pershing Road, Kansas City, Mo. 64108.
Quarterly. 1966 to date.

----

*See Chapter 16 for a detailed explanation of this index.

14.53 Research in Nursing & Health. John Wiley & Sons, Inc.,
       605 Third Avenue, New York, N.Y. 10016. Quarterly.
       1978 to date.

14.54 Western Journal of Nursing Research. Western Journal of
       Nursing Research, 1330 South State College Boulevard,
       Anaheim, Ca. 92806. Quarterly. 1979 to date.

II

LIBRARY INFORMATION

15

Organization of the Library

The nursing profession plays an integral part in the delivery of health care. Since health care is a constantly changing and dynamic field, the nurse must keep abreast of new developments in order to participate in providing optimum health care delivery. The nursing profession looks at both the well and the ill adult throughout the life cycle. To this end, the nurse's task is to be involved as much as possible in the study of the individual not only as a patient, but as a person. The necessity for keeping abreast in nursing demands a familarity with libraries, the storers of valuable information. For it is in the contemporary literature of medicine and nursing that new developments in patient care delivery are reported.

As a nurse in any setting, you have access to a variety of libraries. On one end of the spectrum is the highly specialized research library which is used by a select clientele, and on the other end is the broad-based library which collects every variety of subject material and is open to the public. Depending on your situation, you may have access to any or all categories of the libraries we will discuss below and there is material in each of them which can be useful to you.

TYPES OF LIBRARIES

The main categories of libraries are (1) public, (2) academic, and (3) special. Public libraries are designed to

serve the communities in which they are located and are
supported by local and state and/or federal funds. Academic
libraries are those which serve institutions of learning.
Generally, they are supported fiscally by the institutions
which they serve and their clientele are the students, staff,
and faculty of the institution. A special library houses a
collection of materials on a specific subject or array of subjects (e.g., music, art, rare books, state materials) or
may be designed to fill the specific needs of a particular organization or group (e.g., a bank, an industry). Special
libraries can be found in institutions of learning and in other
public or private settings. All three categories of libraries—
public, academic, special—can be any size depending on the
clientele they serve. Each library must try to serve its
users' needs within the limits of its resources.

FUNCTIONS OF LIBRARIES

Regardless of a library's size or category, there are certain tasks which all libraries perform so that materials can
be acquired, found by users of the library, and checked out
of the library. In order for libraries to obtain materials
and to make such materials available to their clientele,
there are numerous operations which must take place. For
purposes of discussion, we will talk about printed materials
throughout this chapter, realizing that libraries must perform the same types of operations with nonprint materials
as well, though the routines may be altered in some cases.

Acquisitions

Before a library can buy materials, it must have an idea of
what is available in the area in which it wishes to acquire
materials. Such is the function of the Acquisitions Department of a library. It selects items which are to be added to
a particular library's collection. This is done systematically by checking library materials, such as acquisitions lists
of large libraries; publishers' magazines, flyers, and

catalogs; and journal advertisements, to mention only a few. In addition, most libraries welcome requests from their users (in library jargon: patrons). The Acquisitions Department, then, with the help of the library users and staff, decides on the items to be ordered. Items are ordered directly from the publisher, or they can be obtained through a "jobber"—usually a commercial firm which acts as a distributor of books available from various publishers. Using a jobber can be quite convenient for an Acquisitions Department, since it may be able to order many books through one source, instead of having to place separate orders through individual publishers.

Cataloging

Once an item has been received by the Acquisitions Department, it must be added to the library's collection and made available to the library's clientele. The idea of a Catalog Department in a library might seem strange to you until you think of what would happen were a library simply to place books as they are received on the shelf randomly. It would make finding the specific book you needed at any given time extremely difficult.

Enter the cataloger. This person takes all the books which a library receives and makes both a number and word description for the item. The cataloger uses a specific scheme which has been developed or is used by the library and involves placing the call number (classifying) and the description of the book (cataloging) on a "catalog card" (usually 3" x 5"). This card becomes the library's permanent record of the item and is kept in the card catalog. The Catalog Department also places the call number on the book itself and sees that the catalog cards are filed in the card catalog. (See page 376 for further discussion of the card catalog.)

The acquisitions and cataloging functions of the library are behind-the-scenes operations which you do not usually see, yet they are vital in helping you locate the type of information you need. These two departments are called, in library jargon, the Technical Services component of the library.

Once a book has been acquired and cataloged, it is the job of the Public Services (sometimes called Readers' Services) Department to help you, the patron, find what you are seeking. The Public Services Department is comprised of the Circulation Department, the Reference Department, and the Interlibrary Loan Department. The first two are probably the most well-known departments of the library from your standpoint.

Reference

The Reference Department in any library is there to help you get the particular piece of information you are seeking. You should not hesitate to consult a member of the Reference Department at any time if you cannot locate what you are looking for or if you are unsure as to where to go in the library. The Reference Department staff tries to be as familiar as possible with the library collection and operations in order to give the best service. Reference Departments can help you in a number of ways besides locating specific information. Many Reference Departments, for example, compile bibliographies on specific subjects for their patrons, or conduct computerized literature searches of specific subjects.

Circulation

The Circulation Department is probably the first thing that comes to mind when you think of a library and a librarian. The Circulation Department is, if you will, the sergeant-at-arms of the library collection. This department is basically there to help you check out library materials and to assure that both you and the library materials are protected. It determines when an item is due and the parameters for using library materials. This department keeps track of the items which are checked out and sees that they are returned when they should be returned. Most libraries have a one-month or two-week check-out period for their books. Journals either do not circulate, or circulate for varying periods, ranging from an hour or a day up to a week or more.

Interlibrary Loan

The Interlibrary Loan Department is one which many library patrons do not realize exists. This department attempts to locate books or articles in journals which are not in your particular library's collection. There are networks set up between libraries with specific regulations and forms which make it possible for the library to perform this service. When you cannot gain access to a particular book or journal in your area, tell the Interlibrary Loan Department exactly what you need and, most importantly, give them a verification of the item: where you obtained your information. If the verification is done, it avoids duplication of effort by the library staff and saves time for both you and the library.

LIBRARY PERSONNEL

We have discussed the various departments of a library. How about the people who make it possible for these departments to perform their functions? The personnel in a library are basically in two categories: the support (library technical assistants, nonprofessional or subprofessional) staff, and the professional staff. The former outnumber the professional staff and perform many important clerical and technical tasks. The professional staff are people who have studied, usually for a year or more beyond college, in order to obtain a master's degree in library science (usually called a M.L.S. or a M.S.L.S.). These professional personnel have studied about libraries and their workings and many of them have either a second master's degree in a subject field or an undergraduate degree in a specific subject. Professional medical librarians have usually had some course work specifically designed for medical librarians or have passed an examination in order to be considered qualified

for such positions. In the medical library field, the Medical
Library Association (MLA) certifies medical librarians on
various levels depending on their background and/or experience. Though all medical librarians are not certified by
the MLA, many are. Within the professional staff there are,
of course, heads of the various departments such as Acquisitions, Reference, and there may be a head of Public Services or a head of Technical Services. Over the entire
library is a professional librarian who is designated the
Head Librarian or the Director or some similar appellation.
Of course the extent to which such people are necessary is
totally dependent on the size of the library.

COLLECTIONS

Having looked at the departments in a library and its personnel, let's talk a little about library collections, the kinds of
things in a library. Most libraries are made up basically of
books and journals. Another component of many library collections is audiovisual material. Just what constitutes a
book or a journal or an audiovisual?

A book is usually defined as a work, published only one
time, which is authored, edited, or compiled by a specific
person or set of persons. We know that in many instances
books are published in new editions, but a book of this nature
undergoes revision and is considered for all intents and purposes a new book. A book with scholarly pretensions on a
specific or limited subject is usually dubbed a monograph.
A journal, on the other hand, comes out several times a
year and has articles by any number of persons. It is usually published year after year, issue after issue, under the
same title, simply by adding enumeration or a designation
which distinguishes one issue from another. Another word
for journal is periodical. Serial is a broader term which
includes journals but which also encompasses regular annual
publications (which, we will see, some libraries treat as
books and others as journals).

Generally, it is simple to tell the difference between a
book and a journal. Obviously, the book, A Guide for the

Beginning Researcher, is different from Nursing Research, the journal which comes out bimonthly and has been published since 1952. However, there are certain publications which are difficult to fit into either of these categories. Take, for example, a yearly publication such as the Physicians' Desk Reference. Librarians might treat this type of publication as a book or as a journal, since it meets the qualifications of both in one way or another. It only comes out once a year, but it comes out each and every year, in the same format and with the same title. To add further confusion to the matter, there are some journals which are really published like books, for example, the journals which publish conference proceedings as a special issue of the subscription. In this case, the library may catalog and/or classify the journal just as it would a book. In most cases cataloging is not done for journals, since periodical indexes are available to perform the cataloging function for journals. This problem is significant only if you use a library where books and journals are listed in different catalogs, as is the case with many medical libraries. In this situation, it would be important to check both the book catalog and the journal catalog for this type of publication.

Many libraries collect audiovisual (A.V.) equipment and programs, dubbed hardware and software respectively. This is a relatively new development and some libraries are just getting into developing this type of collection. A.V.'s may be defined broadly to encompass all non-print materials, including microfilm, microfiche, computer assisted instruction, models, charts, etc. The scope and breadth of any A.V. collection, of course, depends on the library's clientele, but for our purposes we will discuss some of the more conventional categories of audiovisuals. Audiovisual software can be of many varieties: 16-mm motion pictures, records, reel-to-reel audiotape; audiocassette tape; slides (of varying sizes and shapes, most popularly 2 x 2); slide/tape sets often including scripts; filmstrip (35mm) with or without audiotape or record; motion picture cartridges of varying shapes and sizes (Super 8mm, 8mm, most popularly); reel-to-reel videotape; or videocassette (usually 3/4" U-matic), to mention only some of the formats. Since many subjects can be understood better by means of visuals with audio than by audio or visual alone, libraries have added such materials to their collections. Usually these materials are stored in a separate facility within or adjacent to the library; however, some libraries choose to house such materials on shelves with the book and/or journal collection. Users generally have the same access to A.V.'s as they have to books or journals, limited only by the availability of equipment.

Reference Collections

Within a library collection, there may be certain special collections of materials, e.g., reference, reserve, newspaper, government document, or rare book collections. Regardless of size, most libraries have a reference collection.

Reference materials consist of items which have high usage and also which are used primarily to gain a specific piece of information. They are not to be read from cover to cover like most books or even journals. Webster's Third Unabridged Dictionary, The Encyclopaedia Britannica, Readers' Guide to Periodical Literature are examples of reference books. Such sources are available for you or a reference librarian to "refer" to in order to get a specific piece of information—a fact, a definition, a spelling, or the title of an article or book or audiovisual dealing with a particular subject. For this reason, most libraries sort out this kind of material and place it in the reference collection. Reference collections can be organized in different ways depending on the library. These books usually do not leave the library building so that they are available at all times for consultation.

Reference collections can include books or journals or indexes (really a specific type of journal). There are other more specific categories of books in reference collections— dictionaries, encyclopedias, atlases, handbooks, gazetteers, yearbooks, etc. See Chapter 1 for a more detailed discussion of reference materials.

Reserve Collections

Another special collection found in many libraries is the reserve collection. This section usually consists of items (books, journals, journal articles) which will be used heavily by students or some other part of the library clientele and for that reason are taken out of regular circulation. In many cases, these items can be used only in the library, or can be checked out for just a few hours so that a maximum number of people will have access to them. Depending on the volume of reserve books which a library has, there can be an entire floor, a room, or shelf space behind the circulation desk specifically for this type of collection.

Other Collections

Other types of special collections within libraries might include newspaper collections, government document collections, rare book collections. Such special collections are usually created when a library has a large number of such items or anticipates a large number and believes they are more useful in a specifically designated place.

USING THE LIBRARY

Just how do you go about locating what you need when you go into a library? It may be a small library where all the functions outlined earlier are carried out by one person who may not be a trained professional librarian, or it may be a huge library which employs hundreds of professional librarians to keep it functioning efficiently. Regardless of the size, each and every library has some sort of catalog listing what is available within its facilities (on cards, in a book, or on an on-line computer). We will discuss the card catalog for purposes of simplicity, since it is by far the most popular and standard format currently used in libraries of all sizes and types.

The Card Catalog

The card catalog usually includes all the books in the
library's collection, organized by author, title, and subject. A card catalog may or may not list the journals which
a particular library owns. In any event, most libraries
have a separate journal catalog, called the "kardex," in
which they check in journal issues as they are received.
We will discuss the kardex shortly.

A card catalog can be of two types—a split (or divided)
catalog or a dictionary catalog. A split catalog usually contains authors and titles in one section, and subjects in another, or separates all three categories. A dictionary catalog interfiles author, title, and subject together in one alphabet. This means that if you are looking for a book by
John Smith you need to look under Smith, John in the author/
title section of a split catalog, or in the alphabetic sequence
of Smith in a dictionary catalog. A book entitled Smoking
for Adults would be filed after Smith in both catalogs, but
books cataloged under the subject "smoking" would be filed
either in the subject section in the split catalog or together
with the titles and authors in the dictionary catalog. It is
important to know which system is being used; otherwise it
is possible to miss an item completely.

In either type of catalog, the basic arrangement is alphabetic, i.e., Smathers before Smith before Smythe, etc.
However, there are numerous filing rules which sometimes
make it difficult to locate items. For example, most catalogs file by the principle of "nothing before something"
rather than strictly letter-by-letter when filing alphabetically, i.e., North Carolina and North Dakota would come before Northampton, for though the "a" in Northampton comes
before the "c" or the "d" in Carolina or Dakota, the space
files before the letter "a." Another filing rule involves Mc
or Mac or variables of this. Mc and Mac are usually filed
under Mac in the card catalog, so you will find MacDonald
before McGovern before MacManus before McReedy before
Magruder. Or an "a" with a circle over it, such as ård-
vark or åborg, is often filed as two a's, e.g., aardvark and
aaborg. An umlaut, e.g., schöne, is usually filed as the

vowel with an e after it, as schoene. Hyphenated names or
names with several parts (de Los Angeles, diStefano, Obras
y Maja, etc.) may be filed by any of the three parts of the
name, so be sure to check under all three. Usually the same
library will file the same author in the same place, but where
that place is can vary from library to library. Also a word
about corporate authors, such as the National League for
Nursing or the American Nurses' Association. A book
authored by one of these associations is usually filed under
the name of the association. However, if the book is by a
department or council or agency of the association, you
should look first under the name of the association, then
under the name of the department or council, e.g., National
League for Nursing Council of Baccalaureate and Higher Degree Programs and not just National League for Nursing.
Rules like this may seem picky, but they were generally established for good reasons. Be sure to ask if you cannot
locate something in the card catalog, and remember if you
do not find it listed under the first place you check, since
there are several cards filed for each item, you can look
under title, joint author or editor or compiler, subject, etc.,
for the same book.

Catalog Cards

The author, title, and subject cards in a card catalog are
called catalog cards, and constitute the library's permanent
record of items it has received or purchased. A standard
catalog card is illustrated on page 378. Notice that it
contains both a number and a word description. The word
description is the descriptive cataloging and the number is
the call number. In most libraries, the call number is in
the upper left hand corner of the catalog card and consists
of at least two lines. The first line is the class number and
places the book in a broad subject category according to a
predesigned classification scheme. The second line of the
call number is the cutter number and places books in the
same subject category in alphabetical order by author. In
medical libraries, because of the necessity for current in-

```
WY          Bullough, Vern L.
11              The emergence of modern nursing  by
B938e       Vern L. Bullough  and  Bonnie Bullough.
1969        2d ed.  New York  Macmillan; London,
            Collier-Macmillan    c1969
                vii, 277 p.  illus.

                Authors' names listed in reverse order
            on title page of 1964 edition.

                1.  History of Nursing  I.  Bullough,
            Bonnie                   II.  Title
8-25-70c
```

formation, there is usually a third line added to the call
number which gives the year of publication of the item.
While dates are used by many medical libraries, few general public or even academic libraries use them. Some
libraries may place the class number on two lines, as $\frac{WY}{100}$
instead of WY100, but the principle is still the same.
    The other part of the catalog card is the descriptive
cataloging and comprises the bulk of the information on a
particular item. It is also what you see at first glance when
you look an item up in the card catalog. The descriptive
cataloging is made up of "paragraphs." The first includes
the author(s), editor(s), or compiler(s), as well as the title,
place, publisher, and date of publication. The number of the
edition is also given here if it is beyond the first or if this is
the first edition and other editions are foreseen. On the very
top line of the catalog card is the first author or editor or
compiler who is listed on the title page. For purposes of
appellation, the top line of a catalog card (not including
typed-in headings in red, black, or capital letters) is called
the main entry. This is the entry under which the cataloger
thinks you are most likely to look for the book, assuming
you know the specific book you are looking for and aren't
looking by subject. After the bibliographic paragraph on the

catalog card, comes the <u>collation</u> line, the second paragraph
on the card. This line usually stands out because it is in-
dented under the title and includes the number of pages (preliminary pages are listed in either small Roman numerals
or Arabic numerals depending on how the book itself is numbered), whether or not the book has plates, diagrams, illustrations or the like, and whether or not they are in color.
You will note on some catalog cards there is also a series
statement in this paragraph, e.g., if the book is part of a
specific series, this is noted. On some catalog cards there
is a <u>notes paragraph.</u> Such a paragraph will note the inclusion of a lengthy bibliography, earlier titles of the book, and
so forth. The last paragraph on the catalog card contains
what are called the <u>added entries.</u> While a book itself can
only be put in one place on the shelf, use of added entries
allows the patron to find it under several alternate entries
in the card catalog. Take, for example, a book on the pediatric nurse practitioner. The cataloger can list it under
several subject categories such as pediatric nursing, nurse
practitioners, etc. Within the added entry paragraph on the
catalog card, you will notice that items are typed after
Arabic numerals in the first case and Roman numerals in
the second case. The Arabic numerals delineate subject
headings which help you access the book by specific topic.
In some libraries, subject headings are typed in red, and in
others they are typed in capital letters. The Roman numeral
headings are usually typed in black in small letters except
for the initial letters and consist of alternate authors or co-
authors, title, etc. Note that authors can be individual as
well as corporate, e.g., John Doe or U.S. One word of
caution: many large libraries do not put common title entries in their card catalog; e.g., <u>Fundamentals of</u> . . . or
<u>Textbook of</u> . . . so you may not find added entry cards for
such titles. If this is the case, check under subject or a
truncated title. If the title is <u>Textbook of Internal Medicine</u>
try under "I" for Internal rather than under "T" for Textbook. With the book we used as an example here, cards are
filed under three different places in the card catalog besides
the main entry "Bullough, Vern L." They are filed under
"History of nursing" as subject; "Bullough, Bonnie" as joint
author; and "Emergence of modern nursing" as title.

Remember, the card catalog is there to give you the information necessary to locate the item you are seeking. Looking carefully at a catalog card can save you time if you have a specific type of book in mind, if you want a book of a special length, or if you need a book which is illustrated, to mention only a few examples.

If you don't find something listed in the card catalog, you might think that a particular library doesn't own it. This might be the case, or the book might be on order or you may have the title or author or subject slightly wrong. If a book is on order or has just been received, some libraries file a special card, usually under the title. This card gives a minimum of information, just enough so that you will know the item is either on order or just received. If you are not sure of the author or title of a specific book, or if you cannot locate the book in a library which you think should have it, you can try to verify (make sure of) the information you have by checking Books in Print (BIP, a yearly publication of books currently available for sale through various publishers). If you can't locate your item in BIP, or if your library doesn't own it, you can ask for an Interlibrary Loan (ILL) so that your library can try to get the material for you from another library. Your ILL Department can give you the appropriate forms to fill out and tell you the guidelines for this type of service.

Classification Schemes

The call numbers which libraries most commonly use come from three separate classification schemes, or schedules. These schemes are the Dewey Decimal Classification System, a strict number system; the Library of Congress Classification System, a letter-number designation developed by the Library of Congress; and the National Library of Medicine Classification System, a letter-number system developed by the National Library of Medicine.

The Dewey Decimal Classification System has ten categories from 0 to 9 and has placed all knowledge into these categories. Within each category, the more specific the subject area, the longer the class number. The Dewey system has been widely accepted and is used by many old and established libraries. Catalogers, of course, argue over the pros and cons of using a specific classification system and recently there has been a trend toward usage of the Library of Congress (LC) Classification System instead of the Dewey.

The LC schedules encompass the letters of the alphabet with number designations following, e.g., BF789. Many librarians believe they allow for more growth of subject coverage and also that the alpha-numeric designations make it easier to remember categories of numbers.

The National Library of Medicine Classification System (NLM) was designed to be used either alone or in conjunction with the LC schedules. Though the LC schedule itself has a category designation for medicine (class R) and for science (class Q), this is generally not sufficient for large or extensive medical collections. The NLM schedule, however, does use letters in its scheme which were not used by the LC schedule or which were not fully developed if they were used. For example, W, the main component of the NLM schedule, is not used in LC, nor are QS through QZ. Therefore, many large medical libraries use NLM with LC as a supplement in non-health-related areas. Brief outlines of these three schedules appear in Chapter 16, with a more detailed breakdown for the WY category, which is the nursing category in the NLM schedule.

Familiarity with a specific classification scheme is not mandatory for the library user. However, if you are somewhat familiar with it, you will be able to browse more freely when attempting to locate information.

There are many classification schemes other than the three just described; we have merely tried to tell you of the major ones. Also, in cataloging, libraries try to be as exact as possible. To this end, catalogers often do not agree with classification schemes at times and may make minor, or even major, alterations. For example, a library may think that using only WY18 for nursing education (which encompasses undergraduate, graduate, and continuing education

in all types of programs) is not satisfactory and this might
alter it. When using any library, you will quickly become
attuned to its inclinations in this direction.

Standardized Subject Heading Lists

Just as libraries have standardized classification schemes
which they use in placing call numbers on books, they also
have standardized subject heading lists. Each of the three
classification schemes we have discussed has a specific set
of subject headings which a library can use with it. For the
NLM scheme it is MeSH (or Medical Subject Headings), for
LC, it is the LC List of Subject Headings, and for Dewey it
can be the LC list or some other standardized list.

Using the card catalog to find a book is usually quite
simple if you know the author and title, but determining the
exact subject heading under which it might be filed can be
more difficult. The need for a standardized subject listing
will become clear when you think of the problem of looking
for books on cancer, for example. You go to the card catalog and find nothing under "cancer" except a book or two beginning with cancer as its title in a dictionary catalog. Then
you decide to try "carcinoma," and still you find nothing but
books beginning with that word in the title. Finally, you try
"neoplasms" and you find many books on that subject in that
one place under that one subject heading. The idea of always
using a particular word or group of words to delineate a particular concept may seem unnecessary until you imagine how
annoying and endless it could be to think of every cancer
term and to search for items under the various headings,
eliminating duplicates. It would mean you would have to
think the way a particular cataloger or author was thinking
at a given time. Because of this, most libraries have standardized subject heading listings which they employ in as-
signing subject terms. Such a listing is usually available to
you at the card catalog and tells you the term or terms
under which items on a variety of topics have been listed.
Our discussion of MeSH in Chapter 16 will give you an
idea of how the concept of listing by specific subject headings
is applied.

Journals

Suppose the item which you want to locate is not a book but a
journal. Many libraries catalog their journals and put a
card for them in the card catalog. However, such libraries
usually do not check in on the catalog card each issue they
receive. Whether or not a library catalogs its journals, it
will have what is called a "kardex" to check in issues as they
are received and in which the library records the volumes
which it owns. The kardex is usually arranged in alphabetical order by the title of the journal and gives the location of
the journal in the library, as well as the volumes and current issues received. A word of warning—most large medical libraries arrange their journals on the shelves and in the
kardex by title, but many large academic libraries arrange
journals by corporate author. Hence, Journal of the American Medical Association would be filed under "J" for Journal
in a medical library, but in an academic library might be
under "A" for American Medical Association (as corporate
author).

CITATIONS

Suppose you want to find specific books or articles in journals which you have been told about, either by an instructor
or which appeared in a bibliography. Many people become
confused by the format used for citing materials in bibliographies. A citation or a reference, in library jargon,
means a listing of an article or a book which gives you all
the information needed to locate the material, e.g., author
and title of article, title of journal, volume, pages, date
(in the case of a journal article), or author or editor or
compiler, title, place of publication, publisher and date of
publication (in the case of a book). You are probably most
familiar with citations or references from bibliographies or
footnotes. When people become confused as to how to locate
a particular book or journal article which they see listed in
a bibliography, it is usually because they either do not understand the format for citing materials or because the

reference is incorrect. On the left below is a standard journal reference and on the right a standard book reference from a bibliography.

Journal	Book

Miller, R. L. "Antici-   Jucius, M. J. Personnel Man-
pate Questions, Seek   agement. 6th ed. Homewood,
Answers for Adept Labor   Ill., Irwin, 1967.
Relations Efforts."
Hospitals 50(13): 50-54,
1976.

Of course, the method of citing varies from journal to journal or book to book and the punctuation may differ, but these are the basic components necessary for a good, reliable reference.

Look at some examples below and try to figure out the best way to look for the specific items.*

Strudel, A. (1960) "The genesis of the fruit," Nature 25-30.
This is a journal reference. You will note the position of the date and the difference in punctuation. Also, the volume number of the journal is not given nor is the issue number. Even if the journal is not paged continuously (i.e., there are several page 25's in 1960), you should still be able to find the article if the year and author or title are correct. Note that journal references usually underline the title of the journal and that the title of the article is usually in quotes. Also, no place of publication or publisher is given. Having determined that this reference is to a journal, you need only go to your library's kardex or journal section to determine whether or not it takes this journal and, if so, its location.

Queen, Frank. The Ranch I Knew. Boston, Mass., 1976.
This is a book reference. Note that the title of the book is underlined and a place of publication is given

---

*Please note that all examples used are fictitious.

even though the publisher is left out. You need only go to your library's card catalog and check under author (Queen, Frank), or title (Ranch I Knew), or subject heading after determining an appropriate one. If you still can't locate the item, you might check Books in Print to see if you have the correct information, and if you still cannot locate the item, check with the reference librarian.

Mesmer, Sir F. G. S., "Sassafras," Botany 1974-75.
This appears to be a journal reference because a title is in quotes and the journal title is underlined. However, the use of two years makes one suspect that it may be a yearly or a biyearly publication as discussed earlier, which could be treated as a book or a journal. You should check the kardex under Botany to see if perhaps the article is in a journal by that name, and also the card catalog to see if perhaps Botany is some sort of book publication. It should be noted that if Botany is a book publication and Mesmer is the author of a chapter in the publication, there would not be a card in the catalog under "Mesmer," since each chapter in each book which a library owns cannot be listed. If you cannot locate this reference using these approaches, you should consult the reference librarian for additional ideas and help.

Bruce, Clarence, "Naval insignias," In The British Navy, 1900-1950, ed. by J. M. Noughton. N.Y.: Pantheon, 1971.
This is a reference to an article in a book. By bibliographic convention, the first author listed is the author of the article in the book. However, he would not be listed in the card catalog and neither would the title "naval insignias" for the reason given in Mesmer, above. But the use of the word "in" signifies that this is an article in a book with the title underlined and edited by "Noughton, J. M." Further evidence that this is a book is given by the designation of the place of publication and the publisher. Therefore, you would look in the library's card catalog under either

"Noughton, J. M." (editor), or "British Navy . . ." (title), or appropriate subject.

The basic thing to remember about a library is that it is arranged scientifically and items can be located scientifically. Above all, if you can't find what you are looking for, ASK!

POSTSCRIPT

Obviously, we cannot cover everything in this very brief chapter. So, in keeping with the rest of the book, we have included here a brief annotated bibliography of just a few of the many good books for library users who are interested in reading a little further than this chapter.

15.1 Gates, Jean Key. Guide to the Use of Books and Libraries, 4th ed. New York: McGraw-Hill, 1979.
    292 pp. Cloth.
    A good, basic introduction to the library and library materials. Gives some historical treatment of libraries as well as explanations of library arrangement and specific reference materials within the library. Last chapter is called "The Undergraduate Research Paper."

15.2 Lolley, John L.; Marino, Samuel J. Your Library—What's in It for You? [Wiley Self-Teaching Guide.] New York: Wiley, 1974.
    152 pp. Paper.
    A self-instructional booklet which goes step-by-step into many library basics in entertaining ways. States objectives before each chapter. Also has an appendix on "Writing a Research Paper."

15.3 McCormick, Mona. The New York Times Guide to Reference Materials. New York: Popular Library, 1971. (Original title: Who-What-When-Where-How-Why Made Easy.)

230 pp. Paper
A brief, concise, readable book. Goes into reference
books and collections and using materials in a library
as the two books above. Gives a sample term paper.

15.4 Morton, Leslie T. How to Use a Medical Library, 5th ed.
London: Heinemann, 1971.
120 pp. Cloth.
A concise, useful guide to medical library resources
with a more technical orientation than the other books
listed above. Besides dealing with indexes, reference
books, and such materials, discusses historical and
bibliographical sources.

15.5 Morton, L. T., ed. Use of Medical Literature, 2d ed.
London: Butterworths, 1977.
462 pp. Cloth. Index.
"A comprehensive guide to the general and specialist
literature covering the medical sciences." (Preface,
1st ed.) Chapters cover using libraries; primary information sources; indexes, abstracts, bibliographies,
reviews; mechanized information retrieval; historical
and biographical sources; and specific subjects (anatomy and physiology; public health; pharmacology and
therapeutics; surgery and anesthesia). By a noted
British librarian.

16
Miscellaneous Library Information

In this chapter, we will give some examples of library
catalog cards, discuss computerized retrieval systems,
and present some library classification schemes and information on medical subject headings (MeSH) as well as on indexes and abstracts.

PARTS OF THE CATALOG CARD

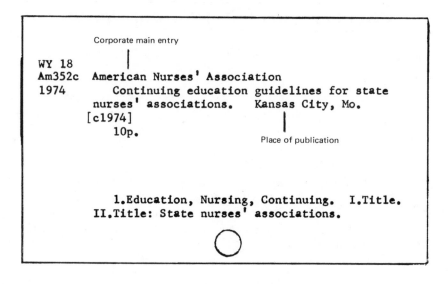

```
                    Corporate main entry

WY 18                   │
Am352c   American Nurses' Association
1974          Continuing education guidelines for state
         nurses' associations.    Kansas City, Mo.
         [c1974]                        │
             10p.
                                 Place of publication



             1.Education, Nursing, Continuing.    I.Title.
         II.Title: State nurses' associations.
```

```
                    National League for Nursing

WY 18.5
Oz5b     Ozimek, Dorothy.
1974          The baccalaureate graduate in nursing: what
         does society expect?  New York, National League
         for Nursing [c1974]
             8p.   (NLN publication no.15-1520)
                                                      Publisher
                 │
            Series statement


             1.Education, Nursing, Baccalaureate.   2.
         Students, Nursing.   3.Delivery of health care.
         I.National League        for Nursing.   II.Title.
```

Class No.
(subject)

Nurse-patient relations ——— Added entry (subject)—in
red or all capital letters

WY 160 ——— Cutter No. (author)
R561
1974   Robinson, Lisa.
              Liaison nursing: psychological approach to
          patient care. Philadelphia, Davis [c1974]
              xiii,238p.

Year of publication

              1.Psychiatric nursing. 2.Nurse-patient
          relations. I.Title

QU 120
D13i
1970   Dagley, S
              An introduction to metabolic pathways by
          S. Dagley and Donald E. Nicholson. Oxford,
          Blackwell Scientific Publications [c1970]
No. of pages, —— xi,343p. charts.
illustrations, etc.

              Colored chart of "Metabolic pathways" in
          pocket.
              Bibliography: p. 251 -320.   Notes about book

Alternate access points   Subject heading

              1.Metabolism.   I.Nicholson, Donald E
          joint author.   II.Title: Metabolic path-
          ways.   ways.

                                   Alternate title

A SET OF CATALOG CARDS FOR ONE BOOK

```
WY        Hall, Joanne E.                    Main entry card (author)
87            Nursing of families in crisis.  Edited
H177n     by Joanne E. Hall and Barbara R. Weaver.
1974          Philadelphia, Lippincott  [c 1974]
```

```
                                              Coauthor card
              Weaver, Barbara R.

WY            Hall, Joanne E.
```

```
              CRISIS INTERVENTION - NURSING TEXTS

WY            Hall, Joanne E.
87                Nursing of families in crisis.  Edited
```

```
                                              Subject cards—in red
              FAMILY - NURSING TEXTS          or all capital letters

WY            Hall, Joanne E.
87                Nursing of families in crisis.  Edited
H177n         by Joanne E. Hall and Barbara R. Weaver.
```

```
                                              Title card
              Nursing of families in crisis

WY            Hall, Joanne E.
87                Nursing of families in crisis.  Edited
H177n         by Joanne E. Hall and Barbara R. Weaver.
1974          Philadelphia, Lippincott  [c1974]
                  x, 264 p.

              Includes bibliographical references.


                  1.  Crisis intervention - nursing texts
              2.Family-nursing      texts  3. Nursing care
              I.  Weaver,        ◯      Barbara R.  II.  Title
```

COMPUTERIZED RETRIEVAL SYSTEMS

Through the use of the computer for storing and retrieving information, libraries are able to offer extensive service to patrons who are seeking specific types of information. There are a wide variety of data bases now available for searching, either on-line (direct interaction with a computer through the use of a cathode ray tube or a hard copy printer), or off-line (processing at a computer center with information mailed to a patron or a library).

In general, data bases contain information available in a printed index or in a series of printed indexes. Data bases are available in all areas from medical and nursing to non-medical areas. Libraries subscribe to specific data bases, depending on their user population. Generally, they charge a fee which will recover the costs incurred in subscribing to the data base.

The major data bases in the nursing and medical fields are available through the National Library of Medicine, one of the world's largest research libraries, whose holdings include over 2,500,000 books, journals, audiovisuals, and other materials.

The National Library of Medicine computer system includes a variety of data bases, some of which are listed below.

MEDLINE covers nursing, medicine, dentistry, and allied health for the current two years. It includes journals indexed in the International Nursing Index, the Hospital Literature Index, and Index Medicus, as well as some monographs and symposia. This is available on-line at a subscribing library or institution. A detailed explanation of MEDLINE follows this section.

MEDLARS covers the same indexes as above except that access is off-line and covers from 1966.

AVLINE indexes non-print materials in the health sciences.

BIOETHICSLINE indexes English-language material in

philosophy, law, ethics, and health-related fields
from 1973 to the current year.

SDILINE is a monthly search of MEDLINE for the most current month and as such is a current awareness service.

Also available are CANCERLIT, CANCERPROJ, CHEMLINE,
CLINPROJ, EPILEPSYLINE, TOXLINE, among others.
 A hospital or library can become an on-line center by
completing an application available through a Regional Medical Library. However, the United States has been divided
into 11 regions which coordinate requests for on-line acces-
sibility as well as for needed medical information via the
Biomedical Communications Network. There are also international centers cooperating with this service, which is coordinated through the National Library of Medicine.
 In addition to the data bases of the National Library of
Medicine, there are three major organizations or companies
to which a library or agency can subscribe. In subscribing
to one or more of these companies, a library or agency
agrees to pay a specific fee in return for access to the data
bases which are offered. Since these are commercial companies and the National Library of Medicine data bases are
partly subsidized by the U.S. government, fees of the commercial companies are higher and are perhaps much more
subject to increases.
 Bibliographic Retrieval Services, Inc. (BRS), Lockheed Missiles and Space Company, Inc. (Lockheed), and
System Development Corporation (SDC) are all commercial
companies which offer a variety of data bases to subscribers.
Among data bases that are available are ASI (American Statistics Index), BIOSIS (Biological Abstracts), Dissertation
Abstracts International, ERIC (Educational Resources Information Center), Sociological Abstracts, Excerpta Medica
Online, and many, many others. It is important to note
that not all of the above commercial companies supply the
same data bases and that while there is overlap, they each
supply some data bases which are unique to them alone.
 For further information contact:

1. Office of Inquiries and Publications Management, National
   Library of Medicine, 8600 Rockville Pike, Bethesda,
   Md. 20014

2. Bibliographic Retrieval Services, Inc., 702 Corporation
   Park, Scotia, N.Y. 12302. [518) 374-5011]

3. Lockheed Missiles & Space Co., Inc., Code 5020/201, 3251
   Hanover Street, Palo Alto, Calif. 94304. [(800) 227-
   1960; (800) 982-5838 (California)]

4. System Development Corporation, 2500 Colorado Avenue,
   Santa Monica, Calif. 90406. [(800) 336-0496]

Medline *(Medical* Literature Analysis and Retrieval System On *Line)**

Definition

A computerized information retrieval system through which
health professionals, at their own locations, can obtain references to current biomedical literature. Originated by the
National Library of Medicine (NLM), 8600 Rockville Pike,
Bethesda, Md. 20209. Available in the United States and
abroad.

Scope

Citations for articles in some 3,000 journals and for papers
in published congress or symposium proceedings (the latter
beginning in May 1976) can be retrieved. The data base contains more than half a million references which are also
found in Index Medicus, Cumulated Index Medicus, and the
NLM recurring bibliographies (e.g., International Nursing
Index) for the current year and the two immediately prior
years.

---

*Compiled in cooperation with Kathryn W. Kruse, Head,
Reference and Bibliography, Duke University Medical Center Library, Durham, N.C.

At the present time, retrospective literature searching to obtain references as early as the 1966 CIM (Cumulated
Index Medicus) is possible by using auxiliary files.

Mode of Operation

A local telephone call gives a user, at a typewriter-like
terminal in a subscribing library, access to computer files
at either NLM or the State University of New York in Albany.
Each publication represented in the computer files has been
assigned (indexed under) those MeSH headings which best
describe its subject content. A MEDLINE search is executed
when the computer compares the MeSH terms chosen and entered at the terminal by a user with the ones assigned to references in its files. Each time there is a match or "hit,"
the appropriate citation can be printed out at the terminal
(on-line). References retrieved through BACKFILE
searches, however, cannot be printed on-line, but must be
mailed from the computer installation (off-line).

A search statement can consist of a single MeSH heading or of several headings linked together by the Boolean op-
erators—AND, OR, AND NOT. Even if MeSH does not contain a term suitable to the user's need, a subject search can
still be run by having the computer check for specific words
in publication titles or abstracts.

MEDLINE is not limited to subject searches. Citations
can be retrieved by specifying an author, language, publication date, or journal title.

Example

The requests best suited for MEDLINE searching are the
multifaceted topics; i.e., those of two or more parameters.

If you need a list of references on the Nurse Practitioners, it would be advisable (at least in terms of expense)
to photocopy the appropriate pages from the subject section
of IM or CIM. Suppose, however, that you are interested
in material which discusses the Pediatric Nurse Practitioner

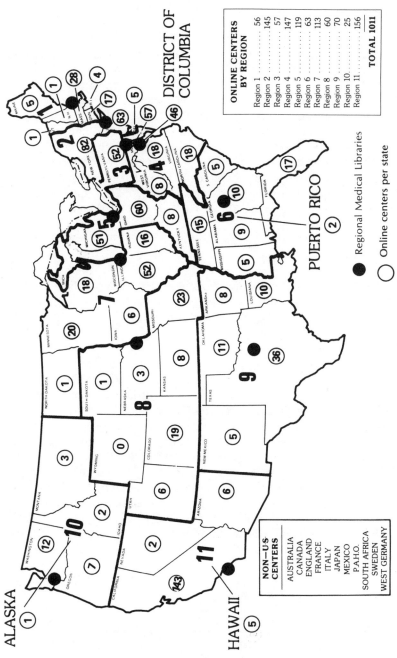

ONLINE CENTERS
BY REGION

Region 1	56
Region 2	145
Region 3	57
Region 4	147
Region 5	119
Region 6	63
Region 7	113
Region 8	60
Region 9	70
Region 10	25
Region 11	156
TOTAL	**1011**

DISTRICT OF
COLUMBIA

PUERTO RICO

● Regional Medical Libraries

○ Online centers per state

ALASKA

HAWAII

NON–US
CENTERS
_____
AUSTRALIA
CANADA
ENGLAND
FRANCE
ITALY
JAPAN
MEXICO
P.AHO.
SOUTH AFRICA
SWEDEN
WEST GERMANY

Map of online centers with access to NLM data bases. (From Public Health Service, National Institutes of
Health. MEDLARS: The Computerized Literature Retrieval Services of the National Library of Medicine.
NIH publication no. 80–1286. Bethesda, Md.: NLM, 1980.)

in North Carolina. It would be a tedious job to read through
all the titles in the printed index under the subject heading
NURSE PRACTITIONERS. Furthermore, a title does not always reveal the full contents of a publication. Here, then,
is a topic suitable for a MEDLINE search. By entering the
search statement—NURSE PRACTITIONER AND PEDIATRIC
NURSING AND NORTH CAROLINA—a user is directing the
computer to retrieve only those references which are indexed under all three of these MeSH terms. For this particular example it is important to note that geographic terms,
while available for computer searching, do not appear as
printed headings in the IM or CIM subject sections.

Charges

Users may be charged for searches depending on how their
library handles this. However, charges for this search are
usually less than for commercial data bases.

Additional Points

MEDLINE is updated monthly. This update portion of the
file, SDILINE, can be queried for current awareness
searches.

Remember, that while a citation in the computer files
has been assigned any number of MeSH headings, this same
reference will be printed in the IM or CIM subject section,
generally, under no more than three headings.

The success of a MEDLINE search is directly propor-
tional to the thoughtfulness with which the search terms are
selected and, subsequently, formulated into a search statement.

LIBRARY CLASSIFICATION SCHEMES

Sections of the National Library of Medicine, the Library of
Congress, and the Dewey Decimal Classification schemes

are reproduced in the next few pages. These are intended to be a guide to these three classification schemes in a general sense. As previously noted, libraries may have modified these systems to suit their user population and/or their book collection. In addition, for a fuller understanding of each of the systems, the complete sets of schedules should be consulted.

National Library of Medicine Synopsis of Classes*

Preclinical Sciences

QS	Human Anatomy
QT	Physiology
QU	Biochemistry
QV	Pharmacology
QW	Bacteriology and Immunology
QX	Parasitology
QY	Clinical Pathology
QZ	Pathology

Medicine and Related Subjects

W	Medical Profession
WA	Public Health
WB	Practice of Medicine
WC	Infectious Diseases
WD 100	Deficiency Diseases
WD 200	Metabolic Diseases
WD 300	Diseases of Allergy
WD 400	Animal Poisoning
WD 500	Plant Poisoning
WD 600	Diseases Caused by Physical Agents
WD 700	Aviation and Space Medicine

*From National Library of Medicine Classification....4th ed., 1978, p. xliii.

WE   Musculoskeletal System
WF   Respiratory System
WG   Cardiovascular System
WH   Hemic and Lymphatic Systems
WI   Gastrointestinal System
WJ   Urogenital System
WK   Endocrine System
WL   Nervous System
WM   Psychiatry
WN   Radiology
WO   Surgery
WP   Gynecology
WQ   Obstetrics
WR   Dermatology
WS   Pediatrics
WT   Geriatrics. Chronic Disease
WU   Dentistry. Oral Surgery
WV   Otorhinolaryngology
WW   Ophthalmology
WX   Hospitals
WY   Nursing
WZ   History of Medicine

National Library of Medicine Nursing Classification*

WY 1   Societies
WY 5-7   General Collections
WY 11   History
WY 16   Nursing as a Profession. Peer Review. Quality
            Control
WY 17   Atlases. Pictorial works
WY 18   Education. Outlines. Questions and Answers.
            Teachers' Instruction. Catalogs and Discussions
            of Audiovisual Materials. Computer Assisted
            Instruction
WY 19-20 Schools of Nursing

----

*Adapted from National Library of Medicine Classification
. . ., 4th ed., 1978, pp. 209-13.

WY 20.5   Research
WY 21   Licensure. Certification
WY 29   Employment. Placement Agencies
WY 31   Statistics. Surveys
WY 32-33   Laws. Jurisprudence
WY 44   Malpractice. Liability. Liability Insurance
WY 77   Economics of Nursing
WY 85   Nursing Ethics
WY 86   Nursing Philosophy
WY 87   Psychology Applied to Nursing. Psychological
           Aspects of Nursing. Relations to Patients,
           Physicians, Public
WY 90   General Referral and Consultation
WY 100   General Works on Nursing Procedures
WY 100.5   Nursing Records. Nursing Audit

Special Fields of Nursing

WY 101   General Works. Primary Nursing Care
WY 105   Administrative Work. Supervisory Nursing.
           Teaching
WY 106   Community Health Nursing
WY 108   Public Health Nursing
WY 109   Office Nursing
WY 113   School Nursing
WY 115   Home Care Services (Including Visiting Nursing
           and Visiting Nurse Associations)
WY 125   Institutional Nursing. Team Nursing
WY 127   Private Nursing
WY 128   Nurse Practitioners. Nurse Clinicians
WY 130   Governmental Nursing Services
WY 137   Red Cross Nursing
WY 141   Industrial Nursing
WY 143   Transportation Nursing
WY 145   Nursing by Religious Orders

Nursing Technics in Special Fields of Medicine

WY 150   General Works
WY 151   Nurse Anesthetists

WY 152 Geriatric and Chronic Disease Nursing. Long-
      Term Care. Terminal Care

WY 152.5 Cardiovascular Nursing. Hemic and
      Lymphatic Disease Nursing

WY 153 Communicable Disease Nursing

WY 154 Critical Care. Intensive Care. Recovery Room
      Care

WY 154.5 Dermatological Nursing

WY 155 Endocrine Disease Nursing

WY 156 Cancer Nursing

WY 156.5 Gastroenterologic Nursing

WY 156.7 Gynecological Nursing

WY 157 Obstetrical Nursing

WY 157.3 Maternity Nursing. Maternal-Child Nursing

WY 157.6 Nursing of Diseases of the Musculoskeletal
      System

WY 158 Ophthalmic Nursing. Otorhinolaryngological
      Nursing

WY 159 Pediatric Nursing

WY 160 Psychiatric Nursing. Neurological Nursing

WY 161 Surgical Nursing

WY 162 Operating Room Technics

WY 163 Nursing of Diseases of the Respiratory System

WY 164 Urological Nursing

  Other Nursing Services

WY 191 Male Nurses

WY 193 Nurses' Aides, Ward Attendants, and Orderlies

WY 195 Practical Nursing

WY 200 Home Nursing

  By Country

WY 300 Nursing by Country

Library of Congress Classification Schedules: Synopsis*

A	General Works
B-BJ	Philosophy. Psychology
BL-BX	Religion
C	Auxiliary Sciences of History
D	History: General and Old World (Eastern Hemisphere)
E-F	History: America (Western Hemisphere)
G	Geography. Maps. Anthropology. Recreation
H	Social Sciences
J	Political Science
K	Law (General)
KD	Law of the United Kingdom and Ireland
KE	Law of Canada
KF	Law of the United States
L	Education
M	Music
N	Fine Arts
P-PA	General Philology and Linguistics. Classical Languages and Literatures
PA Supplement	Byzantine and Modern Greek Literature. Medieval and Modern Latin Literature
PB-PH	Modern European Languages
PG	Russian Literature
PJ-PM	Languages and Literatures of Asia, Africa, Oceania. American Indian Languages. Artificial Languages
P-PM Supplement	Index to Languages and Dialects
PN, PR, PS, PZ	General Literature. English and American Literature. Fiction in English. Juvenile Belles Lettres
PQ Part 1	French Literature
PQ Part 2	Italian, Spanish, and Portuguese Literatures

---

*From <u>LC Classification Outline</u>, 4th ed. Washington, D.C.: Library of Congress, 1978.

PT Part 1	German Literature
PT Part 2	Dutch and Scandinavian Literatures
Q	Science
R	Medicine
S	Agriculture
T	Technology
U	Military Science
V	Naval Science
Z	Bibliography. Library Science

Library of Congress Classification Schedule: Medicine*

R		Medicine (General)
	131–684	History of medicine
	735–847	Medical education
	895	Medical physics. Electronics. Radiology, radioisotopes, etc.
RA		Public aspects of medicine
	5–418	Medicine and the state Including medical statistics, medical economics, provisions for medical care, medical sociology
	421–790	Public health. Hygiene. Preventive medicine Including environmental health, disposal of the dead, transmission of disease, epidemics, quarantine, personal hygiene
	791–954	Medical geography. Medical climatology and meteorology
	960–998	Medical centers. Hospitals. Clinics
	1001–1171	Forensic medicine
	1190–1270	Toxicology
RB		Pathology

---

*From <u>LC Classification Outline</u>, 4th ed. Washington, D.C.: Library of Congress, 1978, p. 24.

RC		Internal medicine. Practice of medicine
		Including diagnosis, individual diseases and special types of diseases, diseases of systems or organs
	86–88	First aid in illness and injury
	321–576	Neurology and psychiatry
	952–954	Geriatrics
	955–962	Arctic and tropical medicine
	963–969	Industrial medicine
	970–1015	Military medicine
	1030–1097	Transportation medicine
		Including automotive, aviation and space medicine
	1200–1245	Sports medicine
RD		Surgery
	92–96	Wounds and injuries
	701–796	Orthopedics
RE		Ophthalmology
RF		Otorhinolaryngology
RG		Gynecology and obstetrics
RJ		Pediatrics
RK		Dentistry
RL		Dermatology
RM		Therapeutics. Pharmacology
	214–258	Diet therapy. Diet and dietetics in disease
	270–282	Serum therapy. Immunotherapy
	283–298	Endocrinotherapy
	300–666	Drugs and their action
	695–890	Physical medicine. Physical therapy
	845–862	Medical radiology
RS		Pharmacy and materia medica
RT		Nursing
RV		Botanic, Thomsonian, and eclectic medicine
RX		Homeopathy
RZ		Other systems of medicine
	201–265	Chiropractic
	301–397	Osteopathy
	400–408	Mental healing

Dewey Decimal Classification—Second Summary*

000	Generalities
010	Bibliography
020	Library & information sciences
030	General encyclopedic works
040	
050	General serial publications
060	General organizations & museology
070	Journalism, publishing, newspapers
080	General collections
090	Manuscripts & book rarities
100	Philosophy & related disciplines
110	Metaphysics
120	Epistemology, causation, humankind
130	Paranormal phenomena & arts
140	Specific philosophical viewpoints
150	Psychology
160	Logic
170	Ethics (Moral philosophy)
180	Ancient, medieval, Oriental
190	Modern Western philosophy
200	Religion
210	Natural religion
220	Bible
230	Christian theology
240	Christian moral & devotional
250	Local church & religious orders
260	Social & ecclesiastical theology
270	History & geography of church
280	Christian denominations & sects
290	Other & comparative religions
300	Social sciences
310	Statistics

---

*From Dewey Decimal Classification and Relative Index, 18th ed., Vol. 1. Lake Placid, N.Y.: Forest Press, 1971.

320	Political science
330	Economics
340	Law
350	Public administration
360	Social problems & services
370	Education
380	Commerce (Trade)
390	Customs, etiquette, folklore
400	Language
410	Linguistics
420	English & Anglo-Saxon languages
430	Germanic languages German
440	Romance languages French
450	Italian, Romanian, Rhaeto-Romanic
460	Spanish & Portuguese languages
470	Italic languages Latin
480	Hellenic Classical Greek
490	Other languages
500	Pure sciences
510	Mathematics
520	Astronomy & allied sciences
530	Physics
540	Chemistry & allied sciences
550	Sciences of earth & other worlds
560	Paleontology
570	Life sciences
580	Botanical sciences
590	Zoological sciences
600	Technology (Applied sciences)
610	Medical sciences
620	Engineering & allied operations
630	Agriculture & related technologies
640	Home economics & family living
650	Management & auxilliary services
660	Chemical & related technologies
670	Manufactures
680	Manufacture for specific uses
690	Buildings

700	The arts
710	Civic & landscape art
720	Architecture
730	Plastic arts Sculpture
740	Drawing, decorative & minor arts
750	Painting & paintings
760	Graphic arts Prints
770	Photography & photographs
780	Music
790	Recreational & performing arts
800	Literature (Belles-lettres)
810	American literature in English
820	English & Anglo-Saxon literatures
830	Literatures of Germanic languages
840	Literatures of Romance languages
850	Italian, Romanian, Rhaeto-Romanic
860	Spanish & Portuguese literatures
870	Italic literatures Latin
880	Hellenic literatures Greek
890	Literatures of other languages
900	General geography & history
910	General geography Travel
920	General biography & genealogy
930	General history of ancient world
940	General history of Europe
950	General history of Asia
960	General history of Africa
970	General history of North America
980	General history of South America
990	General history of other areas

MEDICAL SUBJECT HEADINGS (MeSH)*

Part I.   Alphabetic MeSH: Contains legitimate subject
headings + cross-references.
 A.   Types of cross-references (see page 410 for
examples):
  1.   "See": Directs Index Medicus user from a
term which is not used as a subject heading to a synonymous or closely related one
which is. Referred from designation = X.
  2.   "See under": Directs Index Medicus user
from a specific term which is not used as
a heading to a broader, more general one
which is. Referred from designation = XU.
  3.   "See related": Links related terms which
are both headings, but which, usually, appear in different categories and do not
stand together alphabetically. Referred
from designation = XR.

Part II.   MeSH Trees: A rearrangement of the legitimate
headings and "see under" terms from the alphabetic
section into 14 subject categories. Categories are
divided into subcategories, each of which has been
assigned an alphanumeric designation. Within each
subcategory, entries are listed hierarchically,
from the general to the specific. Subcategories may
may have as many as seven levels.

---

*Compiled (1976) by Kathryn W. Kruse, Head, Reference
and Bibliography, Duke University Medical Center Library,
Durham, N.C.

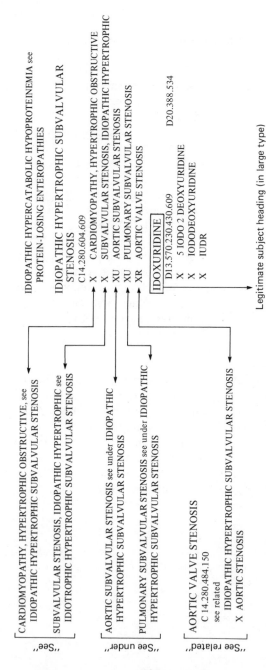

Examples of cross references in Medical Subject Headings (MeSH).

410

Subcategory C14

| CARDIOVASCULAR DISEASES | C14 |
| HEART DISEASES | C14.280 |

MYOCARDIAL DISEASES, PRIMARY   C14.280.604
ENDOCARDIAL FIBROELASTOSIS   C14.280.604.282
ENDOMYOCARDIAL FIBROSIS   C14.280.604.407   Tree number
IDIOPATHIC HYPERTROPHIC SUBVALVULAR
STENOSIS   C14.280.604.609
AORTIC SUBVALVULAR STENOSIS •   C14.280.604.609.203
PULMONARY SUBVALVULAR STENOSIS •   C14.280.604.609.715
MYOCARDIAL DISEASES, SECONDARY   C14.280.629
MYOCARDITIS   C14.280.629.554
PERICARDIAL EFFUSION   C14.280.695   A12.393.594
HEMOPERICARDIUM •   C14.280.695.463   C23.510.000
PERICARDITIS   C14.280.720
PERICARDITIS, CONSTRICTIVE   C14.280.720.595

"See under" term marked with a "bullet"

Another tree location for the
subject heading PERICARDIAL EFFUSION

Example of MeSH trees.

ABRIDGED INDEX MEDICUS

History   Began publication in 1970.

Frequency   Monthly. Cumulated yearly.

Scope   Contains citations from 125 English-language
journals especially selected from the biomedical journal literature because of particular interest for practicing physicians
and other health professionals.
Provides more selective coverage than Index
Medicus, and all items in AIM are indexed
in IM.

Format   Includes separate subject and author sections.

Sample Citations

Subject Index

CHILD DEVELOPMENT

Child abuse. Its relationship to birthweight, apgar score, and developmental testing. Goldson E, et al. **Am J Dis Child** 132(8)-790–3 Aug 78

Newborn head size and neurological status. Predictors of growth and development of low birth weight infants. Gross SJ, et al. **Am J Dis Child** 132(8)-753–6, Aug 78

Developmental surveillance in general practice [letter] **Br Med J** 2(6129):52, 1 Jul 78

Author Index

Goldring RM see Jayamanne DS

Goldring S: A method for surgical management of focal epilepsy, especially as it relates to children. J Neurosurg 49(3):344–56, Sep 78

Goldson E, Fitch MJ, Wendell TA, Knapp G: Child abuse. Its relationship to birthweight, apgar score, and developmental testing. Am J Dis Child 132(8):790–3, Aug 78

Goldstein B see Wofsy C

Goldstein DA see Massry SG

AMERICAN STATISTICS INDEX

History   Began publication in 1973.

Frequency   Monthly with annual cumulations. The base (retrospective) edition covers publications from the early 1960s through January 1, 1974.

Scope   An index and guide to the statistical publications of the U.S. government. Covers over 400 federal statistical, research, administrative, regulatory, and other government agencies which produce statistics.

Format

Includes abstract and index volumes. Index volumes provide access to the abstracts using subject, name, geographic, economic, demographic parameters. Abstracts are numbered for easy reference.
Document availability information is included.
Searchable via computer through SDC.

Sample Citations

Numbered Abstract

4118   (HRA)
BUREAU OF HEALTH
MANPOWER
                          Special and
                          Irregular Publications

4118 – 3   PREDICTION OF
           SUCCESSFUL NURSING
           PERFORMANCE, Part III and
           Part IV
           1979. v + 138 p.
           HRA 79-15, ●Item 507-J-I.
           GPO $3.25   ASI/MF/4
           S/N 017-022-00650-2.
           ●HE20.6602:N93/21/pt. 3, 4.
By Patricia M. Schwirian. Report on the success of nursing schools in predicting effective clinical performance by their graduates, 1976.
    Report is in 4 parts. Parts I and II, published in a single volume, presented bibliographic sources and results of a survey on nursing schools' student admission and evaluation practices; they are described in ASI 1978 Annual under this number. Parts III and IV, also published in a single volume, are described below.

Subject Index

Nurses and nursing
    Developing countries socioeconomic
    indicators, 92 countries, selected years
    1960-76,   (4) 7208-16.5

Nursing home employees, by demographic,
    education, work, and nursing home
    characteristics, 1973 - 74,
    (4) 4147 –14.21
Performance of nurses related to nursing
    school predictions, type of school, and
    nurse characteristics, 1976
    (6)4118 – 3

4118 – 3.3: Part III. Evaluation and Prediction of the Performance of Recent Nurse Graduates.
    (p.1 - 94) Report on nursing performance of 1975 graduates nominated "promising" or "most promising" by school administrators and faculty. Based on 1976 surveys of 914 nurses and 687 of their supervisors. Surveys covered nurses' and supervisors' characteristics, and self- and supervisor-assessed nursing performance.

CUMULATIVE INDEX TO NURSING & ALLIED HEALTH LITERATURE

History

First published in 1956 by the Seventh-Day Adventist Hospital Association, Glendale Sanitarium and Hospital, Glendale, California.
Title before 1977: <u>Cumulative Index to Nursing Literature.</u>

Frequency

Five issues per year plus annual cumulation.

Scope

Indexes major English language nursing periodicals. Since 1977, has expanded coverage to include selected periodicals for certain allied health professions.
The only index to nursing literature from 1960-65.
Since 1967, has indexed all serials published by the National League for Nursing. Since 1972, has indexed state nursing association journals. Also indexes American Nurses' Association publications.

Format

References are entered in separate subject and author sections. In addition, appendixes are separate and list book reviews; films, filmstrips, recordings; pamphlets.
Yearly cumulation includes "List of Nursing Subject Headings" (subject headings used in CINAHL) in the back of the volume on yellow pages.

Sample Citations

Subject Index

Bunions See: HALLUX

BURNS

Nursing care of burn patient... US
Army Institute of Surgical Research,
Ft Sam Houston, Tex (McGranahan
BG) AORN J 20:787-93, Nov 74

Skin coverage for burn injury
(Murphy WL) (pictorial) AORN J
20:794-6+, Nov 74

Author Index

McGranahan BG: Nursing care of
burn patient...US Army Institute
of Surgical Research, Ft Sam
Houston, Tex. AORN J 20:787-93,
Nov 74

McGrath A See: LANG C

McGrath P, LALIBERTE EB: Level
of basic venereal disease knowledge
among junior and senior high school
nurses in Massachusetts: A survey
(research, nurs) NURS RES 23:31-
7, Jan/Feb 74

EDUCATION INDEX

History	Began publication in 1929.
Frequency	Published every month except July and August. Cumulates yearly.
Scope	Author/subject index to educational materials in the English language. Subject areas/ fields include: administration; counseling; teaching; health; rehabilitation and the like. Primarily a periodicals index, but includes

some proceedings, yearbook, bulletin, monographic materials, etc.

Includes author listing of book review citations after the main part of the index.

Format   Author and subject indexes are arranged in one alphabet.

Searchable by computer via BRS, Lockheed, SDC

Sample Citations

Subject Index

NURSING education
   Curriculum
Credit for consciousness raising. N. F. Fasano.
   J Nurs Educ 16:3-6 O '77
Crisis intervention in basic nursing education.
   D. Dunlop and others. J Nurs Educ 17:37-41
   Ap '78
Educating the nurse-community health educator
   to educate. P. Heit. J Nurs Educ 17:21-3 Ja
   '78
Guided independent study program for nurses.
   A. L. Jones and E. Kerwin Com Coll Front
   6:24-8 Wint '78
Identification and analysis of core courses in
   nursing education . R. O. Podratz and others.
   il J Nurs Educ 16:24-9 O '77

Author Index

JONASSEN, Ellen O. and Stripling, R. O.
   Priorities for community college student personnel services during the next decade. J Coll
      Stud Personnel 18:83-6 Mr '77
JONES, A. Louise and Kerwin, Ellen
   Guided independent study program for nurses.
      Com Coll Front 6:24 - 8 Wint '78
JONES, Anton
   Multicultural neighbourhood comprehensive.
      Forum 20:14-17 Aut '77
JONES, Arnold
   Choral tone quality and blend. Sch Mus 49:64-5
      O '77
   High school operetta. Sch Mus 49:58-60 D '77

EXCERPTA MEDICA ABSTRACTING JOURNALS

History
Began publication at varying intervals (see next pages).

Frequency
Varying rate of publication, from one to three volumes annually. Indexes are cumulated for each volume which normally comprises ten issues.

Scope
Over 40 sections abstract the international literature of the biomedical sciences. A major resource for research.

Format
Includes separate subject and author indexes as well as an abstract section arranged by subject classification.
MALIMET (Master List of Medical Index Terms) is available for terminology information.
Searchable via computer via Lockheed.

Sample Citations

Numbered Abstract

Author Index

827 Herms V.
1120 Herms V.
1404 Hernandez L.
256 Herold F.
781 Herold E.S.
2303 Herrera A.
42 Herrmann Ch.
1182 Herter U.
456 Herz Z.

781. Attitudes of nurses to providing contraceptive services for youth-Herold E.S. and Thomas R.E.-Dept. Family Studies, Univ. Guelph, Ontario CAN-CAN. J. PUBL. HEALTH 1977 68/4 (307-310)-summ in FREN
The attudes of 200 nurses and nursing students in Southwestern Ontario toward the provision of contraceptive services to youth and related issues were surveyed. Although strong support was found for providing contraceptive services, one-half of the respondents indicated they did not feel adequately trained to work in the area of contraception and many desired more education in this area.

Subject Index

nullipara, cancer epidemiology, endometrium carcinoma, pregnancy, 549
nursing, attitude, contraception, youth, canada, 781
nutrient, congenital malformation, fetus, malnutrition, short review, 307
nutrition, behavior, growth, intrauterine growth, low birth weight, mental develop

SECTION LISTING
(currently being published)

Section 1: Anatomy, Anthropology, Embryology, and
Histology
1947 to date. 10 issues (1 volume) annually.

Section 2: Physiology
1948 to date. 30 issues (3 volumes) annually.

Section 3: Endocrinology
1947 to date. 20 issues (2 volumes) annually.

Section 4: Microbiology, Bacteriology, Mycology, and
Parasitology
1948 to date. 20 issues (2 volumes) annually.

Section 5: General Pathology and Pathological Anatomy
1948 to date. 30 issues (3 volumes) annually.

Section 6: Internal Medicine
1947 to date. 20 issues (2 volumes) annually.

Section 7: Pediatrics and Pediatric Surgery
1947 to date. 20 issues (2 volumes) annually.

Section 8: Neurology and Neurosurgery
1948 to date. 30 issues (3 volumes) annually.

Section 9: Surgery
1947 to date. 20 issues (2 volumes) annually.

Section 10: Obstetrics and Gynecology
1948 to date. 20 issues (2 volumes) annually.

Section 11: Otorhinolaryngology
1948 to date. 20 issues (2 volumes) annually.

Section 12: Ophthalmology
1947 to date. 10 issues (1 volume) annually.

Section 13: Dermatology and Venereology
1947 to date. 10 issues (1 volume) annually.

Section 14: Radiology
1947 to date. 20 issues (2 volumes) annually.

Section 15: Chest Diseases, Thoracic Surgery, and
Tuberculosis
1948 to date. 20 issues (2 volumes) annually.

Section 16: Cancer
1953 to date. 30 issues (3 volumes) annually.

Section 17: Public Health, Social Medicine, and Hygiene
1955 to date. 20 issues (2 volumes) annually.

Section 18: Cardiovascular Diseases and Cardiovascular
Surgery
1957 to date. 20 issues (2 volumes) annually.

Section 19: Rehabilitation and Physical Medicine
1958 to date. 10 issues (1 volume) annually.

Section 20: Gerontology and Geriatrics
1958 to date. 10 issues (1 volume) annually.

Section 21: Developmental Biology and Teratology
1961 to date. 10 issues (1 volume) annually.

Section 22: Human Genetics
1963 to date. 20 issues (2 volumes) annually.

Section 23: Nuclear Medicine
1964 to date. 20 issues (2 volumes) annually.

Section 24: Anesthesiology
1966 to date. 10 issues (1 volume) annually.

Section 25: Hematology
1967 to date. 20 issues (2 volumes) annually.

Section 26: Immunology, Serology, and Transplantation
1967 to date. 20 issues (2 volumes) annually.

Section 27: Biophysics, Bio-engineering, and Medical
Instrumentation
1967 to date. 10 issues (1 volume) annually.

Section 28. Urology and Nephrology
1967 to date. 10 issues (1 volume) annually.

Section 29. Clinical Biochemistry
1948 to date. 30 issues (3 volumes) annually.

Section 30: Pharmacology and Toxicology
1948 to date. 30 issues (3 volumes) annually.

Section 31: Arthritis and Rheumatism
1965 to date. 10 issues (1 volume) annually.

Section 32: Psychiatry
1948 to date. 20 issues (2 volumes) annually.

Section 33: Orthopedic Surgery
1956 to date. 10 issues (1 volume) annually.

Section 34: Plastic Surgery
1970 to date. 10 issues (1 volume) annually.

Section 35: Occupational Health and Industrial Medicine
1971 to date. 10 issues (1 volume) annually.

Section 36: Health Economics and Hospital Management
1971 to date. 20 issues (2 volumes) annually.

*Section 37: Drug Literature Index
1969 to date. 24 issues (1 volume) annually.

---

*A drug literature bibliography. Although it is given a sec-
tion number, it is not considered a part of the abstract
journal series.

*Section 38: Adverse Reactions Titles
1966 to date. 12 issues (1 volume) annually.

Section 40: Drug Dependence
1972 to date. 12 issues (1 volume) annually.

Section 46: Environmental Health and Pollution Control
1971 to date. 20 issues (2 volumes) annually.

Section 47: Virology
1971 to date. 10 issues (1 volume) annually.

Section 48: Gastroenterology
1971 to date. 20 issues (2 volumes) annually.

Section 49: Forensic Science
1975 to date. 10 issues (1 volume) annually.

Section 50: Epilepsy
1971 to date. 12 issues (1 volume) annually.

Section 51: Leprosy and Related Subjects
1979 to date. 10 issues (1 volume) annually.

Address: Excerpta Medica, P.O. Box 1126, 1000 B C
Amsterdam, The Netherlands [Tel.: (020) 264438;
Telex: 14664]

Editorial and subscription information (North America):
Journals Department, Excerpta Medica, Inc.,
P.O. Box 3085, Princeton, N.J. 08540
[Tel. (609) 896-9450; Telex: 843-344]

HOSPITAL LITERATURE INDEX

History   Began in 1945. Compiled in the Library of
the American Hospital Association. Since
1978, done in cooperation with the National

Library of Medicine using the MEDLARS
computer retrieval system.

Frequency   Quarterly with annual cumulation.

Scope   Covers English language journals all over the
                 world pertaining to health care administra-
                 tion in hospitals and other health care insti-
                 tutions.

Format   Arranged by author and subject in two sepa-
                 rate sections.
                 Uses MeSH (Medical Subject Headings).
                 Includes a list of recent acquisitions in the
                 AHA Library at the end of each issue.

Sample Citations

Subject Index

NURSING SERVICE, HOSPITAL

Recognizing contributions to nursing [editorial]
  Am Nurse 10(5):4, 15 May 78

A small - town nurse is still a nurse——and a lot more.
  Fahey PL. **RN** 41(5):60 −1, May 78
The situation of nursing administrators in hospitals for
  the mentally handicapped: problems in measuring
  and evaluating the quality of care.
  Alaszewski A. **Soc Sci Med** 12(2A):91−7, Mar 78
The organization of nursing services. A model for the
  future. Porter-O'Grady T. **Superv Nurse** 9(7):30−8,
  Jul 78

Author Index

J Assoc Care Child Hosp 7(1):23 −7, Summer 78
Ajemian I see **Wilson DC**
Alamin EM see **Wren GR**
Alaszewski A: The situation of nursing administrators
  in hospitals for the mentally handicapped: problems
  in measuring and evaluating the quality of care.
  Soc Sci Med 12(2A):91−7, Mar 78
Albanese M see **Barnes HV**
Alcena V: Medical students, practitioners hold health

INDEX MEDICUS

History   Began publication in 1960. Published from
                        1879-1927 as Index Medicus; 1927-1956 as
                        Quarterly Cumulative Index Medicus; 1957-
                        1959 as Current List of Medical Literature.

Frequency   Monthly. Cumulated annually as Cumulated
                        Index Medicus.

Scope   The major medical index. The National Li-
                        brary of Medicine's computer-produced
                        index to the international literature of bio-
                        medicine. Covers over 2500 biomedical
                        journals in English and other languages.
                        Since 1976 has covered selected monographs
                        and symposia proceedings.

Format   Separate author and subject sections as well
                        as a Bibliography of Medical Reviews sec-
                        tion at the beginning of each monthly number
                        and yearly cumulation.
                        Medical Subject Headings (MeSH), the subject
                        listing used, as well as the List of Journals
                        Indexed in Index Medicus are published an-
                        nually as part of the index and are available
                        separately.
                        Foreign language references are listed in
                        brackets at the end of each subject listing.
                        Searchable via the National Library of Medi-
                        cine computerized retrieval system.

Sample Citations

Subject Index

NURSING CARE

STANDARDS

What you should know about malpractice insurance. Mancini
M. **Am J Nurs** 79(4):729−30, Apr 79

Clinical research: translation into nursing practice. Cuddihy
JT. **Int J Nurs Stud** 16(1):65−72, 1979

Author Index

Mancini M: What you should know about malpractice
insurance. Am J Nurs 79(4):729−30, Apr 79

Manczak M see **Nowicka J**

Manczak M see **Schlesinger D**

**Mandal AK, Oleinick SR, James TM, Wise W, Long H,
Nordquist JA, Bell RD, Yunice AA, Parker D**:
Glomerular thrombosis in spontaneously hyperten-

INTERNATIONAL NURSING INDEX

History   First published in 1966 by the American
              Journal of Nursing Company in cooperation
              with the National Library of Medicine.

Frequency   Issued quarterly with annual cumulations.

Scope   Indexes over 200 nursing journals received
              from all over the world as well as nursing
              articles in more than 2,200 non-nursing
              journals currently indexed in Index Medicus.

Format   Article references are entered in separate
              subject and author sections.
              Special sections include listings of current
              nursing publications of organizations and
              agencies as well as selected nursing books.
              Doctoral dissertations by nurses for the
              current year are included only in the yearly
              cumulation.

Nursing Thesaurus (listing of subject headings in INI) is issued as part 2 of the first issue of each year and is also included in the annual cumulation.

Foreign language articles are included at the end of each subject listing in brackets.

Searchable by computer via the National Library of Medicine computerized retrieval systems.

Sample Citations

Nurs Times 69:1292-3, 4 Oct 73

GERIATRIC NURSING

The role of the geriatrician in mental hospitals. Hall
MR. et al. **Age Ageing** 3:36-42, Feb 74

Caring for the aged: reaction time in the elderly.
Greenberg B. **Am J Nurs** 73:2056-8, Dec 73

An incentive contract for nursing home aides. Sand P.
et al. **Am J Nurs** 74:475-7, Mar 74

Editorial: Speaking of response. Schorr TM. **Am J
Nurs** 73:2043, Dec 73

Subject Index

Author Index

the knowledge, attitudes, and practices of rural poor
homemakers. Am J Public Health 64:722-4, Jul 74

Green MD: Changing attitudes.
Occup Health (Lond) 26:175-8, May 74

Greenberg B: Caring for the aged: reaction time in the
elderly. Am J Nurs 73:2056-8, Dec 73

Greenberg JS: Learning games. Perceptions of me. Sch
Health Rev 5:44-5, Jul-Aug 74

Greenberg RA, Loda FA, Pickard CO, et al: Primary

MONTHLY CATALOG
OF U.S. GOVERNMENT PUBLICATIONS

History
Published since 1950. Published from 1895–1907 as Catalogue of the United States Public Documents; July 1907–1939 as Monthly Catalog, United States Public Documents; 1940–1950 as United States Government Publications: Monthly Catalog.

Frequency
Monthly. Cumulated yearly.

Scope
The major index to the publications of all branches of the United States government.

Format
Documents are arranged by department and/or agency with author, title, subject and series/report indexes.
Uses Library of Congress—Subject Headings (8th ed. and supplements) for entering subjects in the index as well as the Anglo-American Cataloging Rules.
Includes all government document numbers, Library of Congress catalog card numbers as well as OCLC (Ohio College Library Center) computer data base numbers.

Sample Citations

Subject Index

Nutrition – Research – United States.
  Nutrition and cancer research: hearings
    before the Subcommittee on Nutrition
    of the Committee on Agriculture, Nu-
    trition, and Forestry, United States
    Senate, Ninety-fifth Congress, second
    session...June 12 and 13, 1978, 79 –
    8765

Nutrition – Statistics.
  Future of the national nutrition intelli-
    gence system: study/, 79 – 7823

Main Document Listing

79 – 7823
        GA 1.13:CED – 79 – 5
United States General Accounting Office.
      Future of the national nutrition intelligence system: study
  / by the staff of the U.S. General Accounting Office. –
  Washington: General Accounting Office. 1978.
      v, 39 p.: 27 cm.
      "CED – 79 - 5."
      Issued Nov. 7, 1978.
      ● Item 546-D (microfiche)
      pbk
      1. Nutrition policy – United States. 2. Nutrition –
  Statistics. I. Title.

  OCLC 4611833

79 – 7824
        GA 1.13:CED – 79 – 10
United States General Accounting Office.
      Commercial safety regulations are avoided by some large

PSYCHOLOGICAL ABSTRACTS

History   Began publication in 1927.

Frequency   Monthly, cumulated twice per year. Three-
               year cumulative indexes are available as
               well.

Scope   Provides summaries which are nonevaluative
               of the literature in psychology and related
               fields published worldwide. Covers over
               950 journals, books, book chapters, govern-
               ment reports, dissertations, etc.
               Includes materials from the areas of educa-
               tion and business not usually found in indexes
               available at health sciences libraries.

Format   References, most with abstracts, are listed
               under 16 categories which can be divided
               into subcategories. Thesaurus of Psycho-
               logical Index Terms (2d ed., 1977) provides
               a guide to the subject vocabulary of PA.
               Abstracts are numbered for easy reference.
               Computer searching of PA is available via
               BRS, Lockheed, SDC.

Sample Citations

Subject Index

Nurses [See Also Psychiatric Nurses]
102, 1197, 1198, 1292, 1514, 1756, 1778,
2090
Nursing 1292, 1508
Nursing Students 230
Nurturance [See Animal Maternal Behavior, Parent Child Relations]
Nutrition 507, 1990
Nutritional Deficiencies [See Also Vita-
min Deficiency Disorders] 782, 787, 820
1411, 1942

Author Index

Seifert, Keith, 1823
Seiler, Nikolaus, 474
Seipel, Magnus, 1025
Seitz, Pauline M. 1508
Seitz, Victoria, 1848
Singell, Larry D. 1950
Singer, Greta, 1891

Numbered Abstract

1508. Seitz, Pauline M. & Warrick, Louise H. (New
York Hosp. New York) Perinatal death: The grieving
mother. *Americal Journal of Nursing,* 1974 (Nov), Vol
74(11), 2028 – 2033.—Discusses nursing help for the
mother whose newborn or fetus dies. Suggestions are
made for dealing with both parents according to their
differing needs. The stages through which the mother
passes are described. Establishing contact with her is felt
to be essential in the delivery room where the full reality
of the death falls on her for the 1st time. After separation
from the baby, during the postpartum period, more
active grieving occurs. At this time the nurse should
provide an atmosphere in which the mother can cry,
remain silent, or speak. The particular problem of per-
mitting contact between the dead fetus or the dying newborn and the mother is addressed. The special problems
of a subsequent pregnancy are also cited.—*R. S. Albin*

READERS' GUIDE TO PERIODICAL LITERATURE

History   Published since 1900.

Frequency   Published semimonthly from September to
                 January and from March to June, monthly
                 in February, July, and August. Cumulated
                 annually.

Scope   Index by author and subject to general inter-
                 est periodicals in the United States. Good
                 for lay materials, information.
                 Includes author listing of book review cita-
                 tions after the main part of the index.

Format   Author and subject references are arranged
                 in one alphabet.

Sample Citations

Subject Index

MARRIAGE counseling
   Baby talk: E. Whelan's counseling service. B.
      Carter. il pors Newsweek 90:73 Ag 8 '77
   Can this marriage be saved? D.C. Disney, See
      issues of Ladies' home journal
   Making marriage work. D. R. Mace. Parents Mag
      52:80 My '77
   Marriage counseling for unwed couples. A. Gross
   N Y Times Mag p52+ Ap 24 '77
   Marriage: minefields on the way to paradise P.
      Yancey. il Chr Today 21:24−7 F 18 '77

Author Index

GROSMAN, Tatyana
   Goldilocks' cosmic teach - in. M. Hoelterhoff. il
      pors Art N 76:19 -21 Mr '77
GROSS, Amy
   Marriage counseling for unwed couples. N Y
      Times Mag p52+ Ap 24 '77
   Verbal sex − the world's greatest noncontact
      sport. Mademoiselle 83:149+ Je '77
   Weekend at the heart of the Human Potential
      Movement. il Mademoiselle 83:202+ Ap '77
   Your friends, my friends, our friends. Redbook
      149:76+ My '77

Appendix
Addresses of Selected Medical and Nursing Publishers

Addison-Wesley Publishing Co., Inc., Medical-Nursing
Publishers, 2727 Sand Hill Road, Menlo Park, Calif.
94025

American Nurses' Association, 2420 Pershing Road, Kansas
City, Mo. 64108

Appleton-Century-Crofts, 292 Madison Avenue, New York,
N.Y. 10017

Aspen Systems Corporation, 20010 Century Blvd.,
Germantown, Md. 20767

R. R. Bowker Co., P.O. Box 1807, Ann Arbor, Mich. 48106

F. A. Davis Co., 1915 Arch Street, Philadelphia, Pa. 19103

Harper & Row Publishers, Inc., Medical Department,
2350 Virginia Ave., Hagerstown, Md. 21740

Intermed Communications, Inc., 132 Welsh Road, Horsham,
Pa. 19044

Lange Medical Publications, Drawer L, Los Altos, Calif.
94022

Lea & Febiger, 600 S. Washington Square, Philadelphia,
Pa. 19105

---

*For further listings of publishers' addresses see Medical
Books and Serials in Print, 1979.

J. B. Lippincott Co. , East Washington Square,
    Philadelphia, Pa. 19105

Little, Brown & Co. , 200 West Street, Waltham, Mass.
    02154

McGraw-Hill Book Co. , 1221 Avenue of the Americas, New
    York, N. Y. 10020

Macmillan Publishing Co. , Inc. , Riverside, N. J. 08075

Medical Examination Publishing Co. , Inc. , 969 Steward
    Avenue, Garden City, N. Y. 11530

C. V. Mosby Co. , 11830 Westline Industrial Drive,
    St. Louis, Mo. 63141

National League for Nursing, 10 Columbus Circle, New
    York, N. Y. 10019

Prentice-Hall, Inc. , Englewood Cliffs, N. J. 07632

W. B. Saunders Co. , W. Washington Square, Philadelphia,
    Pa. 19105

Springer Publishing Co. , Inc. , 200 Park Avenue So. ,
    New York, N. Y. 10003

Superintendent of Documents, Washington, D. C. 20402

John Wiley & Sons, Inc. , 605 Third Avenue, New York, N. Y.
    10016

Williams & Wilkins Co. , 428 E. Preston Street, Baltimore,
    Md. 21202

Year Book Medical Publications, Inc. , 35 E. Wacker Drive,
    Chicago, Ill. 60601

Author Index

Abdellah, Faye G., 14.1
Abels, Linda F., 4.32
Abu-Saad, Huda, 11.1
Acri, Michael J., 8.33
Adams, George L., 4.54
Adams, John E., 6.17
Adams, Raymond D., 3.18
Adler, Diane C., 4.33
Adler, Gerhard, 6.15
Affonso, Dyanne D., 9.16
Aguilera, Donna Conant, 7.1,
    7.19, 7.45
Aiken, Eula, 12.70
Aker, J. Brooke, 8.40
Aker, Saundra, 4.1
Aladjem, Silvio, 10.74
Albrecht, Gary L., 3.46
Alexander, Edythe L., 3.20, 13.1
Alexander, Mary M., 10.21
Allen, Robert D., 8.93
Altschule, Mark D., 5.30
Alyn, Irene Barrett, 11.64
American Academy of Pediatrics,
    10.39
American College of Surgeons,
    3.33
American Hospital Association,
    1.38, 2.56, 14.37
American Journal of Nursing
    Company, 1.8, 14.2
American Medical Association,
    12.59

American Nurses' Association,
    13.58
American Nurses' Foundation, 1.19
American Pharmaceutical Associa-
    tion, 5.48
American Public Health Association,
    8.94
Anderson, Betty Ann, 9.10
Anderson, C. L., 8.13
Anderson, Diann Laden, 3.36
Anderton, J. L., 4.78
Andreoli, Kathleen G., 4.15
Annas, George J., 11.24
Anthony, Catherine P., 5.3
Anyan, Walter R., Jr., 10.40
Anzalone, Joseph T., 9.34
Applied Management Sciences, Inc.,
    13.59
Archer, Sarah E., 8.1
Arcilla, Rene A., 10.52
Arena, Jay M., 10.56
Argondizzo, Nina T., 8.24
Arieti, Silvano, 7.41
Arms, Suzanne, 9.46
Arndt, Clara, 13.2
Arnold, W., 6.13
Aroskar, Mila A., 11.26
Ash, Joan, 12.25
Association of American Medical
    Colleges, 12.60
Ashley, Jo Ann, 11.4
Asperheim, Mary K., 5.49

Title Index

Subject Index

Abortion, 8.70, 8.71, 9.94. See
  also Family planning
Abstracts
  natural science, 5.67, 5.68
  psychology, 6.63
  sociology, 6.65
  on stress, 6.22
Adaptation, 2.23, 6.26. See also
  Coping; Stress
Administration
  educational, 12.21-12.24
  general, 8.14, 8.86, 8.118,
    13.16, 13.24-13.41, 13.88,
    13.90, 13.91
  nursing, 13.1-13.23, 13.92-
    13.95
Adolescent. See also Pediatric
  nursing
  developmentally disabled, 10.63
  dying, 10.53
  growth and development, 10.94
  hospitalized, 10.67
  medicine, 10.40
  nursing, 10.28, 10.30
  psychology, 6.19, 10.11, 10.15
  visually impaired, 10.82
Aging. See Geriatric nursing and
  geriatrics
Alcoholism, 7.4, 7.21, 7.25
Allied health. See also Health
  careers; specific profession
  and aging, 8.59
  and anthropology, 6.50

and cancer rehabilitation, 4.8
and child development, 10.2, 10.6
and childbearing, 9.15
and communication, 6.45, 10.68
and community health, 8.13, 8.19
and critical care, 4.38
and evaluation, 12.50
and family, 8.15, 8.75
and family planning, 8.68
and hospitalized children, 10.68,
  10.71
and human sexuality, 8.65
and marriage, 8.75
and mathematics, 5.26
and mental health, 7.4, 7.16,
  7.44, 7.45
and nursing skills, 2.31, 2.49
and psychology, 6.3, 6.11, 6.18
and renal disease, 4.84
and research, 14.25
and respiratory care, 4.88, 4.89
and role theory, 11.13
and statistics, 5.21, 5.24
and sociology, 6.62
and suicide, 7.29
Almanac, 1.52
  mental health, 8.93
  nurses', 11.22
Ambulatory care. See Primary care
American Nurses' Association,
  11.50, 11.53
Anatomy. See Physiology
Anorexia nervosa, 7.54

Supplement

CHAPTER 2:
FUNDAMENTALS OF NURSING

S2.1 Berger, Karen J.; Fields, Willa J. Pocket Guide to Health
Assessment. Reston, Va.: Reston Publishing, 1980.
>146 pp. Paper (spiral). Bibliography.
>This convenient guide to health assessment provides a
>clinical support in outline format for both the learner
>and practitioner. Organized according to the usual
>steps of a physical examination, each chapter has sec-
>tions on history questions, clinical examination, life-
>cycle variations in physical findings, and abnormal
>conditions. Has helpful diagrams and growth charts.
>The final pages outline health history and physical ex-
>amination.

S2.2 Bower, Fay Louise; Bevis, Em Olivia. Fundamentals of
Nursing Practice; Concepts, Roles, and Functions. St.
Louis: Mosby, 1979.
>602 pp. Cloth. Index. References. Glossaries.
>Written by two nurses, "this book reflects [a] new
>spirit as it presents concepts, processes, and skills
>truly <u>fundamental</u> to all levels of nursing today."
>(p. ix) Chapters discuss nursing today and its evolu-
>tion; the health care system and nursing; the nursing
>process; the various nursing roles (communicator,
>planner, protector, healer, teacher, rehabilitator,
>coordinator, collaborator); and the future. Each
>chapter has a summary and study questions.

S2.3 Diekelmann, Nancy; Bennett, Patricia H.; Shauger,
Margaret; et al. Fundamentals of Nursing. New York:
McGraw-Hill, 1980.
>621 pp. Cloth. Index. References. Glossary.
This text for the beginning student includes content
basic to the practice of nursing. The six modules
focus on health care, nursing, and the nursing process; psychosocial and sexual needs; nutrition and
elimination; oxygen and carbon dioxide exchange; activity and rest; and safety and security. A systems
approach is used. Each chapter has objectives, student activities, and study questions. Appendixes include units of measurement, dietary allowances, and
the ANA Code for Nurses.

S2.4 Pivar, William. Survival Manual for Nursing Students.
[Saunders Survival Series.] Philadelphia: Saunders, 1979.
>180 pp. Paper. Index. Bibliography.
This book is written for nursing students and those
considering nursing as a profession. Topics range
from Nursing and You to Employment During and After
College. Students will find helpful chapters on planning their programs, how to study and take tests, and
how to write reports. The chapter on Adjustment to
Nursing includes information specific to nursing but
much of the material is appropriate for any college
student.

S2.5 Shortridge, Lillie M.; Lee, E. Juanita, eds. Introduction
to Nursing Practice. New York: McGraw-Hill, 1980.
>588 pp. Cloth. Index. Bibliography. Glossary.
A text for an introductory course in nursing that uses
a systematic approach. Part I looks at professional
nursing practice including the nursing process. Part
II considers the application of the nursing process in
a variety of diagnostic areas including Pain, Inadequate Nutrition, Inadequate Elimination, Anxiety, and
Inadequate Health in Communities. Chapters have
objectives, discussion of application of content and
a case study, a care plan for that diagnostic category,

and review questions. Client focus includes individuals, families, and communities.

CHAPTER 3:
MEDICAL-SURGICAL NURSING

S3.1 Barber, Janet M.; Budassi, Susan A. Mosby's Manual of
      Emergency Care; Practices and Procedures. St. Louis:
      Mosby, 1979.
      652 pp. Paper. Index. Bibliography.
      Written for advanced students and practitioners of life
      support skills, this book is both a basic text and a
      technical reference. Persons involved in prehospital
      care and in emergency room care will find it useful.
      Includes practical considerations, clinical considera-
      tions, and procedures for classic emergencies. Ma-
      terials in the appendixes focus primarily on pharmaco-
      logic data. Well illustrated.

S3.2 Brand, Janet Coogan; Tolins, Stephen H. The Nursing Stu-
      dent's Guide to Surgery. Boston: Little, Brown, 1979.
      457 pp. Paper (spiral). Index. Bibliography.
      Glossary.
      Provides a useful introduction to the surgical ex-
      perience using a physiologic approach. Focuses on
      basic considerations and then on specific situations.
      Uses an outline format.

S3.3 Cousins, Norman. Anatomy of an Illness as Perceived by
      the Patient; Reflections on Healing and Regeneration. New
      York: Norton, 1979.
      173 pp. Cloth. Bibliography.
      This book is an expansion of the author's article,
      which appeared in the Saturday Review and the New
      England Journal of Medicine. It describes his illness
      and his involvement and partnership with his physician
      in its resolution. Reflects the ideas underlying holis-
      tic health.

S3.4 Fry, John. Common Diseases; Their Nature, Incidence

and Care. 2d ed. Philadelphia: Lippincott, 1979.
413 pp. Cloth. Index. References.
"This book deals with common diseases as seen by a
British family physician." (p. 11) The first part of
the book looks at disease in general; the second part
discusses a large number of common diseases. Written largely for the family physician, primary care
physician, or general practitioner.

S3.5 Vander Salm, Thomas J.; Cutler, Bruce S.; Wheeler, H.
Brownell, eds. Atlas of Bedside Procedures. Boston:
Little, Brown, 1979.
408 pp. Paper. Index. Bibliography.
Describes selected diagnostic and therapeutic procedures that can be carried out at the bedside. Includes 40 procedures with an equipment list, specific
steps, indications, complications, and treatment.
Uses an outline format with line drawings. Examples
of procedures included are intravenous cannulation,
pericardiocentesis, sigmoidoscopy, and liver biopsy.

S3.6 Werner-Beland, Jean A., ed. Grief Responses to Long-
Term Illness and Disability: Manifestations and Nursing
Interventions. Reston, Va.: Reston Publishing, 1979.
219 pp. Paper. Index. References.
Looks at the grief response in patients and their significant others. It also discusses the "burnout" syn-
drome in nurses. Part 1 looks at theoretical explanations; Part 2, grief responses of persons at various
ages; and Part 3, the nurse. One of the few books to
focus on the loss of bodily functions and parts; the experience of chronic illness.

CHAPTER 4:
MEDICAL-SURGICAL NURSING SPECIALTIES

S4.1 Disch, Joanne Marilyn. Diagnostic Procedures for Cardio-
vascular Disease. [Continuing Education in Cardiovascular
Nursing. Series 2: Surgical Aspects of Cardiovascular
Nursing.] New York: Appleton-Century-Crofts, 1979.

99 pp. Paper. References.
Discusses the purposes, patient preparation, and
nursing care regarding selected diagnostic procedures.
Includes EKG, pulse wave tracings, sonic studies,
dynamic studies, radiography, and angiography. A
post-test concludes the book.

S4.2 Gutch, C. F.; Stoner, Martha H. Review of Hemodialysis
for Nurses and Dialysis Personnel, 3d ed. [Mosby's Comprehensive Review Series.] St. Louis: Mosby, 1979.
241 pp. Paper. Index. References.
Using a question-and-answer format, this book provides basic information for persons involved in
dialysis, both the health professional and the patient.
Chapters include discussions of the dialysis team
members, principles, equipment, monitoring, medical management, and maintenance dialysis.

S4.3 Jackle, Mary; Rasmussen, Claire. Renal Problems; A
Critical Care Nursing Focus. Bowie, Md.: Brady, 1980.
346 pp. Paper.
A programmed instructional text for nursing students
and graduates focusing on renal problems in critical
care. Reviews anatomy, physiology, and causes of
renal disease; examines renal mechanisms and assessment; and presents case materials that delineate
major renal problems and nursing care. Discusses
transplantation and dialysis. Appendixes include a
form for admission assessment.

S4.4 McBride, Helena; Moses, Dorothy. Acute Myocardial Infarction. [Continuing Education in Cardiovascular Nursing.
Series 1: Myocardial Infarction.] New York: Appleton-
Century-Crofts, 1979.
79 pp. Paper. Bibliographies.
The Standards of Cardiovascular Nursing Practice are
used as the format for discussing 1) coronary arteries,
2) myocardial infarction and electrical and mechanical
disturbances associated with the sites of the infarction, and 3) the associated nursing care.

S4.5 Nursing Critically Ill Patients Confidently. [Nursing Skillbook Series.] Horsham, Pa.: Intermed Communications,
1979.
>   192 pp. Cloth. Index. Bibliography. Glossary.
>   Following a discussion of assessment this monograph
>   focuses on Supporting Faltering Vital Systems and
>   Managing Special Problems. Included are renal,
>   respiratory, cardiovascular, neurologic, hepatic sys-
>   tems, multiple trauma, lethal crises, endocrine im-
>   balances, and others. Skillchecks are included. Writ-
>   ten for advanced students and nurses in practice.

S4.6 Schroeder, John Speer; Daily, Elaine Kiess. Techniques in
Bedside Hemodynamic Monitoring. St. Louis: Mosby, 1976.
>   212 pp. Paper. Index. References. Glossary.
>   This text focuses on the monitoring of the cardiovascu-
>   lar patient based on physiologic concepts and treat-
>   ment rationale. It is written for medical, nursing,
>   and other personnel involved with patients requiring
>   monitoring of cardiovascular function. Both invasive
>   and non-invasive techniques are discussed. A useful
>   reference in patient care units. Second edition due
>   1980.

S4.7 Seal, A. Lucy. Cardiogenic Shock. [Continuing Education
in Cardiovascular Nursing. Series 1: Myocardial Infarction.] New York: Appleton-Century-Crofts, 1980.
>   96 pp. Paper.
>   Designed for continuing education and self-instruction,
>   this brief publication covers heart physiology and
>   pathophysiology, pharmacology and cardiac assist,
>   and nursing care of cardiogenic shock patients. Each
>   chapter has objectives and self-examination questions
>   (with answers provided). Includes post-test, with
>   answers.

S4.8 Vinsant, Marielle Ortiz; Spence, Martha I.; Hagen, Dianne

Chapell.   A Commonsense Approach to Coronary Care: A
Program, 2d ed. St. Louis: Mosby, 1975.
> 228 pp. Paper (spiral). References.
> A programmed text that focuses on the major problems
> of acute myocardial infarction faced by nurses in the
> coronary care unit. The first units cover anatomy and
> physiology followed by basic electrophysiology and
> chemical imbalance. Subsequent units include diag-
> nosis, complications, and interventions in acute myo-
> cardial infarction. Nursing care is stressed. The
> text is written for the beginner as well as for the ex-
> perienced nurse.

S4.9 Wang, Rosemary Y.; Kelley, Ann Manchester. Self-
Assessment of Current Knowledge in Oncology Nursing;
1,061 Multiple Choice Questions and Referenced Answers.
Garden City: Medical Examination, 1979.
> 210 pp. Paper (spiral). Bibliography.
> Uses a multiple choice question and answer format
> with answers cited in the literature. Contents include
> information on cancer in general, the nurse's role,
> psychosocial aspects, treatment modalities, and nurs-
> ing care in specific cancer disorders.

CHAPTER 5:
THE NATURAL SCIENCES AND NURSING

S5.1 Davidson, Sir Stanley; Passmore, R.; Brock, J. F.; et al.
Human Nutrition and Dietetics, 7th ed. Edinburgh: Churchill
Livingstone, 1979.
> 641 pp. Cloth. Index. References. Glossary.
> A medical text which covers the field of nutrition "at a
> moderately advanced level" (p. v) for those who work
> with the problems of human nutrition in both health
> and disease. Part I: Physiology; Part II: Food; Part
> III: Primary Nutritional Diseases; Part IV: Diet and
> Other Diseases; Part V: Public Health; and Part VI:
> Diet and Physiological Status. Uses an international
> approach since three of the authors live in different
> countries.

S5.2 Guthrie, Helen Andrews. Introductory Nutrition, 4th ed.
      St. Louis: Mosby, 1979.
            693 pp. Cloth. Index. Bibliographies. Glossary.
            A text for a basic college course in nutrition, this
            book provides an introduction to the principles of nutri-
            tion. Major sections cover basic and applied nutrition.
            A number of appendixes provide additional useful
            material including diabetic exchange lists, height-
            weight charts, and a table of food composition.

S5.3 Hodges, Robert E.; Adelman, Raymond D. Nutrition in
      Medical Practice. Philadelphia: Saunders, 1980.
            363 pp. Cloth. Index. Bibliographies.
            This text provides nutritional information needed by
            physicians. Topics include evaluation of nutritional
            status; nutrition in pregnancy, heart disease, and in-
            fection; nutrition and specific body systems; food
            fads; and drug-food interactions.

S5.4 Srivastava, Probodh K. Basic Genetics for Health Profes-
      sionals. Littleton, Mass.: PSG Publishing, 1979.
            199 pp. Cloth. Index. References. Glossary.
            A textbook that provides a "short, simple guide for
            new students of medical genetics." (p. ix) Focuses
            on causes and clinical manifestations. Written for
            all health professional students.

S5.5 Trounce, J. R.; et al. Clinical Pharmacology for Nurses,
      8th ed. Edinburgh: Churchill Livingstone, 1979.
            383 pp. Paper. Index.
            Discusses drugs according to body systems, desired
            effects, and drug categories. A brief introduction
            covers administration, dosage, distribution, and
            elimination of drugs. Within each unit the drugs are
            discussed by generic name. Includes some drugs not
            available in the United States.

S5.6 Wiener, Matthew B.; Pepper, Ginette A.; Kuhn-Weisman,
      Gail; et al; eds. Clinical Pharmacology and Therapeutics
      in Nursing. New York: McGraw-Hill, 1979.

895 pp. Cloth. Index. References.
Provides the principles of drug use and serves as a
reference for drug data in a clinical setting. Major
units look at the nursing process as applied to pharmacology in a clinical setting, general pharmacologic
principles, neuropharmacology, therapy for disease
manifestations, pharmacologic therapy for common
disorders, cardiovascular disorders, and pharmacology in clinical specialty areas (surgery, drug abuse,
and women's health). Includes list of drug information
centers by state.

CHAPTER 6:
THE BEHAVIORAL SCIENCES AND NURSING

S6.1 Golden, Charles J. Clinical Interpretation of Objective
Psychological Tests. New York: Grune & Stratton, 1979.
234 pp. Cloth. Index. References.
In one volume the author presents basic clinical knowledge and strategies needed for the competent use of
the tests most used in adult clinical psychology. Tests
included cover four areas: intellectual evaluation,
achievement, personality, and organic brain dysfunction. The level of approach makes it suitable for undergraduate or graduate psychology students or for
professionals outside psychology, such as psychiatrists, social workers, physicians, and rehabilitation
professionals. Well-known tests covered include the
Wechsler Adult Intelligence Scale, Minnesota Multiphasic Personality Inventory, and Bender-Gestalt.
Includes purpose, administration, scoring, and clinical interpretation information for each test.

CHAPTER 7:
MENTAL HEALTH AND PSYCHIATRIC NURSING

S7.1 Dixon, Samuel L. Working with People in Crisis; Theory
and Practice. St. Louis: Mosby, 1979.
203 pp. Paper. Index. Bibliography.
This book provides a basic guide to helping people in

crisis. Part I is a conceptual base for crisis intervention; Part II focuses on application. It is written for
students and beginning practitioners in the helping professions who work in crisis intervention centers, suicide prevention centers, and mental health clinics.

S7.2 Pothier, Patricia C., ed. Psychiatric Nursing; A Basic
Text. Boston: Little, Brown, 1980.
292 pp. Cloth. Index. References. Suggested
Readings.
Uses an eclectic theory base to introduce nursing students to the skills nurses use in the field of psychiatric
nursing. Reflects an emphasis on respect and caring
as important themes in nursing. Part I describes the
field of psychiatric nursing; Part II looks at tools of
practice; Part III focuses on age groups; and Part IV
considers cultural, ethnic, socioeconomic, ethical,
and professional issues. Appendixes include the ANA
Standards of Psychiatric and Mental Health Nursing.

S7.3 Stoltzfus, Doris J. Self-Assessment of Current Knowledge
in Mental Health Nursing; 1,011 Multiple Choice Questions
and Referenced Answers. [Self-Assessment Books.] Garden
City: Medical Examination, 1979.
202 pp. Paper (spiral). References.
For the nurse or student to use in review of mental
health nursing. Multiple choice questions cover basic
skills in mental health nursing (interviewing, nurse-
patient communication, etc.); assessment; psychophysiologic disorders; psychosociologic disorders;
psychologic disorders; therapy; rehabilitation; and
ethics and legal ramifications. Answers are given
as well as references to pertinent literature.

CHAPTER 8:
COMMUNITY HEALTH

S8.1 Atchley, Robert C. The Social Forces in Later Life; An Introduction to Social Gerontology, 3d ed. [Lifetime Series
in Aging.] Belmont, Calif.: Wadsworth, 1980.

467 pp. Cloth. Index. Bibliography. Glossary.
Provides an introduction to aging from the social and
social-psychological view. Uses a multidisciplinary
perspective. After an introduction, the author discusses the effects of age on biologic and psychologic
functioning, special situations facing the aging person,
and society's treatment of the aged. Uses case material and research illustrations.

S8.2 Benson, Evelyn Rose; McDevitt, Joan Quinn. Community
Health and Nursing Practice, 2d ed. Englewood Cliffs:
Prentice-Hall, 1980.
370 pp. Cloth. Index. Bibliography.
A text for nursing students that discusses the concepts
of community health and community health nursing.
Includes community health sciences basic to nursing
practice as well as current health problems and trends
in health care delivery. Describes nursing intervention in the community focusing on family health and
uses case studies to discuss the use of the nursing
process and the problem-oriented record.

S8.3 Burnside, Irene Mortenson, ed. Psychosocial Nursing Care
of the Aged, 2d ed. New York: McGraw-Hill, 1980.
346 pp. Paper. Subject and name indexes.
References. Bibliography.
Focuses on the psychosocial nursing care of the aged
through nurses' descriptions of their experiences with
aged clients. For students and practitioners in most
health care settings in which aged clients receive care.
After an introduction and discussion of initial approaches, the contributions are organized by settings:
community, acute, and long-term care. The last section looks at special concerns such as wandering behavior and incontinence.

S8.4 Dubois, Paul M. The Hospice Way of Death. New York:
Human Sciences Press, 1980.
223 pp. Cloth. Index. Bibliography.
Describes the hospice movement for the professional

and non-professional audience. Addresses issues regarding how hospices fit into the current health care
system and analyzes the movement's potential impact
on the "quality of dying in this country." (p. 20) Includes chapters on causes of death, components of
care, and case studies of three hospices including St.
Christopher's in London.

S8.5 Family Health in an Era of Stress. [General Mills American
Family Report, 1978-79.] Minneapolis: General Mills,
Inc., 1979.
192 pp. Paper. Bibliography.
Focuses on adult family members, teenagers, and
spouses. Major topics include the impact of inflation
on family health attitudes and concerns, barriers to
good health, personal values and their impact on health
attitudes and behaviors, preventive versus crisis
health care, physical fitness, health parenting, mental
illness, health issues, and levels of information about
health practices. Study was conducted by Yankelovich,
Skelly, and White, Inc.

S8.6 Frank-Stromborg, Marilyn; Stromborg, Paul. Primary
Care Assessment and Management Skills for Nurses: A
Self-Assessment Manual. Philadelphia: Lippincott, 1979.
329 pp. Paper. Index. References.
Provides nurse practitioners in adolescent or adult
care settings with "a self-assessment of skills in physical assessment, medical management of diseases,
health counseling and coordination of community resources for health promotion." (p. ix) Uses a case
study format that includes learning goals, suggested
readings, questions with answers, references, and
patient education resources. Authors are a nurse
practitioner and a physician. Case situations are organized according to major body systems. Includes a
list of abbreviations and patient education resources.

S8.7 Helvie, Carl O. Self-Assessment of Current Knowledge in
Community Health Nursing; 1,093 Multiple Choice Questions

and Referenced Answers. [Self-Assessment Books.]
Flushing, N.Y.: Medical Examination, 1975.
> 149 pp. Paper (spiral). References.
> For practitioners and students to help them review and
> assess knowledge. Multiple choice questions cover
> the nursing process in community health nursing and
> selected areas for applying the nursing process (with
> individuals, families, suicide, etc.). Answers are
> given as well as references to pertinent literature.

S8.8 Hymovich, Debra P.; Chamberlin, Robert W. Child and
Family Development: Implications for Primary Health Care.
New York: McGraw-Hill, 1979.
> 474 pp. Cloth. Index. Bibliography.
> Combines knowledge of individual development with
> family development to present guidelines for health
> professionals in primary health care settings. Blends
> concepts, theories, and applications. Each chapter
> considers individual and family development by stages
> (infancy, toddler, etc.), effects of selected variables,
> and clinical applications. Covers the prenatal period
> through middle childhood.

S8.9 McCary, James Leslie. McCary's Human Sexuality, 3d ed.
New York: Van Nostrand Reinhold, 1978.
> 500 pp. Cloth. Index. References. Glossary.
> Presents an approach to human sexuality reflecting
> "the most current thought and analysis concerning the
> physiological, psychological, and sociological param-
> eters." (p. ix) A readable text suitable for a college
> course. Debunks sexual myths and fallacies; explores
> the human sexual system, the sexual act and attitudes,
> as well as sexual complications.

S8.10 Poe, William D.; Holloway, Donald A. Drugs and the Aged.
New York: McGraw-Hill, 1980.
> 209 pp. Paper. Index. References.
> Identifies potential problems regarding the use of
> drugs with aged persons. Written for physicians,

pharmacists, nurses, social workers, and students, as well as patients and their families. Focuses on "the overuse, misuse, or abuse of drugs" (p. 4) as a frequent cause of illness in the older person. Major topics include an overview of drug metabolism, undesirable drug effects, discussion of several categories of drugs, drug costs, and pharmacy roles and procedures in settings for older persons.

S8.11 Willgoose, Carl E.; Blank, Theodore; et al. Environmental Health: Commitment for Survival. Philadelphia: Saunders, 1979.

476 pp. Cloth. Index. Bibliography. Glossary. This text seeks to awaken individuals to the close association between the environment and human activity. Chapters cover the environment and the quality of life; ecology; aspects of environmental health (urban problems, climate, housing, violence, etc.); nutrition and population control; pollutants (air, water, etc.); disease control; nuclear energy; conservation of environment; aging; safe living; health services; welfare and the law; and health education.

CHAPTER 9:
WOMEN'S HEALTH

S9.1 Bishop, Barbara E., ed. The Maternity Cycle: One Nurse's Reflections. Philadelphia: Davis, 1980.

325 pp. Paper. Index. Bibliography. A different kind of a book on maternity nursing. One nurse's practice, assessment, and intervention are described in detail. The ambulatory care aspects are the focus as well as prenatal and postnatal care. The author speaks of the nine months before birth and the nine months after it as the maternity cycle. Places strong emphasis on the social and physical environment as well as on individual and family life styles. The appendix contains useful charts on discomforts with their causes and ways to relieve them and as a list of warning signs. Although the book is not

meant to be comprehensive, it is useful for graduates
and nursing students.

S9.2   Smith, David W.; Knights, Jean. Mothering Your Unborn
Baby. Philadelphia: Saunders, 1979.
> 97 pp. Paper. Index. References.
> For all women planning to have children. Points out
> that "good mothering" begins at conception. Discusses
> fetal development, labor and delivery, nutrition, haz-
> ards to fetal life, and others. Well illustrated.

CHAPTER 10:
CHILD HEALTH

S10.1   Allmond, Bayard W., Jr.; Buckman, Wilma; Gofman,
Helen F. The Family Is the Patient; An Approach to Behavioral Pediatrics for the Clinician. St. Louis: Mosby,
1979.
> 387 pp. Paper. Index. References.
> Written by two physicians and a social worker for
> pediatricians to help them learn the skills of family
> therapy and deal with common behavioral problems
> in well children, children with chronic illness, and
> hospitalized children. Uses case examples and focuses
> on the psychosocial issues of child health care.

S10.2   Heagarty, Margaret C.; Glass, Geraldine; King, Helen;
et al. Child Health: Basics for Primary Care. New York:
Appleton-Century-Crofts, 1980.
> 454 pp. Paper. Index. Bibliographies.
> A systematic presentation of material necessary for
> quality pediatric care. Six sections cover the normal
> growth and development of the child, the pediatric his-
> tory, the pediatric examination, laboratory and screen-
> ing procedures, signs and symptoms in pediatrics, and
> nutrition. Chapters include data and clinical objec-
> tives. Well illustrated.

S10.3   Howe, Jeanne, ed. Nursing Care of Adolescents. New
York: McGraw-Hill, 1980.

524 pp. Cloth. Index. Bibliography.
A multiauthored text written on a specialty that the
editor believes should receive more emphasis in educational programs. The chapters focus on the adolescents themselves (growth and development, nutrition, assessment, for example) and on health care
delivery settings (general hospital, rehabilitation setting, free government clinics, and college health programs). Includes a chapter on the nurse-adolescent
relationship.

S10.4 Randolph, Judson G.; Ravitch, Mark M.; Welch, Kenneth
J.; et al., eds. The Injured Child: Surgical Management.
Chicago: Year Book, 1979.
420 pp. Cloth. Index. References.
This medical text "is an authoritative and up-to-date
review of basic surgical principles in the care of the
injured child." (p. v) The book opens with a chapter
on children as accident victims. Includes chapters on
such general topics as fluid and nutritional support
and psychological considerations as well as on specific
areas of injury (abdominal, thoracic, musculoskeletal).
The last chapter looks at the battered child. Uses
charts and illustrations. Especially useful for physicians and surgeons in pediatrics, family practice,
and emergency care.

S10.5 Van Eys, Jan, ed. Research on Children: Medical Im-
peratives, Ethical Quandaries, and Legal Constraints.
Baltimore: University Park Press, 1978.
152 pp. Paper. Index. References.
Proceedings of a workshop held in Houston in April
1977 and sponsored by the University of Texas System
Cancer Center, the Institute of Religion, and the University of Texas Health Science Center in Houston.
Focuses on better ways of treating childhood disorders while protecting the rights of pediatric patients.
Directed to researchers working with children.

CHAPTER 11:
NURSING AS A PROFESSION

S11.1 American Nurses' Association, Committee for the Study of Credentialing in Nursing. The Study of Credentialing in Nursing: A New Approach. Vol. II, Staff Working Papers. Kansas City, Mo.: ANA, 1979.
> 507 pp. Paper. Bibliographies.
> The introduction discusses the development of the framework for the study and definitions and descriptions. The next sections include The Politics of Credentialing in Nursing, Credentialing and Job Market Issues, Credentialing in the Preparation for Nursing Practice, and Outcomes and Bases for Recommendations. Of special interest is background material for the report in Volume I, The Report of the Committee. Includes the minority opinions on the recommendations made by the Committee for the Study of Credentialing in Nursing.

S11.2 Hoy, Ronald; Robbins, Joy. The Profession of Nursing. [McGraw-Hill Nursing Studies Series.] New York: McGraw-Hill, 1979.
> 166 pp. Paper. Index. Bibliography. References.
> For nursing students in courses that consider the development of nursing, the nurse's roles, practice settings, and the management of care. The focus, including legislation, is on the United Kingdom rather than the United States.

S11.3 Newman, Margaret. Theory Development in Nursing. Philadelphia: Davis, 1979.
> 94 pp. Paper. Index. References.
> This small book will be very useful to persons concerned with nursing as a discipline. Discusses requisites to theory development in nursing. Includes conceptualizations of nursing as frameworks for theory development, the process of specifying a testable theory, and methods suggested for research. Com-

pares conceptual models of Johnson, Rogers, and Roy. The author's approach to theory development in nursing is also included.

S11.4   Quimby, Charles W., Jr.   Law for the Medical Practitioner.   Washington, D.C.: AUPHA [Association of University Programs in Health Administration] Press, 1979.
187 pp.   Cloth.   Index.   Additional Readings.
Provides a basis for physicians to identify potential problems requiring competent legal services.   Looks at the adversary system, malpractice in medicine, informed consent, contracts, confidentiality, and other topics.   Uses case reports and includes a table of pertinent cases.

CHAPTER 13:
ADMINISTRATION AND NURSING

S13.1   Beyers, Marjorie, ed.   Leadership in Nursing.   [The Management Anthology Series.   Theme Two: Management Functions.]   Wakefield, Mass.: Nursing Resources, 1979.
178 pp.   Paper.   Index.   Bibliography.
This volume reprints selected articles on leadership theories, definitions, style, the leader, and leadership in the organization.   The editor provides an introduction to each section and a series of thought-provoking questions at the end.

S13.2   Clark, Carolyn Chambers.   The Nurse as Continuing Educator.   [Springer Series on the Teaching of Nursing, vol. 6.]   New York: Springer Publishing, 1979.
310 pp.   Paper.   Index.   References.
A helpful guide for nurse educators involved in continuing education and for those involved with adult learners.   Chapters focus on the problems of continuing education, the adult learner, assessment of teacher attitudes and learner needs, evaluation, and the conduct of workshops.   Chapters include exercises for the reader.

S13.3 Williams, Stephen J., ed. Issues in Health Services. [Wiley Series in Health Services.] New York: Wiley, 1980.

> 371 pp. Cloth. Index. References.
> Provides a collection of previously published articles useful for students and practitioners involved in health services. The major units provide an introduction, discussion of factors associated with the use of health services, and a look at health care providers, resources, and evaluation.

DATE DUE

69716